VETERINARY CLINICS OF NORTH AMERICA

FOOD ANIMAL PRACTICE

Beef Cattle Nutrition

JOHN MAAS, DVM, MS, GUEST EDITOR

VOLUME 7 • NUMBER 1 • MARCH 1991

W. B. SAUNDERS COMPANY
Harcourt Brace Jovanovich, Inc.
PHILADELPHIA LONDON TORONTO MONTREAL SYDNEY TOKYO

W. B. SAUNDERS COMPANY
Harcourt Brace Jovanovich, Inc.

The Curtis Center
Independence Square West
Philadelphia, PA 19106-3399

The *Veterinary Clinics of North America: Food Animal Practice* is also published in translated editions by the following:

Spanish—Editorial Inter-Medica, Casilla Correo 4625, Buenos Aires, Argentina

THE VETERINARY CLINICS OF NORTH AMERICA
FOOD ANIMAL PRACTICE   ISSN 0749-0720

March 1991   Volume 7, Number 1

Authorization to photocopy items for internal or personal use, or the internal or personal use of specific clients, is granted by the W. B. Saunders Company for users registered with the Copyright Clearance Center (CCC) Transactional Reporting Service, provided that the base fee of $00.00 per copy, plus $0.20 per page, is paid directly to CCC, 27 Congress St., Salem, MA 01970. For those organizations that have been granted a photocopy license by CCC, a separate system of payment has been arranged. The fee code for users of the Transactional Reporting Service is: 0749–0720/90 $00.00 + $.20. All fees are subject to change without notice.

The following information is published in accordance with the requirements of the United States Postal Code.

The Veterinary Clinics of North America: Food Animal Practice (ISSN 0749–0720) is published in March, July, and November by W. B. Saunders Company. Corporate and Editorial Offices: The Curtis Center, Independence Square West, Philadelphia, PA 19106-3399. Accounting and Circulation Offices: One East First Street, Duluth, MN 55802. Second-class postage paid at Duluth, MN 55806, and additional mailing offices. Subscription price is $51.00 per year (U.S. individuals), $61.00 per year (U.S. institutions), and $67.00 per year (foreign). There is a postage charge of $6.00 for subscriptions billed to U.S. addresses and shipped outside the U.S. POSTMASTER: Send address changes to *The Veterinary Clinics of North America: Food Animal Practice*, W. B. Saunders Company, Customer Service, P.O. Box 6467, Duluth, MN 55806–9854.

The editor of this publication is Maureen O'Gibney, W. B. Saunders Company, The Curtis Center, Independence Square West, Philadelphia, Pennsylvania 19106-3399.

GUEST EDITOR

JOHN MAAS, DVM, Case Supervisor, California Veterinary Diagnostic Laboratory System, University of California, Davis, Davis, California

CONTRIBUTORS

C. D. ALLISON, PhD, Professor of Range Science, New Mexico State University, Las Cruces, New Mexico.

WILLIAM FRANCIS CATES, BSc, DVM, PhD, Professor, Herd Medicine and Theriogenology, University of Saskatchewan, Western College of Veterinary Medicine, Saskatoon, Saskatchewan, Canada

LARRY R. CORAH, PhD, Professor, Department of Animal Science, Kansas State University, Manhattan, Kansas, Member of American Society of Animal Science

THOMAS M. CRAIG, DVM, PhD, Professor, Department of Veterinary Pathobiology, College of Veterinary Medicine, Texas A & M University, College Station, Texas

TIMOTHY DELCURTO, PhD, Assistant Professor, Department of Animal Science, Oregon State University, Eastern Oregon Agricultural Research Center, Burns, Oregon

T. M. FRYE, PhD, Group Leader, Technical Services, Department of Animal Health and Nutrition, Roche Vitamins and Fine Chemicals, Nutley, New Jersey

THOMAS W. GRAHAM, DVM, MPVM, Assistant Veterinarian, Department of Nutrition, University of California, Davis; Davis, California

JEFFERY O. HALL, DVM, Research Associate, Department of Veterinary Biosciences, University of Illinois at Urbana-Champaign, Urbana, Illinois

DAVID P. HUTCHESON, PhD, Professor, Texas Agricultural Experiment Station, Texas A & M University, Amarillo, Texas

SAM IVES, DVM, Private Practitioner, Veterinary Clinic Inc., Mexico, Missouri

BILL JOHNSON, DVM, Diplomate, American College of Veterinary Pathologists; Pathologist, California Veterinary Diagnostic Laboratory System, University of California, Davis; Davis, California

GAVIN L. MEERDINK, DVM, Diplomate, American Board of Veterinary Toxicology, Clinical Toxicologist, Laboratories of Diagnostic Veterinary Medicine, University of Illinois at Urbana-Champaign, Urbana, Illinois

S. D. PARSONS, PhD, President, Ranch Management Consultants, Inc., Albuquerque, New Mexico

LAWRENCE E. RICE, DVM, MS, Diplomate, American College of Theriogenologists, Professor, Department of Medicine and Surgery, Boren Veterinary Teaching Hospital, Oklahoma State University College of Veterinary Medicine, Stillwater, Oklahoma

LARRY J. THOMPSON, DVM, Diplomate, American Board of Veterinary Toxicology; Clinical Toxicologist, Diagnostic Laboratory, New York State College of Veterinary Medicine, Cornell University, Ithaca, New York

HARLEY A. TURNER, PhD, Associate Professor, Department of Animal Science, Oregon State University, Eastern Oregon Agricultural Research Center, Burns, Oregon

STEVEN E. WIKSE, DVM, Diplomate, American College of Veterinary Pathology, Associate Professor, Large Animal Medicine and Surgery, College of Veterinary Medicine, Texas A & M University, College Station, Texas

SCOT N. WILLIAMS, PhD, Senior, Technical Services Manager, Department of Animal Health and Nutrition, Roche Vitamins and Fine Chemicals, Nutley, New Jersey

CONTENTS

Some Nutritional and Genetic Considerations in the Performance Testing of Beef Bulls 59
William Francis Cates

Performance testing of bulls provides an opportunity to compare the rate of gain of prospective breeding animals to their contemporaries. However, careful nutritional management is needed to assure good growth rates without risk of impaired spermatogenesis or any degree of laminitis. The performance testing program should help the participating contributors to identify and eliminate undesirable heritable characteristics that may exist in their herds. It should also emphasize the selection of desirable characteristics that will contribute to both productivity and reproductive soundness.

Grazing Management as it Affects Nutrition, Animal Production and Economics of Beef Production 77
S. D. Parsons and C. D. Allison

Profitable beef production is highly dependent upon low cost nutrition, which for all practical purposes is supplied by grazing. Grazing management for nutritional purposes has, surprisingly, been ignored by animal and range scientists alike. Controlled grazing, which avoids both overgrazing and over-resting, is beneficial to both plant and animal. To achieve desired production levels, some supplementation is required for most grazing situations.

Nutritional and Managerial Considerations for Range Beef Cattle Production 95
Harley A. Turner and Timothy DelCurto

Nutritional and managerial schemes are presented to optimize range livestock production. Forage quality, animal requirements, and the animal's ability to meet their requirements from the forage is presented. After inventorying the nutritional value of the forages and determining animal requirements, a prescription supplementation program is presented. Management alternatives to compensate for poor quality forage on range late summer and early fall, such as selling market animals, moving to better feed, chemical curing of forages, time of calving, time of weaning and using the range as a feedlot are presented. Winter-feeding programs using native flood meadow hay as a base are also presented for both growing animals and mature cows. Material presented illustrates a philosophy of range nutrition with methods and procedures that are adaptable to grazing systems in all parts of the world.

Polyether Ionophores — Effect on Rumen Function in Feedlot Cattle 127
Larry R. Corah

For the cattle industry to continue to produce excellent quality, competitively priced beef, the cost of production is of paramount economic importance. Thus, additives that can improve feed efficiency and/or rate of gain have merit.

Nutritional and Dietary Interrelationships with Diseases of Feedlot Cattle
Bill Johnson

High concentrate feedlot rations are incriminated in the development of several problems in feedlot cattle. Discussions of ruminal lactic acidosis, mycotic rumenitis, hepatic abscesses, cauda vena cava thrombosis, pulmonary arterial thromboembolism, bloat and acute bovine pulmonary emphysema (atypical interstitial pneumonia) are presented.

Nutritional and Dietary Interrelationships with Diseases of Grazing Beef Cattle
Steven E. Wikse, Thomas M. Craig, and David P. Hutcheson

This article describes current methods of controlling acute bovine pulmonary emphysema (ABPEE) and edema, lungworm and gastrointestinal nematodes, and bloat in grazing beef cattle. Success in handling outbreaks of these conditions and in their prevention depends on an understanding of their epidemiology and pathogenesis. Supplementation with ionophore antibiotics is effective in prevention of ABPEE and bloat and may also prevent other diseases of cattle that graze lush pastures.

Trace Element Deficiencies in Cattle
Thomas W. Graham

Trace element deficiencies in beef cattle are important causes of production loss. Primary mineral deficiencies typically occur because of environmental conditions that reduce soil nutrients or impair nutrient availability to plants. Thus, the plants contain low concentrations of essential nutrients in the feed. In contrast, primary vitamin deficiencies typically occur because of seasonal changes in forage concentration or because of loss during storage. Secondary deficiencies occur because of concurrent disease states that impair nutrient uptake, retention or function. Another important cause of secondary nutrient deficiencies are the interactions among nutrients. Properties, metabolism, and function of cobalt, copper, iodine, iron, molybdenum, manganese, selenium, and zinc are discussed. Clinical parameters associated with deficiency of these nutrients, an approach to estimating nutrient adequacy/ status, and forms of dietary and parenteral therapy are discussed with each nutrient.

FORTHCOMING ISSUES

July 1991

DAIRY NUTRITION MANAGEMENT
Charles J. Sniffen, MS, PhD, and
Thomas Herdt, DVM, *Guest Editors*

November 1991

APPLIED PHARMACOLOGY AND THERAPEUTICS
K. W. Hinchcliff, BVSc, MSc, and
A. D. Jernigan, DVM, PhD, *Guest Editors*

March 1992

PHYSICAL EXAMINATION
Julia Wilson, DVM, *Guest Editor*

PREVIOUS ISSUES

November 1990

ADVANCES IN SHEEP AND GOAT MEDICINE
Mary C. Smith, DVM, *Guest Editor*

July 1990

SURGERY OF THE BOVINE DIGESTIVE TRACT
David C. Bristol, *Guest Editor*

March 1990

FLUID AND ELECTROLYTE THERAPY/BOVINE
HERD VACCINATION PROGRAMS
Allen J. Roussel, Jr, DVM, MS, and
Charles A. Hjerpe, DVM, *Guest Editors*

PREFACE

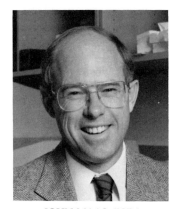

JOHN MAAS, DVM
Guest Editor

This issue is devoted to topics that focus on the nutritional aspects of common diseases and clinical problems of beef cattle. Today's veterinarians are asked to address problems such as reproductive inefficiency, respiratory disease, failure to thrive, and a host of other disorders. Many clinical and subclinical conditions have multiple causes and often involve nutrition and feeding of the herd. Veterinarians oriented toward preventive medicine find they must frequently consider nutrition as an integral part of their approach to diagnosis, therapeutics, and prevention. It is increasingly important to consider nutrition as part of their routine clinical activity.

Dr. Rice leads this issue with two articles concerning nutrition and reproductive performance in cows and heifers. He emphasizes the efficiency of optimum nutrition from an economic as well as biologic perspective. Drs. Corah and Ives focus on the effects of trace element deficiencies on reproductive performance of cattle. The next article, by Dr. Cates, considers nutritional aspects of reproductive performance and genetic evaluation of bulls.

Drs. Parsons and Allison introduce us to intensive grazing management, a relatively new concept in beef cattle nutrition. This article engages us to reconsider many of our basic assumptions regarding nutrition, performance, and management. The next article addresses beef cattle nutrition on arid and semi-arid rangelands. Drs. Turner and DelCurto have included a considerable amount of new data gained from years of observations.

Dr. Corah's discussion of polyether ionophores provides background information of daily importance. Dr. Johnson outlines tools for monitoring feedlot diseases and their relationship to the diet. While veterinarians are asked to explain morbidity and mortality in feedlots, the computerized feed sheet is too often considered unquestionable. Dr. Johnson's article explores the clinical significance of post mortem findings in a clear and concise manner. The important relationships between diet and disease in grazing cattle is summarized by Drs. Wikse, Craig and Hutcheson and manipulations to the diet to prevent or control these conditions are reviewed.

Dr. Graham presents a comprehensive article on trace element deficiencies in beef cattle full of the latest clinical and research information on this topic. The article on vitamin nutrition, by Drs. Frye, Williams, and Graham is a natural compliment to the previous article and contains useful information not often found in the clinical literature. The last article, by Drs. Thompson, Hall, and Meerdink, discusses trace element toxicities in beef cattle. With the present emphasis on supplementation, the risk of trace element toxicity has increased.

This issue does not attempt to duplicate nutrient requirement information such as that found in Nutrient Requirements of Beef Cattle, published by the National Academy of Sciences' National Research Council. Additionally, two recent Veterinary Clinics of North America: Food Animal Practice issues (Vol 4:2 and Vol 4:3) contain valuable review articles on ruminant metabolic diseases and nutrition of stressed cattle. I would refer the reader to these sources to compliment this issue.

The authors of these manuscripts have discussed the important relationships between nutrition and many common problems seen in beef cattle production. They have searched the literature and added their years of experience to bring clinically important facts into focus for the reader. This issue reflects the authors' expertise and will be a valuable reference. I would like to personally thank the authors for a job well done.

JOHN MAAS, DVM
Guest Editor

California Veterinary
Diagnostic Laboratory System
P.O. Box 1770
Davis, California 95617-1770

Beef Cattle Nutrition 0749–0720/91 $0.00 + .20

The Effects of Nutrition on Reproductive Performance of Beef Cattle

Lawrence E. Rice, DVM, MS*

Controlling nutrition at critical times of the reproductive cycle and critical times of the year is most important in ensuring good reproductive performance in beef cows. Veterinarians involved with beef cow reproductive management face two important challenges: (1) recognizing the relationship between nutrition and reproduction and (2) making timely recommendations on nutritional management that will indeed have a positive impact on the reproductive performance. Nutritional requirements and ration balancing are well covered in the Nutritional Requirements of Beef Cattle from the National Research Council (NRC),[26] and other texts[30] and therefore will not be treated here. Readers are also referred to previous issues of the *Veterinary Clinics of North America*, including March 1983, November 1987, July 1988, and November 1988 for articles on reproductive management,[37] reproduction and nutrition,[14] metabolic diseases,[10] malnutrition,[17] and thermal stress feeding.[1]

This article reviews the onset of postpartum estrus in beef cows briefly, then documents the relationship between body condition and reproduction. Finally, cost-effective approaches to correction of reproductive/nutritional problems through body condition evaluation and nutritional improvement are discussed.

NUTRITIONAL PHILOSOPHY

One economic importance of beef cows is that they harvest and convert to animal protein forages that have little value as nutrients for

*Diplomate, American College of Theriogenologists, Professor, Department of Medicine and Surgery, Boren Veterinary Teaching Hospital, Oklahoma State University College of Veterinary Medicine, Stillwater, Oklahoma

other animals or people. Such forages vary greatly in nutritional quality and palatability. While the NRC nutritional requirements are well explained in the tables, we usually have little control over nutrient density and dry matter intake. We therefore cannot evaluate compliance with requirements by ration evaluation in the manner we do for dairy cows or brood sows.

Energy

Ruminants use carbohydrates and fats for energy. Complex carbohydrates are used through microfloral fermentation and enzyme breakdown in the rumen. The microbes also synthesize volatile fatty acids (VFAs), which provide a large portion of the energy requirement in the ruminant. There is very little carbohydrate storage in animals, but excess is readily converted to fats for storage, which are easily converted back to carbohydrate to meet energy requirements when necessary. Therefore, fat storage (body condition) is an important source of energy for beef cows.

While the net energy system is quite precise and is most useful for calculating balanced, least cost rations for feedlot cattle, dairy cattle, and swine, it has limitations for beef cows. Each feedstuff has a specific net energy (NE) value for specific functions (i.e., NE_g for gain, NE_l for lactation, NE_m for maintenance, etc.). These values have been determined for feedlot cattle and their feedstuffs but only have been estimated from *TDN* (total digestible nutrient) values for most forages consumed by beef cows. For practical purposes, the TDN system is used by many nutritionists when estimating supplementation programs for beef cows. It may not be as precise, but neither is our estimate of dry matter intake of pastured cattle. The veterinary clinician may use the system that seems the most practical, and most computer programs now available tend to use the net energy system for beef cows.

Protein

Most protein ingested is catabolized and resynthesized as microbial protein, which in turn is digested and absorbed in the small intestine to meet the protein requirements of the ruminant. Bypass proteins are not commonly used in beef cow rations. Therefore, in beef cows, when we are supplementing protein we are really feeding the rumen microflora that are responsible for maintaining proper rumen function. Meeting protein requirements is not only essential for the animal's protein requirements but also is important to meet the rumen microfloral requirements, which in turn are paramount for use of forage carbohydrates.

Nutritional considerations for the beef cow herd should fit around the forages most suited for a particular area. Knowledge of forage characteristics is essential for planning a nutritional regimen for a beef herd. The calving and breeding seasons should be planned so the cows have the highest quality forages when their need is the greatest, keeping supplemental feed to a minimum and costs within reason. Progressive producers often consult range management specialists and agronomists for advice on pasture management and forage harvesting.

Veterinarians should also consult these specialists to become familiar with the best forage production in the local area.

Forage quality greatly influences total dry matter intake[13] (Table 1). Forage quality is seldom a problem during the growing season but does become a problem during the dry season or winter. During these times the available forage usually consists of dry grass, with 40% TDN values and less than 2% protein; grass hay with 50% TDN values and 4–10% protein; or silage with 60–70% TDN and 6–8% protein. Some producers use alfalfa during the winter but the cost of alfalfa and competition from the dairy and horse industries have reduced the use of alfalfa as a winter feed for beef cows.

The type of forage and the class of cattle will determine the dry matter consumption, which in turn will have a great effect on the supplementation plan. The problem is, the cattle most likely to require supplements will be those on a low consumption forage. The dry matter intake will become a limiting factor in meeting the energy requirements. The dry matter intake (DMI) for low quality forages in Table 1 is based on no protein supplementation. Protein supplementation to pregnant, dry cows would increase forage DMI to 1.8 or 1.9% of body weight and would also increase the digestability of the forage from 40% to approximately 45% TDN. For example, 1000 pound cows on non-supplemented dry winter grass would consume 15–16 pounds of dry matter yielding 6.5 pounds of TDN and less than 0.5 pounds of crude protein (both deficient). Supplementing these cows with 2–3 pounds of cottonseed or soybean meal would increase DMI to approximately 18–19 pounds forage and 2–3 pounds of the protein supplement. This would provide approximately 9 pounds of TDN and 1–1.5 pounds of

Table 1. *Estimated Roughage Capacity of Beef Cattle*

ROUGHAGE TYPE	CLASS OF CATTLE*	DRY MATTER CAPACITY† %	AS-FED CAPACITY‡ LB
Low quality roughages (dry grass, straw, etc.)	dry cows	1.5	17–18
	wet cows	2.0	23–24
Average quality hays (Bermuda, native, etc.)	dry cows	2.0	22–24
	wet cows	2.3	25–28
High quality forages (alfalfa hay)	dry cows	2.5	28–30
	wet cows	2.7	30–32
Green pasture	dry cows	2.5	80–100
	wet cows	2.7	100–110
Silages	dry cows	2.5	80–85
	wet cows	2.7	90–95

*900–1100 lb cows
†Capacity as a percent of body weight
‡Total daily capacity
(*Adapted from* Lusby KS: Feeding the cowherd. *In* Oklahoma Beef Cattle Manual, 2nd ed. Cooperative Extension Service, Division of Agriculture Oklahoma State University, 1988, p 57; with permission.)

crude protein (both adequate). Pregnant cows will maintain condition on such pastures if they receive adequate protein supplementation and if the forage is plentiful.[13] Thin or borderline cows will not gain weight on dry winter pastures even with protein supplementation.

If protein becomes deficient dry matter intake will be adequate and the cows will suffer both protein and energy malnutrition. This will likely happen if cows on poor quality forage are fed a nonprotein nitrogen (NPN) source of protein supplement such as urea. NPN supplements require carbon to combine with the nitrogen to form amino acids and sufficient fermentable energy for the bacteria to grow and synthesize the amino acids. This carbohydrate is not available in low quality forages such as winter grass, wheat straw, crop residues or most grass hays.[5,24] Natural protein should be the supplement for cows on low energy forages. Proper protein supplementation will increase forage consumption, but if the pasture becomes depleted, energy will be deficient, with the cows using body fat for energy and perhaps even deamimating protein as an energy source.

High energy supplements are necessary when forages will not meet the energy requirements. Adding concentrates with high starch content to forage diets will somewhat reduce the digestibility of the forage due to lowered rumen pH. Feeds such as corn gluten feed, soybean hulls, wheat midds, or rice midds are low in starch but have highly digestible fiber that does not suppress forage digestibility. These feeds have moderate protein and good energy values. When available and priced fairly, such feeds can be important supplements to provide required weight gains. Knowledge of forage quality, body condition scores, and nutritional requirements is necessary to give recommendations on forage supplementation programs.

POSTPARTUM REPRODUCTIVE PHYSIOLOGY

Probably the most important endocrine event associated with the onset of estrus in the postpartum cow is the establishment of episodic pulsatile LH secretion. As a cow approaches the first postpartum estrus, frequency and amplitude of the LH release increases, which is followed by waves of follicular development and atresia. The episodic LH release is re-established by the tenth to fifteenth day after calving in nonsuckled cows.[18] Suckled cows, however, have a much later and highly variable onset of episodic LH release patterns. Some suckled cows return to estrus by 30 days postpartum but others may not cycle until the calf is weaned.[15] Cows that are suckled more frequently (those with twins or more aggressively nursing calves) have a significantly slower return to estrus than cows that have the calves limited to nursing once or twice a day.[36] Calves weaned at 30–45 days of age resulted in their dams returning to estrus and conceiving earlier than suckled cows.[13]

Studies in postpartum cows indicate that the pituitary gland has adequate gonadotrophin stores and will release LH and FSH when stimulated with exogenous GNRH.[18] Injection of 5 μg GNRH every 2 hours for 48 hours induced an episodic pattern of LH secretion eventually followed by a pre-ovulatory LH surge. Continuous infusion of GNRH produced the same results.[12] These data indicate that the control of cyclicity rests in the hypothalamus or some higher brain center.

Recent research indicates that endogenous opioid peptides may be responsible for the anestrus observed in suckling beef cows. Opioids such as β-endorphin and methionine enkephalin decrease LH levels in humans and laboratory animals.[4] The administration of an opioid inhibitor (naloxone) causes the resumption of LH secretion. The proposed action is that the opioids inhibit GNRH secretion. When naloxone was administered to anestrus suckled beef cows, a significant increase in the frequency and amplitude of LH release occurred.[34] The response seemed to be influenced by the postpartum interval, as cows 42 days postpartum showed a significantly greater response to lower doses of naloxone than cows 14 or 28 days postpartum. The increased LH secretion following naloxone blockage of the opioids is theoretically similar to that seen in cows with early weaned calves or calves that have been removed for 48 hours. Suckling apparently increases the opioid levels, which in turn, inhibits GHRH release.

Calf removal does not consistently initiate cyclicity in anestrus postpartum beef cows. Part of the variability can be explained by the postpartum interval but the other major factors are nutritional status and body condition. Energy restriction during late gestation results in thin body condition at calving and extends the postpartum anestrus interval. Cows in good body condition at calving and maintaining condition after calving overcome the suckling inhibition earlier in the postpartum period.[3,35,40] Cows gaining weight during the breeding season have higher pregnancy rates than those that lose weight.[22,39]

BODY CONDITION

Prepartum weight loss may be due to any number of causes, including, age, general health, parasitism, or nutrition, but is generally due to energy and protein deficiencies. Weight loss occurs when the energy reserves (fat) and protein reserves (muscle) are being depleted. While weight gains or losses have traditionally been considered to be a good measure of well being and productivity, such changes are often confounded by fill or stage of pregnancy in cows. Also, weighing cattle is laborious and seldom done by cow/calf producers. A more useful method in assessing the energy reserve is based on assigning each animal a body condition score (BCS) based on visual observation or preferably palpation of back, ribs, and rear quarters. Several scoring systems have been used but the one most commonly in use in the United States is a nine point scale (1 to 9) and described by Spitzer[30] and Herd[8]: (Figs. 1–8).

Thin Condition

BCS 1. EMACIATED. Cow is extremely emaciated with no detectable fat over spinous processes, transverse processes, hip bones or ribs. Tail-head and ribs project quite prominently.

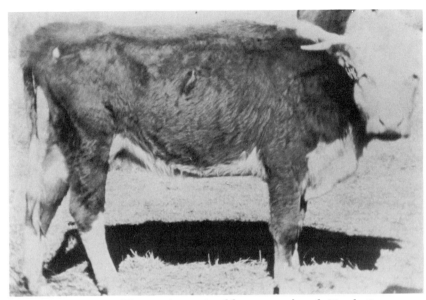

Figure 1. Score 2. The cow is emaciated but not weakened. Muscle tissue seems severely depleted through the hindquarters and shoulder. (*From* Selk GE: Oklahoma Beef Cattle Manual, 2nd ed. Stillwater, Oklahoma, Cooperative Extension Service, Oklahoma State University, 1988; with permission.)

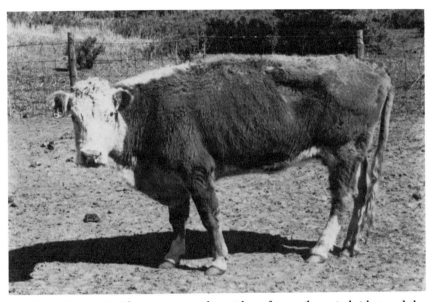

Figure 2. Score 3. The cow is very thin with no fat on ribs or in brisket, and the backbone is easily visible. Some muscle depletion appears evident through the hindquarters similar to BCS 2. (*From* Selk GE: Oklahoma Beef Cattle Manual, 2nd ed. Stillwater, Oklahoma, Cooperative Extension Service, Oklahoma State University, 1988; with permission.)

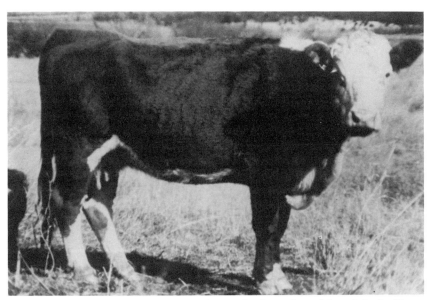

Figure 3. Score 4. The cow appears thin, with ribs easily visible and the backbone showing. Muscle tissue is not depleted through the shoulders. (*From* Selk GE: Oklahoma Beef Cattle Manual, 2nd ed. Stillwater, Oklahoma, Cooperative Extension Service, Oklahoma State University, 1988; with permission.)

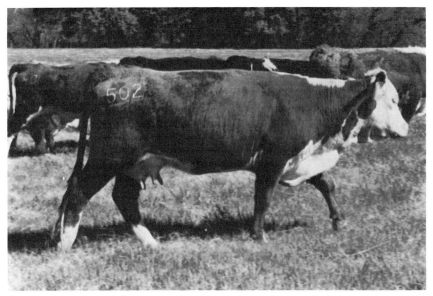

Figure 4. Score 5. The cow may be described as moderate. The last two or three ribs can be seen, and little evidence of fat is present in the brisket, over the ribs, or around the tail head. (*From* Selk GE: Oklahoma Beef Cattle Manual, 2nd ed. Stillwater, Oklahoma, Cooperative Extension Service, Oklahoma State University, 1988; with permission.)

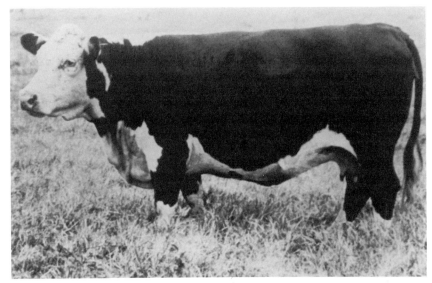

Figure 5. Score 6. The cow exhibits a good smooth appearance throughout. Some fat deposition is present in the brisket and over the tail head. The back appears rounded, and fat can be palpated over the ribs and pin bones. (*From* Selk GE: Oklahoma Beef Cattle Manual, 2nd ed. Stillwater, Oklahoma, Cooperative Extension Service, Oklahoma State University, 1988; with permission.)

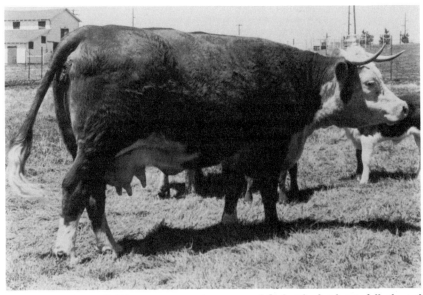

Figure 6. Score 7. The cow appears in very good flesh. The brisket is full, the tail head shows pockets of fat, and the back appears square because of fat. The ribs are smooth and soft to the touch because of fat cover. (*From* Selk GE: Oklahoma Beef Cattle Manual, 2nd ed. Stillwater, Oklahoma, Cooperative Extension Service, Oklahoma State University, 1988; with permission.)

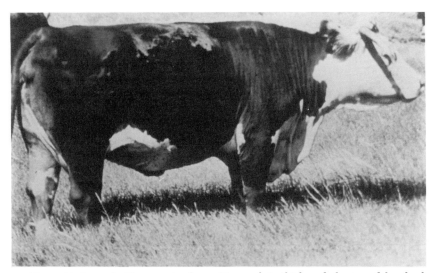

Figure 7. Score 8. The cow is obese. Her neck is thick and short, and her back appears very square because of excessive fat. The brisket is distended, and she has heavy fat pockets around the tail head. (*From* Selk GE: Oklahoma Beef Cattle Manual, 2nd ed. Stillwater, Oklahoma, Cooperative Extension Service, Oklahoma State University, 1988; with permission.)

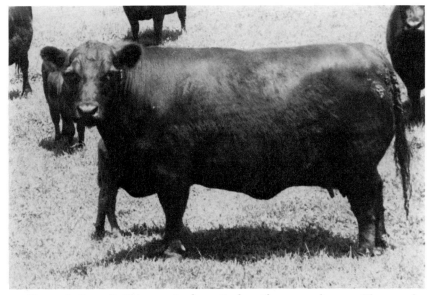

Figure 8. Score 9. This cow is obese. Such cattle are rarely seen. They can be described as similar to 8s but taken to greater extremes. They also have a heavy deposition of udder fat. (*From* Selk GE: Oklahoma Beef Cattle Manual, 2nd ed. Stillwater, Oklahoma, Cooperative Extension Service, Oklahoma State University, 1988; with permission.)

BCS 2. POOR. Cow still appears somewhat emaciated but tail head and ribs are less prominent. Individual spinous processes are still rather sharp to the touch, but some tissue cover exists along spine.

BCS 3. THIN. Ribs are still individually identifiable but not quite as sharp to the touch. There is obvious palpable fat along spine and over tail head with some tissue cover over dorsal portion of ribs.

Borderline Condition

BCS 4. BORDERLINE THIN. Individual ribs are no longer visually obvious. The spinous processes can be identified individually on palpation but feel rounded rather than sharp. Some fat cover over ribs, transverse processes and hip bones.

Optimum Condition

BCS 5. MODERATE. Cow has generally good overall appearance. Upon palpation, fat cover over ribs feels spongy, and areas on either side of tail head now have palpable fat cover.

BCS 6. HIGH MODERATE. Firm pressure now needs to be applied to beef spinous processes. A high degree of fat cover is palpable over ribs and around tail head.

BCS 7. GOOD. Cow appears fleshy and obviously carries considerable fat. Very spongy fat cover over ribs and over and around tail head. In fact, "rounds" or "pones" are beginning to be obvious. Some fat around vulva and in the twist area.

Fat Condition

BCS 8. FAT. Cow very fleshy and overconditioned. Spinous processes almost impossible to palpate. Cow has large fat deposits over ribs, around tail head, and below vulva. "Rounds" or "pones" are obvious.

BCS 9. EXTREMELY FAT. Cow obviously extremely wasty and patchy and looks blocky. Tail head and hips buried in fatty tissue and "rounds" or "pones" of fat are protruding. Bone structure no longer visible and barely palpable. Animal's mobility may even be impaired by large fatty deposits.

Studies have shown BCS is a better predictor of carcass fat content than is body weight and is highly repeatable by scorers and within animals.[7,8,32] A study involving three breeds (Jersey, Brown Swiss, and Simmental) crossed with Hereford or Angus showed the same BCS accurately predicted carcass fat content regardless of breed type.[31] However, the Jersey crosses had higher reproductive performance at lower BCS, indicating some breed types have different biologic responses at different BCS. The system has been used by both experienced scientists and novices trained during trials. It has been found to be the most objective measure of body fat and has major advantages in that cattle do not need to be weighed, merely observed and palpated at a time when other procedures may be performed (i.e., pregnancy palpation). One BCS evaluation can assess a cow's energy status whereas at least two weighings are necessary to record a weight change. There are approximately 80 lb difference in body weight per BCS in average size beef cows, but the very large breeds will have slightly larger weight differences between BCSs.

Cows in good body condition at calving have the greatest probability to return to estrus and become pregnant early in the next breeding season[35] (Tables 2 and 3). These studies also showed there was a negative relationship (R = −.50) between the duration of the postpartum period and prepartum weight change.[6]

Research trials in Texas and Wyoming reported the rebreeding performance of cows in thin (BCS 4 or less), average (BCS 5), or good (BCS 6 or greater) at calving time[27] (Fig. 9). Not only do the BCSs at calving have a marked effect on the average pregnancy rates, but the lower scores have much wider ranges between herds with similar body condition. This is not an indication of subjectivity of the scoring system, but that the lower BCSs are more influenced by postpartum environmental changes that are likely to decrease pregnancy rates. In an Oklahoma State University study, similar results were achieved (Fig. 10). The cows that calved in higher body condition consumed more feed (increased cost = $47/head), but the net return to management and labor was $27–$30 per cow greater than the net return for the thinner cows in a year of relatively low cattle market prices and high interest rates.[33]

Loss of body condition during the last trimester has a greater impact on pregnancy rates in cows with BCS 4 to 6 than in thinner or fatter cows. The reproductive rate of the thinner cows is not likely to be further reduced and the fatter cows have enough energy reserves to withstand some loss of condition and reduced reproductive rates. The goal of the nutritional program should be to assure a BCS of 5 to 6 at calving time. This should be done by making the best use of available forage and necessary supplements.

BODY CONDITION CHANGE AFTER CALVING

Body condition changes from calving through the first few weeks of the breeding season also significantly affect reproductive performance. Lactation greatly increases the energy and protein requirements of beef cows and many of the new breeds and crossbreeds have much

Table 2: *Body Condition at Calving and Percent of Cows Cycling in the Postpartum Period*

BODY CONDITION AT CALVING	NO. COWS	DAYS AFTER CALVING AND % CYCLING					
		50 %	60 %	70 %	80 %	90 %	100 %
Thin	272	34	46	55	62	66	70
Moderate	364	45	61	79	88	92	100
Good	50	42	91	96	98	100	100

(*Adapted from* Whitman RW, Remmega EE, Wiltbank JN: Weight change, condition and beef cow production. J Anim Sci 41:387, 1975; with permission.)

Table 3. *Effect of Body Condition at Calving on Rebreeding*

CONDITION AT CALVING	PREGNANT AFTER BREEDING (%)	
	20 Days	*80 Days*
Thin	25	72
Moderate	35	89
Good	39	92

(*Adapted from* Whitman RW, Remmega EE, Wiltbank JN: Weight change, condition and beef cow production. J Anim Sci 41:387, 1975; with permission.)

greater lactational requirements than more traditional beef breeds. This increased requirement begins at parturition, but like newly freshened dairy cows, beef cows have reduced dry matter intake during the immediate postpartum interval. Often, recently calved beef cows are not separated from the gestating cows, hence they do not receive additional nutrients. A study in Texas evaluated postpartum energy levels of 90%, 100%, and 110% of NRC requirements.[25] Increased nutritional level decreased the postpartum interval to first estrus with a response of 58, 40, and 35 days for the respective energy levels.[25] Regardless of nutritional treatment, cows that maintained weight (and body condition) had a shorter average postpartum interval (32 days) than cows that lost weight (60 days). Again, body condition is a better predictor of reproductive performance than nutritional levels. BCS reflects factors such as lactation, age, and teeth, which may be responsible for variance in body condition within energy level groups.

Most studies indicate prepartum nutrition as reflected by BCS at calving is most important in determining the time of return to first estrus. Cows with body condition of 4 or less at calving are slow to

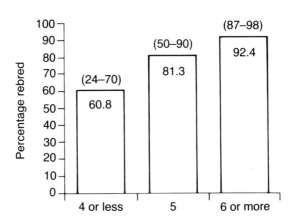

Body condition score at calving

Figure 9. Percentage of cows calving, in different body conditions, that became pregnant during the next breeding season. Summary of five trials (1742 cows). Numbers in parentheses indicate range of values. (*From* Selk GE: Assessing the cowherd condition: Management alternatives and consequences. Proceedings: Cow, Grass, the World, and You. Stillwater, Oklahoma, Cooperative Extension Service, Oklahoma State University, 1989; with permission.)

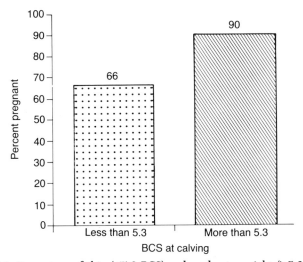

Figure 10. Percentage of thin (<5.3 BCS) and moderate weight (>5.3 BCS) cows pregnant after 90-day breeding season. (*From* Selk GE: Assessing the cowherd condition: Management alternatives and consequences. Proceedings: Cow, Grass, the World, and You. Stillwater, Oklahoma, Cooperative Extension Service, Oklahoma State University, 1989; with permission.)

respond to increased postpartum nutrients.[22,39] The postpartum demand of lactation and the suckling inhibition of GNRH release are simply too much for thin cows to overcome and return to estrus in the same interval as cows with BCS of 5 or greater. The thin cows eventually responded to increased energy levels; however, the response was much later in the breeding season, resulting in an increased calving interval.[39]

Good body condition at calving is even more important for the reproductive performance of first-calf heifers. The combined stresses of calving, first lactation, and continued growth requirements delay their return to postpartum estrus. Heifers must have a BCS of 5 or greater to have acceptable pregnancy rates in less than 120 days postpartum. In an Oklahoma State University study, heifers that calved with BCSs less than 5 and were fed a high energy ration to make good postpartum gains did have higher pregnancy rates than did thin heifers that only maintained body condition. However, the thin heifers that gained postpartum condition still had much lower pregnancy rates than heifers that calved with a BCS 5 or greater[2] (Table 4). The studies also indicated that increasing nutrient levels above the postpartum requirements was of no biologic or economic benefit for cows in acceptable body condition at calving.

Adequate postpartum nutrition is very important for maximum conception rates (Table 5). Cows that have a BCS of 5 or greater at calving but receive inadequate postpartum nutrition will have reduced conception rates even though cycling rates may be near normal. In one study evaluating the effect of postpartum nutrition by maintaining or losing postpartum body condition, even though cows began the last

Table 4. *Effect of Calving BCS and Postpartum Nutrition on Rebreeding Performance of 2-year-old Heifers*

| | BCS AT CALVING | | | |
| | <5 | | >5 | |
Postpartum nutrition	*Maintenance*	*Gain*	*Maintenance*	*Gain*
Calving BCS	4.4	4.4	5.3	5.3
Breeding BCS	4.7	5.3	5.0	5.6
Weight Gain Calving to Breeding (lbs)	25	115	−10	50
Pregnancy Rate (%)				
90 days PP	7	18	35	53
120 days PP	36	66	91	94

(*Adapted from* Bell D, Wettemann RP, Lusby KS: Effects of body condition score at calving and postpartum nutrition on performance of two-year-old heifers. Animal Science Research Report, Stillwater, Oklahoma, Agricultural Experiment Station, Oklahoma State University, 1991; with permission.)

trimester of pregnancy and calved with satisfactory BCS, those that lost one BCS from calving to breeding had pregnancy rates reduced by 21%.[26] These losses are due to reduced conception rates and if the weight loss continues into the breeding, some cows may become anestrus even though they had previous estrous cycles (Fig. 11).

STRATEGIES FOR SPRING CALVING HERDS

Spring calving herds usually calve with lower BCSs than fall calving herds. Calving occurs in late winter to early spring after several months of poor to marginal forage and environmental conditions. Evaluating body condition in midsummer and at weaning are important first steps

Table 5. *Effect of Energy on Post-Calving Pregnancy Rate*

| | PERCENT PREGNANT | | | |
RATION FROM CALVING TIME TO BREEDING	FROM FIRST SERVICE	AFTER BREEDING 20 DAYS	90 DAYS	PERCENT COWS NOT SHOWING HEAT
Losing weight (8 lb TDN)	43	29	72	14
Gaining weight (16 lb TDN)	60	57	82	0
Difference	17	28	10	14

(*Adapted from* Wiltbank JN, Warwick EJ, Vernon EH et al. Factors affecting net calf crop in beef cattle. J Anim Sci 10:409, 1961; with permission.)

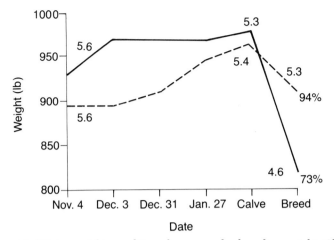

Figure 11. Winter weight, condition changes, and rebreeding weight. Changes in body condition after calving influences rebreeding rates. Cows that maintain body condition (*dashed line*) had a rebreeding rate of 94%. Cows that lost body condition after calving (*solid line*) had a rebreeding rate of 73%. (*From* Selk GE: Assessing the cowherd condition: Management alternatives and consequences. Proceedings: Cow, Grass, the World, and You. Stillwater, Oklahoma, Cooperative Extension Service, Oklahoma State University, 1989; with permission.)

in ensuring proper BCSs at calving. It must be remembered that there are few economical ways to increase body condition once winter has arrived. Thus, good body condition in the winter may depend on nutrition during the previous summer and may be most important during the last trimester, after weaning of the calves. If summer pastures are good and cows are gaining weight as expected, no remedial action is necessary. However, if cows are thin in midsummer to late summer, chances are they will be thin at calving. In these cases, plans must be made to improve body condition while still economically feasible. First, it must be determined why the cows are thin. Is it because of drought, overstocking or parasitism? Whatever the cause, correction and supplementation are necessary to improve body condition. Weaning earlier will certainly help, especially if the situation has adversely affected calf weight gains, in which case both cows and calves would benefit. Supplementation may be helpful. When forage is available, protein supplementation may be all that is needed. Often late summer forage is plentiful, but protein is deficient and the dry matter intake is decreased, resulting in reduced weight gains or weight loss. Protein supplementation will increase dry matter intake and weight gains of 1 to 1.5 pounds per day are not unreasonable for cows not nursing calves.[13] If one waits until fall or winter, large amounts of hay and/or energy supplements will be required to achieve the same goal.

Weaning time is also a good time to evaluate BCS in conjunction with pregnancy palpation, teeth and udder examination and vaccinations. Cows with less than BCS 5 should be separated to be fed to reach at least BCS 5 at calving. Cows with satisfactory BCSs can be fed to maintain body condition. Remember that all cows need to gain approximately 100 lb to allow for fetal and uterine growth, then cows need to gain 80 lb for each increase in BCS (Table 6).

Cows having a surplus of body condition are better able to face severe storms (wet weather with low wind chill factor). When such conditions prevail for long periods, normal feeding regimens may not maintain body condition and increased energy may be necessary. Cows with BCSs 6 and above have "insurance energy stores" to withstand such episodes.

Body condition should be evaluated at calving and before breeding. Shortly after calving, cow-calf pairs should be moved to a different pasture where increased nutrient density feeds can be fed. The postpartum ration will depend on available forages and the most economical supplements. (Consulting a nutritionist or Extension livestock specialist is recommended.) They can develop some novel feeding regimens that are likely more cost-effective than what the producer and veterinarian would ordinarily utilize. The goal is to insure that lactating cows maintain body condition and are gaining weight during the breeding season.

Producers need to develop "what if" programs. Even well planned feeding regimens go awry and cows may calve in thin or borderline body condition. It is very difficult to bring reproductive performance back on schedule and remedial methods need to be considered. One method is "flushing" and 48-hour calf removal. Flushing involves supplying high energy feeds beginning 2 weeks before breeding and continuing through the first 3 weeks of breeding. The energy supplement should be the equivalent of 10 pounds of corn in addition to adequate forage and protein (Table 7). This means an adaptation period of 7 to 14 days to avoid ruminal lactic acidosis. Flushing coupled with 48-hour calf removal at the beginning of breeding has increased cycling and conception rates in borderline (BCS 4–5) cows but is not helpful for cows that have less than BCS 4 or with postpartum intervals less than 45 days.[37]

Table 6. *Weight Needed to Increase Body Condition Score*

		WEIGHT GAIN NEEDED (LB)					
BODY CONDITION AT WEANING	BODY CONDITION AT CALVING	FETUS, FLUIDS AND MEMBRANES	FAT OR MUSCLE	TOTAL	DAYS WEANING TO CALVING	ADG (LB)	RATION TDN REQUIRED (%)
5 (moderate)	5	100	0	100	130	0.77	50
3	5	100	160	260	130	2.00	65
3	5	100	160	260	200	1.30	60
3	5	100	160	260	100	2.60	70
2	5	100	240	340	130	2.60	70
7	5	100	−160	−60	130	−0.46	40

(*Adapted from* Rice LE: Reproductive health management in beef cows. *In* Morrow DA (ed): Current Therapy in Theriogenology. Philadelphia, WB Saunders Co, p 400.)

Table 7. *Pregnancy Rates Following Calf Removal and Flushing*

	CONTROL	F1*	CR+	CR—F1‡
No. cows	18	21	21	21
Pregnant (percent)				
21 Days	28	14	38	57
24 Days	56	52	62	72
63 Days	72	76	62	86

*Flushed with 10 lb corn for 2 weeks before breeding and first 3 weeks of breeding.
+Calf removal for 48 hours at start of breeding.
‡Calf removal+ plus flushing*.
(*Adapted from* Wiltbank JN: Maintenance of a high level of reproductive performance in beef cow herd. Vet Clin North Am 5:41, 1983; with permission.)

Thin cows can only make up time on the reproductive schedule by early weaning of their calves. Early weaning removes the suckling inhibition and eliminates the nutrition requirement of lactation. Research at Oklahoma State University has shown that thin cows (BCS 3 – 4) will respond with high cycling and conception rates soon after weaning of the calves[27] (Table 8). Calves must be weaned at 6 to 8 weeks of age if thin cows are expected to rebreed to maintain a 12-month calving interval. One recommendation is to wean calves every 2 weeks that are from 6 to 8 weeks of age. This meets the physiologic requirements for the cows returning to estrus and the calves are old enough (similar to dairy calves) to consume a complete dry ration. The most critical time for weaning these calves is the first 2 weeks, when they are learning to eat. With good management and small weaning groups, stress can be minimized and early weaning has not been risky. Respiratory and enteric diseases have not been problems, perhaps due to persistent passive immunity at that age. Small pens with shelter plus feed and water accessible to small calves are necessary. The Oklahoma State University early weaning ration is presented in Table 9 and should be fed until calves are approximately 7 months of age. Weight gains have averaged 1.75 pounds per day with a feed conversion ratio of 4.5 pounds of dry matter per pound of gain.[27]
Economically, feeding the calves and salvaging the breeding sea-

Table 8. *Effects of Early Weaning on Cow and Heifer Performance*

	FIRST CALF HEIFERS		MATURE COWS	
	NORMAL WEANED	EARLY WEANED	NORMAL WEANED	EARLY WEANED
Dam weight (lb)				
at early weaning	698	680	816	832
at end of breeding	746	753	922	968
at normal weaning time	788	875	920	1040
Pregnancy rate (%)	59	97	81	100
Days from calving to first estrus	91	73	81	46

(*Adapted from* Lusby KS, Wettemann RP, Turman RJ: Effects of early weaning calves from first-calf-heifers on calf and heifer performance. J Anim Sci 53:1193, 1981; with permission.)

Table 9. *Ration Fed to Early Weaned Calves*

INGREDIENTS	PERCENT (AS FED BASIS)
Cottonseed hulls	30.0
Corn, rolled or ground	46.3
Cane molasses	4.0
Soybean meal	18.0
Calcium carbonate	1.9
Dicalcium phosphate	0.45
Salt	0.30
Vitamin A (30,000 IU/g)	1 lb/ton
Coccidiostat	recommended dosage

(*Adapted from* Lusby KS: Feeding the cowherd. *In* Oklahoma Beef Cattle Manual, 2nd ed. Stillwater, Oklahoma, Cooperative Extension Service, Division of Agriculture Oklahoma State University, 1988; with permission.)

son is far superior to feeding the thin cows while nursing their calves and still having poor reproductive performance. Because the dry cows whose calves were weaned early now have low nutritional requirements and breed well, the net gain after calf feed and labor costs is approximately $90 per cow at 1990 market values.

STRATEGIES FOR FALL CALVING HERDS

In areas where fall calving is a common practice, cows are usually in very good body condition at calving because calving occurs after a summer of grazing good forage. When the breeding season is properly managed, fall calving cows have better reproductive efficiency than spring calving cows. They usually calve with BCS of 6 or greater, and the pasture and environmental conditions are usually favorable for proper postpartum nutrition. It is important to maintain body condition before the breeding season. Unless the producer is in an area that has green forage from November through January, most dry forages, grass hay and silage will be protein deficient. If forage is plentiful the only supplementation required will likely be protein with hay fed as necessary during extremely cold weather.

Fall calving cows entering the breeding season in November– December in good body condition should complete breeding before extreme weather is encountered in January. The largest risk is an unusual cold spell in December or early January. If this happens during the breeding season and radical weight loss occurs over a short time, cycling and conception rates may be drastically reduced.[19] An Oklahoma study reported that breeding activity among cows with BCSs of 5 and 6 was reduced and conception rates of cows that did cycle were reduced. These fall-calving cows losing weight before or during the breeding season had cycling rates reduced 10% and pregnancy rates reduced 19%.[19] Extreme weather usually involves increased environmental moisture, low temperatures and high winds. The wind chill factor and loss of insulation due to moisture greatly increase the energy requirement and are accompanied by marked weight loss unless corrective measures are quickly taken. Additional energy is needed but supplementing large amounts of concentrates risks ruminal lactic acidosis in cows not adapted to a concentrate ration. The best procedure is free choice, good quality hay or silage with a protein supplement. The feeding area should be sheltered, which will reduce the wind chill and therefore the energy requirement.

Critical times for evaluation of body condition in fall calving cows are at the beginning of summer and at weaning. Some producers may wean at the beginning of summer, while others prefer to wean calves at 9 to 10 months of age in July. If cows are thin at the first of June they may not gain sufficiently if calves continue to nurse. In this situation the choice would be to wean the calves, permitting the excess energy from choice forage to be used for weight gain rather than lactation. If forage is maturing at weaning, with decreasing protein content, protein supplementation would be recommended as long as there is an adequate supply of forage.

If fall calving cows go into the breeding season in thin condition, economic options are limited. Early weaning is more of a risk for calf health and weight gain than for cow performance. Greatly increasing feed will be expensive and will more likely increase milk production rather than weight gain. Fall calving cows must be managed to begin calving with BCS 6 or greater and fed to maintain postpartum condition. Strict adherence to a 60 day calving and breeding season is very important to avoid prolonged midwinter periods of bad weather during the breeding season.

REMEDIAL REGIMENS

If we assume a BCS of 5 or 6 at calving and maintaining postpartum body condition plus a slight weight gain immediately before and during the breeding season provides the most cost-effective reproductive performance, we can then assign a ratio of 100 to the performance of such cows. We can assign lower performance ratios for thin cows by interpolating from research data the comparative performance of cows that calve in BCS 4 or less and fail to gain weight after calving (Table 10). The potential calf weaning weight per cow bred ratio will determine

Table 10. *Performance Ratios of Reproductive Parameters with Cows Under Different Nutritional Regimens*

	RATIOS	
VARIABLES	BCS 3–4* MAIN.‡	BCS 5–6* MAIN./GAIN†
Cycling rate 1st 60 days of breeding	72	100
1st service conception rate	70	100
Pregnancy rate 90 day breeding season	74	100
Calf weaning wt.	90	100
Potential calf weaning wt/cow bred	67	100

*BCS at calving.
†Maintain postpartum weight with slight gain during breeding.
‡Maintain postpartum weight.

the gross income producing ability of the cows. We can use this ratio to estimate income lost from cows being in poor body condition at critical times of the reproductive cycle. In this example, if we expect 87 cows from a herd of 100 to wean calves of 500 pounds each under the optimal conditions, the weaning weight per cow bred would be 435 pounds. If the selling price is $0.90 per pound the income per cow bred would be $392. The estimated income from the cows in poor body condition would be 67% of the optimal income or $263, a difference of $129.

Will preventing the loss of income by proper prepartum and postpartum nutrition be cost-effective? First a ration or supplementation program must be developed, then a partial budget determined to assess the cost-effectiveness. The nutritional regimen may be calculated by the use of pocket calculators and the NRC requirements. However, there are numerous inexpensive ration balancing procedures on computer spread sheet programs and the use of such programs is an impressive way to determine the ration. The program used in this example is *Ration Evaluator* developed by the Agricultural Practices section of the Kansas State University College of Veterinary Medicine.[11] In this program, one must put in the animal information and feedstuff information as conditions, feeds or costs change (Tables 11 and 12). In this example, Oklahoma conditions will be used with calves being weaned October 1 and calving starting February 1, 120 days later. An assumption will be made that natural forage will be plentiful and cows will gain approximately 1 lb per day during October and November if protein supplement is provided. If continued gain is expected through December and January, considerable forage and concentrate supplementation will be required. On the other hand, cows will maintain condition until December with no supplementation, but additional forage and protein will be required to maintain condition up to and through calving. Therefore, cows that will be expected to maintain a BCS of 3.5 will receive no supplements until December when approximately half

Table 11. *Animal Information Used in Ration Evaluator Program*

INPUT SCREEN I — ANIMAL INFORMATION	
Current body weight	880 pounds
Current body condition score (1–9)	3.5
Days until calving	120 days
Desired body condition score (1–9)	5
Average weight during feeding period	940 pounds
Average daily gain of feeding period	1 pound per day
Note: This ADG is above and beyond the 0.9 lb/day due to fetal growth	
Number of cows/heifers in the group	100 head
Acclimated temperature	35 °F

(*Adapted from* Lane RJ, Stokka GL, Spire MF: A Lotus 1-2-3 template for formulating and evaluating rations. Section of Agricultural Practices, College of Veterinary Medicine, Kansas State University, 1990; with permission.)

Table 12. *Feed Values and Costs Used in Ration Evaluator Program*

REFERENCE SCREEN II — FEEDSTUFF COST INFORMATION

	As fed $	/unit	lb/unit	$/lb	Daily cost
Alfalfa hay	85.00	ton	2000	0.04	0.00
Prairie hay	50.00	ton	2000	0.03	0.00
CS hulls	150.00	ton	2000	0.08	0.00
Corn grain	2.50	bu	56	0.04	0.18
Milo grain	4.75	cwt	100	0.05	0.00
Wheat midds	100.00	ton	2000	0.05	0.35
Fescue	50.00	ton	2000	0.03	0.30
CS meal	180.00	ton	2000	0.09	0.00
Dical	4.95	bag	80	0.06	0.00
Limestone	2.85	bag	60	0.05	0.00
					$0.83

DM BASIS FEEDSTUFF COMPOSITION VALUES

	DM%	NEm Mcal/kg	NEg Mcal/kg	CP%	Ca%	P%
Alfalfa hay	90.00	1.24	0.68	17.00	1.41	0.24
Prairie hay	92.00	1.00	0.45	5.80	0.43	0.15
CS hulls	90.00	1.03	0.19	4.30	0.16	0.10
Corn grain	88.00	2.24	1.55	10.10	0.02	0.35
Milo grain	87.00	2.06	1.40	10.10	0.04	0.34
Wheat midds	90.00	1.91	1.25	17.00	0.13	1.01
Fescue	90.00	1.15	0.44	6.00	0.50	0.35
CS meal	90.00	1.70	1.06	41.00	0.17	1.31
Dical	97.00	0.00	0.00	0.00	22.00	19.30
Limestone	100.00	0.00	0.00	0.00	34.00	0.00

(*Adapted from* Lane RJ, Stokka GL, Spire MF: A Lotus 1-2-3 template for formulating and evaluating rations. Section of Agricultural Practices, College of Veterinary Medicine, Kansas State University, 1990; with permission.)

Table 13. *Ration Formulation from Ration Evaluator Program*

INPUT SCREEN II — RATION FORMULATION

Feedstuff	Lb of as fed feed/hd/day		Amt req'd	Amt spl'd	Amount oversupplied
Alfalfa hay	0.00	Dry matter	—	20.72	— lb
Prairie hay	0.00	NetEn(M)	10.78	10.78	0.00 Mcal
CS hulls	0.00	NetEn(G)	2.16	2.17	0.01 Mcal
Corn grain	4.00	Crude prt	1.83	2.07	0.25 lb
Milo grain	0.00	Calcium	0.08	0.10	0.01 lb
Wheat midds	7.00	Phosphor	0.05	0.11	0.06 lb
Fescue	12.00				
CS meal	0.00	Cost of ration/day			DM intake
Dical	0.00				
Limestone	0.10		$0.83		2.14% of BW

(*Adapted from* Lane RJ, Stokka GL, Spire MF: A Lotus 1-2-3 template for formulating and evaluating rations. Section of Agricultural Practices, College of Veterinary Medicine, Kansas State University, 1990; with permission.)

the expected forage intake will be hay and all the protein requirement will be supplemented.

The ration may be quickly balanced by trial and error from listed feedstuffs (Table 12). Cows that have a BCS of 3.5 at weaning and are expected to be in BCS 5 at calving will need to gain 1 lb per day (see Table 11). Half of that gain will be made in October and November on fall pasture plus protein supplementation. The ration from December through calving will be hay and concentrates. The example ration in

Table 14. *Report to Client on Ration Formulation and Feed Cost for Cows Fed to Gain Prepartum Body Condition*

KANSAS STATE UNIVERSITY — COLLEGE OF VETERINARY MEDICINE COMMODITY PROGRAM

Prepared for:	Deadpuddle Ranch			04/30/90
	RR 3 Box 12			
	Stillwater, OK 74074			
Prepared by:	Dr. Larry Rice			
	Oklahoma State University			

Cattle Information

	Number of cows	100 head
	Days until calving	60 days
	Initial body weight	940 pounds
	Average body condition score	4.25
	Desired body condition score	5
	Expected average daily gain in addition to fetal growth	1.00 ADG
	Average expected daily temperature	35 °F

Ration Ingredients

Ingredient	Daily Amt Per Head	Daily Amt Per Group
Alfalfa hay		
Prairie hay		
CS hulls		
Corn grain	4.00 lb	400 lb
Milo grain		
Wheat midds	7.00 lb	700 lb
Fescue	12.00 lb	1200 lb
CS meal		
Dical		
Limestone	0.10 lb	10.0 lb
Total As-Fed Feed	23.10 lb	2310 lb
DM Intake	2.14 % of BW	
Cost of Ration	$0.83	$83.33

Daily Nutrient Sufficiency Table

	NEm Mcal	NEg Mcal	CP lb	Ca lb	P lb
Amt Req'd	10.78	2.16	1.83	0.08	0.05
Amt Spl'd	10.78	2.17	2.07	0.10	0.11
Deficiency	Ok	Ok	Ok	Ok	Ok

(*Adapted from* Lane RJ, Stokka CL, Spire MF: A Lotus 1-2-3 template for formulating and evaluating rations. Section of Agricultural Practices, College of Veterinary Medicine, Kansas State University, 1990; with permission.)

Table 13 will be fed only the last 60 days of the prepartum period. (Note that wheat midds, a highly digestable fiber with moderate protein, is the greater portion of the concentrate. It supplies good energy and protein values without reducing forage intake.) A report is developed for the client, including the ration ingredients and daily cost (Table 14). The partial budget must include an estimate of feed costs if the thin cows were not fed to reach the breeding goals; the increased feed costs being the difference between the selected ration and no gain ration (Table 15). The increased income is $8382 or $83.82 per cow bred, a return on investment of 185%.

This plan would be developed in October after weaning, palpating for pregnancy, and determining body condition scores. This is also a good time to determine why some cows had low body condition scores. Next year, can those poor BCSs be avoided, thereby reducing the feed costs necessary to increase BCS for the desired reproductive performance?

Table 15. *Partial Budget: Feeding Cows to Gain 1.5 BCS Calving and Maintain Postpartum Condition with Weight Gain During the Breeding Season*

Assumptions:
1. 100 cows calving in February-March.
2. BCS 5–6 and gaining = 87% weaned calf crop 18 months later.
3. BCS 3–4 and maintaining = 67% of BCS 5–6 weaned 18 months later.
4. Weaning weight = 500 lb.
5. Market price of calves — $.90/lb.
6. Cost of supplement — BCS 5–6
   October-November = $0.23/day/cow
   December-January = $0.83/day/cow
   Postpartum = $0.91/day/cow.
7. Cost of supplement — BCS 3–4
   October-November = $0.0 /day cow
   December-January = $0.48/day/cow
   Postpartum = $0.81/day/cow.

Added Receipts		Added Expenses	
Calf sales		Feed costs	
@ BCS 5–6 — $39,150		BCS 5–6	
@ BCS 3–4 — 26,231		Prepartum $6,360	
		Postpartum 7,280	
Difference	$12,919		$13,640
		BCS 3–4	
		Prepartum $2,880	
		Postpartum $6,480	
			$9,360
		Difference	$4,280
		6 mo. interest @12%	
		$257	
Total Additions: $12,919		Total Subtractions:	$4,537
	Net Change: $8,382	= $83.82/cow.	

SUMMARY

The concept of feeding for optimal reproductive performance is not new. The effects of prepartum and postpartum nutritional levels on return to postpartum estrus and conception rates was reported in 1962.[37] The effect of body condition regardless of nutrition regimen was first reported in 1975.[35] Body condition scoring has become a popular topic for Extension and practitioner sponsored producer meetings. To effectively promote a management change that requires increased cash flow and does not have an immediate return requires demonstration of cost-effectiveness. This requires knowledge of the biologic information and transformation of that knowledge (through partial budget analysis) into additional profit for the producer.

Controlling reproduction through proper nutrition at critical times of the reproductive cycle requires:

1. Calving and breeding seasons of 60 days.
2. Cows to be in moderate to good body condition at calving (BCS 5–7).
3. Cows to be slightly gaining at the beginning of the breeding season.
4. Cows to be bred to fertile bulls.
5. Evaluation and correction of body condition well in advance of the actual impact of BCS on reproductive function.
6. Producer to be prepared to initiate "alternate" plans (i.e., early weaning or 48 hour calf removal).

REFERENCES

1. Ames DR: Adjusting rations for climate. Vet Clin North Am [Food Anim Pract] 4:543, 1988
2. Bell D, Wettemann RP, Lusby KS: Effect of body condition score at calving and postpartum nutrition on performance of 2-year-heifers. Animal Science Research Report, Agricultural Experiment Station, Oklahoma State University, 1990, MP-129 p 23–27, 1990
3. Bellows RA, Short RE: Effects of precalving feed level on birth weight, calving difficulty and subsequent fertility. J Anim Sci 46:1522, 1978
4. Bicknell RJ: Endogenous opiod peptides and hypothalmic neuroendocrine neurones. J Endocrinol 5 170:437, 1985
5. Clanton DC: Non-protein nitrogen in range supplements. J Anim Sci 47:765, 1978
6. Dunn TG, Kaltenbach CC: Nutrition and postpartum interval of the ewe, sow and cow. J Anim Sci 51(suppl 2):29, 1980
7. Dunn TG, Riley ML, Murdoch WJ, et al: Body condition score and carcass energy content in postpartum beef cows. Proc West Sec Am Soc Anim Sci 34:56, 1980
8. Evans DG: The interpretation and analysis of subjective body condition scores. Anim Prod 26:119, 1978
9. Herd DB, Spratt LR: Body condition, nutrition and reproduction of beef cows. Texas Agricultural Extension Service Bulletin 1526, 1986, p 11
10. Herdt TH: Fuel homeostasis in the ruminant. Vet Clin North Am [Food Anim Pract] 4:213, 1988
11. Lane RJ, Stokka GL, Spire MF: A Lotus 1-2-3 template (Winter Wk 1) for formulating and evaluating rations. Section of Agriculture Practices, College of Veterinary Medicine, Kansas St Univ, 1990

12. Lofstedt RM, Mauns JG, Murphy BD, et al: Influence of GNRH infusion on endocrine parameters and duration of postpartum anestrus in beef cows. Theriogenology 15:359, 1981
13. Lusby KS: Feeding the cow herd. In Oklahoma Beef Cattle Manual, ed 2. Cooperative Extension Service, Division of Agriculture Oklahoma State University 1988, pp 1–20
14. Maas J: Relationship between nutrition and reproduction in beef cattle. Vet Clin North Am [Food Anim Pract] 3:633, 1987
15. Morrow DA, Roberts SJ, McEntee K: Review of postpartum ovarian activity and involution of the uterus and cervix in cattle. Cornell Vet 59:134–154, 1969
16. National Research Council (NRC): Nutrient requirements of beef cattle. Washington, DC, National Academy of Sciences, NRC, 1984
17. Oetzel GR: Protein-energy malnutrition in ruminants. Vet Clin North Am [Food Anim Pract] 4:317, 1988
18. Peters AR, Lamming GE, Fisher MW: A comparison of LH plasma concentrations in milked and suckled postpartum cows. J Reprod Fert 62:5677, 1981
19. Rakestraw JD, Lusby KS, Wettemann RP, Wagner JJ: Postpartum weight and body condition loss and performance of fall-calving cows. Theriogenology 26:461, 1986
20. Rice LE: Reproductive health management in beef cows. In Morrow DA (ed): Current Therapy in Theriogenology. Philadelphia, WB Saunders Co, 1986, p 400
21. Randel RD: Nutrition and postpartum rebreeding in cattle. J Anim Sci 68:853, 1990
22. Richards MW, Spitzer JC, Warner MB: Effect of varying levels of postpartum nutrition and body condition at calving on subsequent reproductive performance in beef cattle. J Anim Sci 62:300–306, 1986
23. Riley GM, Peters AR, Lamming GE: Induction of pulsatile LH release, FSH release and ovulation in postpartum beef cows by repeating small doses of GNRH. J Reprod Fert 63:559–565, 1981
24. Rush IG, Totusek R: Supplemental value of feed grade biuret and urea-molasses for cows on dry winter grass. J Anim Sci 42:497, 1976
25. Rutter LM, Randel RD: Postpartum nutrient intake and body condition: Effect on pituitary function and onset of estrus in beef cattle. J Anim Sci 58:265, 1984
26. Selk GE, Wettemann RP, Lusby S, et al: Relationships among weight change, body condition and reproductive performance of range beef cows. J Anim Sci 66:3153, 1988
27. Selk GE, Lusby KS: The management of beef cattle for efficient reproduction. In Oklahoma Beef Cattle Manual, ed 2. Cooperative Extension Service, Division of Agriculture, Oklahoma State University, 1988, pp 40–66
28. Selk GE, Wettemann RP, Lusby KS, et al: The importance of body condition at calving on reproduction in beef cows. Anim Sci Res Report MP118. Oklahoma Agriculture Experiment Station 1986, pp 316–319
29. Somerville SH, Lowman BG, Deas DW: The effect of plane of nutrition during lactation on the reproductive performance of beef cows. Vet Rec 104:95, 1979
30. Spitzer JC: Influence of nutrition on reproduction in beef cattle. In Morrow DA (ed): Current Therapy in Theriogenology ed 2. Philadelphia, WB Saunders Co, 1986, pp 320–351
31. Tinker ED: Evaluation of cow type and body condition score on carcass composition and postpartum return to estrus in two-breed-cross beef cows. PhD Thesis, Department of Animal Science Oklahoma State University, 1990
32. Wagner JJ, Lusby KS, Oltjen JW, et al: Carcass composition in mature Hereford cows: Estimation and effect on daily metabolizable energy requirement during winter. J Anim Sci 66:603, 1988
33. Wettemann RP, Lusby KS, Turman EJ: Relationship between changes in prepartum body weight and condition and reproductive performance of range cows. Oklahoma Agriculture Experiment Station Research Report, MP-112:12, 1982
34. Whisnant CS, Kiser TE, Thompson FN, et al: Opioid inhibition of luteinizing hormone secretion during the postpartum period in suckled cows. J Anim Sci 62:1340–1345, 1986
35. Whitman RW, Remmega EE, Wiltbank JN: Weight change, condition and beef cow production. J Anim Sci Abstr 41:387, 1975

26

LAWRENCE E. RICE

36. Williams GL: Suckling as a regulator of postpartum rebreeding in cattle: A review. J Anim Sci 68:831, 1990
37. Wiltbank JN: Maintenance of a high level of reproductive performance in the beef cow herd. Vet Clin North Am [Food Anim Pract] 5:41, 1983
38. Wiltbank JN, Rowden WW, Ingalls JE, et al: Effect of energy level on reproductive phenomena of mature Hereford cows. J Anim Sci 21:219, 1962
39. Wiltbank JN, Rowden WW, Ingalls JE, et al: Influence of postpartum energy level on reproductive performance of Hereford cows restricted in energy intake prior to calving. J Anim Sci 23:1049, 1964
40. Wright IA, Rhind SM, Russel AJF, et al: Effects of body condition, food intake and temporary calf separation on the duration of the post-partum anoestrous period and associated LH, FSH and prolactin concentrations in beef cows. Anim Prod 45:395, 1987
41. Wright IA, Russel AJF: Partition of fat, body composition and body condition score in mature cows. Anim Prod 38:23, 1984

Address reprint requests to

Lawrence E. Rice, DVM, MS
Boren Veterinary Teaching Hospital
Oklahoma State University
College of Veterinary Medicine
Stillwater, OK 74078

0749-0720/91 $0.00 + .20

Nutrition and the Development of Replacement Heifers

Lawrence E. Rice, DVM, MS*

Uniform calf crops are the result of shortened breeding seasons. Shortened breeding seasons for the entire herd must start with the replacement heifers. Heifers that calve early and over a short period of time tend to repeat that performance throughout their lifetime if they are properly managed.[10,29,47,55] Dams that attain puberty at an early age and calve at a young age have more efficient lifetime production.[13] Such management is not easy or inexpensive. Low input operations depend on heifers calving for the first time at 3 years of age. The development cost is low, but the loss of return becomes very expensive. Most producers now expect heifers to calve for the first time at 2 years of age. Proper nutritional management is the key to the development of high performance replacements.

HOW DO HEIFERS INFLUENCE THE HERD?

The success of managing heifers through the second calving will determine the success of the adult cow herd. To emphasize this concept, let us examine a hypothetical herd drawn from observation of many herds. The example herd has 100 cows that calve during a period of approximately 4 months. The owner adds 10 replacement heifers that calve relatively early during the calving season. The owner also rebreeds selected dry cows (cows that failed to calve during the current calving season) in order to maintain enough pregnant cows. With the exception of the fat dry cows, the cows are in moderate to thin body condition at calving in the late winter and spring. Nutrition improves following calving, especially as new pasture improves and cows are gaining weight during the breeding season. Approximately 100 cows

---

*Diplomate, American College of Theriogenelogists, Professor, Department of Medicine and Surgery, Boren Veterinary Teaching Hospital, Oklahoma State University College of Veterinary Medicine, Stillwater, Oklahoma

and 15 to 20 replacement heifers are bred to maintain 100 pregnant females for the next calving season. Pregnant replacements are pastured and fed with the adults. The calving pattern has been similar for many years (Table 1).

Many of the breeding problems in this herd can be traced directly to the management of heifers. Note that 7 (70%) of the heifers calved in the first 42 days of the calving season but only 41 (46%) of the cows calved during the same period. If the time of replacement heifer calving represents the future calving patterns, 70% of the cows in this herd should calve in the first 42 days. However, first-calf heifers require approximately 20 days more postpartum rest to have cycling rates comparable to those of cows.[57] Therefore, many first-calf heifers lose 20 days between the first and second calving (Table 2). In this case, the second calving actually sets future calving patterns.

Also, the cycling rates in Table 2 are dependent upon the heifers and cows being maintained separately. Replacement heifers have high growth requirements and are suddenly subjected to two new stresses, calving and nursing. The loss of incisor teeth between 18 months and 3 years of age is an added handicap and they cannot compete for available nutrients when maintained with adult cows. Less than favorable conditions will lengthen postpartum anestrus, resulting in delayed calving or possibly open young cows the next year. This partially explains how the breeding program deteriorates between the first and subsequent calvings in the example herd.

One solution to the above problem is to breed replacement virgin heifers for only 45 days, beginning 21 days before the cow herd, and to maintain the replacements separately through the second breeding season when they are nursing their first calves.[49] This provides adequate postpartum rest for all the replacements to cycle and become pregnant to fit into the cow calving schedule. Note in Table 3 that heifers calving in the second and third calving groups are not all cycling until after 60 days of the breeding season.

The long calving season in the example herd presents a problem in initiating an early short calving season for heifers. Many early calving 2-year-old heifers will, in fact, be under 2 years of age at calving if they are expected to calve 20 days before the cows. Consequently, they must be cycling and fertile at 13 to 15 months of age; however, many beef heifers have not reached puberty at 15 months of age. This means that most replacements must come from the heifers that were born

Table 1. *Calving Pattern in 90 Adult Cows and 10 Heifers*

CALVING GROUP*	1	2	3	4	5	6	
DAY OF CALVING SEASON	21	42	63	84	105	126	
	Number of Calves						Total
First-calf heifers	3	4	1	1	1		10
Adult cow	14	27	27	13	6	3	90
Total	17	31	28	14	7	3	100

*Each calving group represents consecutive 21-day periods.

Table 2. *Effect of Age on Return to Estrus in Beef Cows Nursing Calves*

	DAYS AFTER CALVING						
	40	50	60	70	80	90	100
				% Cycling			
Cows	30	53	72	82	89	94	100
Heifers	15	24	47	62	68	79	90

(*Adapted from* Wiltbank JN: Wean more pounds of beef. National Association of Animal Breeders, 1969, p 8; with permission.)

during the first 42 days of the calving season, yet the example herd has only 24 heifer calves born during that time. After normal attrition, it is unlikely that 15% to 20% replacements could be procured from heifer calves born during the first 42 days of the previous calving season. This means that heifers must be managed for early puberty.

ONSET OF PUBERTY

First, what are the endocrine events associated with the onset of puberty? One time-honored theory is that the prepuberal hypothalamus and anterior pituitary are extremely sensitive to the negative feedback of gonadal steroids.[2] The most minute steroid levels would therefore prevent the release of gonadotrophins that are necessary for the onset of estrual activity. Puberty was viewed as a progressive loss of hypothalamic sensitivity to the negative feedback and as the animal matured, increasing amounts of gonadotrophins were released followed by increasing steroids, eventually inducing estrus and ovulation. During prepuberal development in heifers, estrogen becomes less effective in inhibiting LH secretion, finally becoming more effective in causing LH secretion through positive feedback as puberty approaches.[45,51]

Bovine ovaries are responsive at an early age and can be stimulated to ovulate, but cyclic function cannot be maintained.[46] Pituitary responsiveness to exogenous GNRH is maximal before cycling is initiated.[3] However, episodic LH release is low and irregular in prepuberal heifers, probably due to low GNRH production.[21] The frequency and

Table 3. *Estimated Effect of Time of Birth of First Calf on Reproductive Performance*

	PERCENTAGE OF HEIFERS IN HEAT TO BREED FOR SECOND CALF		
TIME OF BIRTH OF FIRST CALF	*by First 21 days of breeding season*	*by First 42 days of breeding season*	*by First 63 days of breeding season*
21 days prior to start of calving	90	100	100
First 21 days of calving season	68	90	100
Second 21 days of calving season	47	68	90
Third 21 days of calving season	15	47	68

amplitude of GNRH and LH episodic releases increase as puberty approaches.

As in the anestrus ewe, the prepuberal heifer requires a priming level of progesterone to act synergistically with estrogens for estrus and ovulation to occur. The gradual increase of the episodic LH release may be primed by progesterone in the 2 months preceding puberty. One study showed progesterone levels were very low (300 pg/ml) in prepuberal heifers, but two distinct perpuberal elevations were observed followed by LH peaks after the progesterone returned to baseline.[22] Progesterone may also sensitize the ovaries to the gonadotrophins.

A theory gaining credibility is that hypothalamic and pituitary activity is controlled by a pulse generator in the central nervous system.[2] The activity of the pulse generator can be modified by a large variety of internal and external stimuli such as gonadal hormone levels, photoperiod, pheromones, and nutritional state. The negative feedback mechanism of the gonadal steroid is probably mediated through the pulse generator. Puberty would be reached following changes in the pulse generator, which would increase the frequency and amplitude of episodic gonadotrophin releases, resulting in estrus and ovulation.[17]

Methods for induction of estrus in prepuberal heifers have been reported with varied success. The most reliable seems to be the use of progesterone priming for 9 days with a progestogen implant such as Norgestromet.[20,48] Failures occur when the exogenous hormones are used on young or light weight heifers. The hypothesis is that exogenous hormone induction would work only when the heifers were in a physiological state that would allow the hypothalamus to respond to progesterone priming.

Photoperiod or season of the year seems to influence the onset of puberty. Fall born Angus-Holstein heifers have been reported to reach puberty at 307 days, whereas spring born heifers reached puberty at 334 days.[25] Also heifers submitted to 18 hours of light reached puberty 27 to 49 days earlier than heifers in natural light in Wisconsin.[23] There were no apparent differences in body condition or fatness. Other studies indicate that good nutrition may minimize the seasonal effect.[24]

Reproductive performance in Zebu (*Bos indicus*) is more influenced by seasonality than in European breeds (*Bos taurus*). Zebu cattle have a lower preovulatory LH surge in winter than in spring or summer and first service conception rates are dramatically reduced in the winter.[41] Anestrus and anovulatory estrus have been reported to be higher in winter than in summer among young Zebu females.[36]

Puberty is a heritable trait that is altered by the environment. Burfening has cautioned that relying on feed additives and hormonal induction could propagate late maturing heifers.[9] There is evidence that early puberty can be selected through proper sire. Bulls with large testicles at 15 months of age reach puberty earlier than those with small testicles and their half-sib heifers also reach puberty earlier. The correlation coefficient between bull scrotal size and heifer puberty was −0.71.[7] The heritability of bull scrotal size is very high (0.67) so with such a close relationship, age of heifer at puberty could be reduced by selecting bulls with large testes.[12]

NUTRITION

The most easily controlled factor in heifer management is nutrition. Heifers should be fed to reach a weight that will ensure puberty at 13–15 months of age. Low average daily gain (ADG) from weaning to breeding has been reported to delay the onset of puberty[58] (Table 4).

This study also showed the breed effect of the onset of puberty. Among heifers fed low energy rations, Angus and crossbred heifers had the highest ADG and reached puberty earlier than Herefords. There were no differences among breeds when fed high energy levels. There is a point at which very high energy levels increase weight more rapidly than skeletal growth or physiological maturity. This results in excessively heavy heifers for their age without appreciably enhancing the onset of puberty.

Another study showed heifers with ADG of 0.6 lb, 1.0 lb, and 1.5 lb had cycling rates of 7%, 31%, and 83% respectively at the beginning of the breeding season. Pregnancy rates during the first 40 days of breeding were 40%, 83%, and 80%, respectively.[47] Depending on weaning weights, days from weaning to breeding, and target weight at breeding, ADG from 1.0 to 1.5 lb should meet the growth requirements for most yearling replacement heifers.

The ration must be balanced to provide the minimum daily requirements of all nutrients. Producers often think protein is the most important nutrient for growth so they overfeed protein to the prepubertal yearlings to increase growth and underfeed late gestation pregnant heifers to reduce fetal growth and dystocia rate. In addition to the basic function for growth and tissue repair, protein increases forage consumption and energy use.[38] Proper protein supplementation will increase the digestibility of poor forages, hence the energy use.[6] From a practical standpoint, protein intake may be more liberal than the

Table 4. *Occurrence of First Heat in Heifers on Two Levels of Feed*

FEED LEVEL	BREED	APPROX DAILY GAIN (LB)	PERCENT IN HEAT BY						
			11 mo.	12 mo.	13 mo.	14 mo.	15 mo.	16 mo.	17 mo.
Low	Angus	0.9	0	0	0	33	82	90	100
	Hereford	0.6	0	11	22	33	38	50	100
	Crossbred	1.0	0	0	12	68	85	100	100
High	Angus	1.6	8	33	58	100	100	100	100
	Hereford	1.3	0	12	50	100	100	100	100
	Crossbred	1.9	0	18	75	94	94	100	100

(*Adapted from* Wiltbank JN, Kasson CW, Ingalls JE: Puberty in crossbred and straight-bred beef heifers on two levels of feed. J Anim Sci 19:602, 1969; with permission.)

stated minimum daily requirements, but gross overfeeding of protein is not cost effective.

Energy is usually the limiting factor in achieving satisfactory ADG and target weights.[27,56] This is usually due to an overestimation of forage quality and intake, plus failure to adequately supplement protein and energy. Replacement heifers require a minimum energy value of 60%–65% TDN and most winter forages or hays will not meet this energy value.[35]

High quality forages such as small grain pastures, legume-grass mixture pastures, sudan-sorghum hybrid pastures, and other improved pastures will meet the protein and energy requirements of heifers, weaning through breeding. The availability of these forages is limited to geographical areas and seasons that favor their production at a reasonable cost. Often, supplementation of available hay or providing a complete mixed ration is necessary. In areas where silage production is common, it is an excellent source of energy but requires protein supplementation. In all circumstances, target weights must be determined, average daily gain calculated, ration balanced and then weight grains monitored through periodic weighing. If the gain is not up to expected levels the ration must be adjusted.

The reproductive requirement for vitamins, minerals and trace minerals does not surpass that of growth, and meeting the ADG requirement should be all that is necessary. The addition of beta-carotene to vitamin A-sufficient diets has been advocated to enhance reproduction, but its actual role is equivocal and definitive use is yet to be determined.[52]

What feed additives or growth stimulants influence growth rate and the onset of puberty? Replacement heifers fed monensin at the rate of 200 mg per head per day from weaning through breeding had higher ADG and reached puberty at an earlier age in several studies.[18,32,34] However, there was no difference in first service conception rates or pregnancy rates.

Monensin is used in feedlot rations to increase feeding efficiency through reduced feed consumption.[18,42] Monensin increases the percentage of propionic acid, which is much more energy efficient than acetic or butyric acid. Increased propionic acid also spares protein from gluconeogenesis, thereby increasing nitrogen retention.[16,37] Cattle on lower energy rations, such as growing rations, do not experience reduced feed intake because rumen capacity rather than energy satiation will limit feed intake. In this case, the increased propionic acid is then used for growth and other metabolic processes.

Addition of monensin to replacement heifer rations is most advantageous when the heifers would be at a borderline age and target weight at the beginning of the breeding season. Some reports indicated that in addition to improved ADG, monensin enhanced pituitary response to GNRH and ovarian response to gonadotrophins.[11,40,50] This mechanism is not known, but the data clearly indicate the inclusion of monensin in replacement heifer rations will enhance the onset of puberty.

Growth-stimulating implants improved growth rates in replacement heifers. While all implants improved growth rates and increased pelvic areas, aberrant cycling rates and reduced pregnancy rates were often associated with the use of growth implants.[33] Apparently, one time implantation of 1 to 2 month-old nursing heifer calves does not harm reproduction but reimplantation at weaning should be avoided.[19]

Weight and age have been reported to influence the onset of puberty in beef heifers.[47] Breed differences, differences within breeds, and environmental factors often make selection of target weights variable and difficult. Note the variation of weights among breeds and expected cycling rates in Table 5.[4]

In recent years genetic selection has been for larger cattle, resulting in heavier weaning and yearling weights as well as heavier adult weights. A guideline that has been cited by this author and others is that 90% of 14 – 15 month old heifers will have reached puberty if they have been fed to reach 65% of their mature weight.[44] While this generalization has some error (Zebu breeds require additional age) it does adjust for changing adult weights and is practical to apply to most herds.

A comment should be made regarding preweaning growth rates and body condition at weaning. Studies have shown that heifers that had excessive preweaning gains, resulting in being overly fat at weaning had reduced milk production as adults. This became known as the "fatty udder syndrome," in which excessive fat was deposited in the udder at the expense of glandular tissue.[26] In one study, every other generation produced reduced weaning weights because the dam's milk production was decreased due to the excessive fat deposition in their udders while they were nursing.[31] With most of the breeds now being selected for growth rates it does not appear this is of great concern in the current nursing heifer calves. The growth rate is great enough that it is unlikely nursing heifer calves will receive more energy than is required for growth; hence excess fat will not be deposited in the udder. However, this information would suggest creep feeding of heifer calves could be contraindicated.

Table 5. *Estimates of Heifers Reaching Puberty at Various Weights*

	HEIFERS REACHING PUBERTY		
BREED	50% in Estrus	70% in Estrus	90% in Estrus
		Weight in lb.	
Angus	550	600	650
Brahman	675	725	750
Brangus	600	650	700
Charolais	700	750	775
Hereford	600	650	700
Santa Gertrudis	675	725	341
Jersey x British	500	550	600
Limousin	650	700	750
Simmental	625	675	750

(*Adapted from* Beverly JR, Spitzer JC: Management of replacement heifers for a high reproductive and calving rate. College Station, Texas, Texas A & M University Agricultural Extension Service Bulletin, B-1213, 1979; with permission.)

Changing a reproductive program should start at weaning time. The adults can be palpated for pregnancy, culled, immunized, and sorted by body condition in preparation for prepartum feeding, and the replacement heifer program can be started correctly.

CONTROLLED THREE YEAR HEIFER PROGRAM

A controlled three year heifer program should be used to set the calving pattern for the cow herd. Control the first two calvings and management of the cow herd is much easier thereafter. What is the controlled three year heifer program?[44] (1) Breed 13 to 15 month old virgin heifers for 42 days, starting 21 days before the regular breeding season. Eighty-five percent of the heifers should be cycling and bred during the first 21 days and 95% cycling by the end of 42 days. Eighty-five percent of the heifers bred are likely to become pregnant. (2) Two-year-old heifers nursing their first calves should be cycling at a rate of 85% to 95% during the first 42 days of the regular breeding season and 85% or more should be pregnant at the end of 63 days' breeding.

To accomplish these breeding goals, three growth requirements should be achieved during specific times: (1) First year (from birth to breeding). Heifers should obtain 65% of their mature weight to ensure 90% cycling at 13 to 15 months of age (see Table 4). (2) Second year (from first breeding to first calving). Pregnant replacement heifers that have been properly managed should have a body condition score (BCS) of 6 and weigh about 85% of their adult body weight at calving. Heifers that are poorly fed during the last trimester will not breed back early the next breeding season, and often will have increased dystocia rates due to small pelvic areas and weakened condition.[15,28] Excessively fattened heifers will have increased dystocia rates due to internal pelvic fat but will not have heavier birth weight calves than properly managed heifers.[56] Excess protein in the diet has had mixed results on calving ability, sometimes being related to increased dystocia and at other times having no effect on dystocia.[1,5] However, protein malnutrition can be a cause of weak calf syndrome.[8,53] Protein requirements should certainly be met and probably the greatest deterrent to excesses would be cost. (3) Third year (from second breeding to second calving). Heifers should reach 95% of their mature weight at three years of age.

The following steps are required to establish a 3-year controlled heifer program: (1) Select approximately one and a half times as many heifers as will actually be needed for replacements. These heifers should be selected on the basis that they will be between 13 and 15 months of age at the beginning of the heifer breeding season. Zebu breeds may require 3–6 months longer to reach puberty. However, there are reports of these cattle reaching puberty as early as English cattle through selection for early puberty.[4] (2) Weigh heifers at weaning and if there are wide ranges between the smaller and the larger heifers, they should be divided into two feeding groups to reach their desired weight by breeding time. Calculate the days between initial weighing and beginning of the breeding season. Determine the average daily gain necessary to reach the desired breeding weight, and feed to attain that average daily gain. The addition of approved levels of monensin to the ration will improve ADG and enhance the onset of puberty.[18,32,34]

Palatability of the weaning ration is very important to ensure proper dry matter intake. The goal at weaning should be to get the calves on feed as quickly as possible with minimal sickness. High energy diets will result in higher gains but morbidity usually increases when calves are weaned on a high energy ration. A good compromise seems to be weaning on a high quality grass hay plus a supplement containing natural protein, vitamins A and E, and a coccidiostat. If a complete milled ration is desired it should contain at least 50% highly palatable fiber feeds such as cottonseed hulls and dehydrated alfalfa. After the calves have become adjusted and have good daily feed consumption, the ration can be switched to the desired growing ration. (3) Weigh a random sample of the heifers every 30 days to check growth rates. If growth rates are not being attained the ration must be adjusted. (4) It may be necessary to cull approximately 10% of heifers at 1 year of age as undesirable for replacement breeding. This also is the proper time for booster immunizations such as IBR and BVD, and when recommended, start vibriosis and leptospirosis immunization.

When evaluating replacement heifers, one trait to look for is pelvic area. It is the maternal trait that is most highly correlated to ease of calving, thus selecting heifers with large pelvic areas should reduce calving difficulty. Heritability of pelvic area is quite high and estimates range from 0.45 to 0.60.[4] In fact, the heritability of pelvic area is greater than that of birth weight. This means that selection based on pelvic area should increase the pelvic area:birth weight ratio.

The best time to measure pelvic areas is just before the breeding season. Keep only those with favorable pelvic areas and market the others. Due to breed differences and the difficulty in controlling birth weights, there is no specific minimum pelvic area. However, there is a research-based rule-of-thumb for use in culling undesirable heifers. For English breeds, weighing 600–650 lb at around 13 months of age, the ratio of pelvic area to birth weight is 2.1:1. For example, if we expect the calves from these heifers to weigh 70 lb at birth, the minimum pelvic area would be 147 square centimeters. For large breed heifers, whose 13-month target weights are 750 to 850 lb, the pelvic area to birth weight ratio is increased to 2.25:1.[14] Larger heifers have heavier calves, hence the need for larger pelvic areas for calving ease. Pelvic measurements are of no value unless the heifers are properly grown by breeding and calving time. First, culling the bottom 20 to 30% from a group of *small* heifers will not significantly reduce the dystocia rate. Second, selecting replacement heifers with large pelvic areas is not helpful if they are bred to bulls with *unknown* calving ease. The use of the pelvimeter is recommended only in herds that are under intensive management and in those instances for which it will provide the additional selection pressure necessary to use the very best replacement heifers. (5) Breed for 42 days, starting 21 days before breeding the cows. Well grown replacement heifers are ideal candidates for estrus synchronization, which facilitates a short breeding season. Preferably, breeding should be by artificial insemination, using semen from a progeny tested bull proven to be an 'easy calving' bull. The use of such a bull, by AI or natural service, will reduce the dystocia rate. (6) The heifers may be tested for pregnancy as early as 35 days following the end of the breeding season. Once the pregnant replacement heifers have been selected, maintain their growth rate to have a BCS 6 and reach 85% of mature cow size at calving. This is an easy task but one often neglected. Adverse conditions such as drought, storms, parasitic infestation, and so on will cause heifers to be thin and weak at calving. A good manager develops "what if" plans for such situations to avoid wasting 2 years of work, as happened in the example herd.

(7) Heifers with body condition scores of less than 5-6 at calving and not gaining weight after calving have very prolonged postpartum intervals to first estrus.[15,54] While all efforts should be made to prevent such an occurrence, it does happen and there are remedial procedures that can be taken. Studies at Oklahoma State University have shown that early weaning of calves (8 weeks of age) markedly improved reproductive performance of beef heifers.[30] Heifers nursing calves had only a 58% pregnancy rate in a 90-day breeding season compared with 97% in heifers that had calves weaned early. The calves were weaned on a high energy starter ration without encountering any sickness and weighed the same at weaning age as the nursing calves. Economic analysis indicated early weaning would be the most cost-effective way to salvage a reproductive program that has been stressed by an unfavorable environment.

SUMMARY

Does the system work? After having been on a controlled heifer replacement program for 3 to 5 years, the entire herd will develop a short calving season resulting in more weaned calf weight per cow exposed to breeding.

Wiltbank has reported on the advantage of feeding heifers for a selected target weight at breeding.[59] Two groups of Brahman-cross heifers were fed to weigh 600 or 700 lbs at the beginning of the breeding season. They were pastured and fed similarly from breeding through weaning their first calves. The heifers that weighed 700 lb at breeding weaned 86 lb more calf per heifer exposed. They bred earlier and more became pregnant. The return above feed costs after 2 years breeding was $52 greater for the heavier heifers. Obviously, the benefits continue through subsequent calvings, emphasizing the importance of managing the replacement heifers for 3 years, through their second breeding and calving.

REFERENCES

1. Anthony RV, Bellows RA, Short RE, et al: Effects of dietary protein level on pre-partum beef heifers. Proc West Sec Am Soc Anim Sci 1982, p 151

2. Austin CR, Short RV: Reproduction in mammals: The hormonal control of reproduction, ed 2, Cambridge. Cambridge University Press, 11–19, 137–141 1984

3. Barnes MA, Bierly ST, Halman RD, et al: Follicle stimulating hormone, luteinizing hormone and estradiol-17_B response in GNRH treated prepuberal Holstein heifers. Biol Reprod 22:459, 1980

4. Beverly JR, Spitzer JC: Management of replacement heifers for a high reproductive and calving rate. TAMU Agricultural Extension Service Bulletin, B-1213, 1979, p 3

5. Bellows RA, Carr JB, Patterson DJ, et al: Effects of ration protein content on dystocia and reproduction in beef heifers. Proc West Sec Am Soc Anim Sci 29:263, 1978

6. Bond J, Wiltbank JN, Cook AC: Cessation of estrus and ovarian activity in a group of beef heifers on extremely low levels of energy and protein. J Anim Sci 17:1211, [Abstract] 1958

7. Brinks JS, McInerney MJ, Chenoweth PJ: Relationship of age of puberty in heifers to reproductive traits in young bulls. Proc West Sec Am Soc Anim Sci 29:28

8. Bull RC, Louchs RR, Edmiston FH, et al: Nutrition and weak calf syndrome. University of Idaho, College of Agriculture Current Information Series 246, 1974

9. Burfening PJ: Induction of puberty and subsequent reproductive performance. Theriogenology 12:215, 1979

10. Burris MJ, Priode GM: Effect of calving date on subsequent calving performance. J Anim Sci 17:527, 1958

11. Bushmich SL, Randel RL, McCartor MM, et al: Effect of dietary monensin on ovarian response following gonadotrophin treatment in prepuberal heifers. J Anim Sci 51:692, 1980

12. Coulter GH, Rounsaville TR, Foote RH: Heritability of testicular size and consistency in Holstein bulls. J Anim Sci 43:9, 1976

13. Davis ME, Rutledge JJ, Cundiff LV, et al: Life cycle efficiency of beef production: VI. Relationship of cow efficiency ratios for progeny slaughtered to growth, condition, fertility, and milk production of the dam. J Anim Sci 60:69, 1985

14. Deutscher GH: Pelvic measurements for reducing calving difficulty. Neb Guide G88–895. Cooperative Extension Service, University of Nebraska, 1988

15. Dunn TG, Ingalls JE, Zimmerman DR, et al: Reproductive performance of two-year-old Hereford and Angus heifers as influenced by pre- and post-calving energy intake. J Anim Sci 29:719, 1969

16. Eskeland BW, Pfander H, Preston FL: Intravenous energy infusion in lambs: Effects on nitrogen retention, plasma free amino acids and plasma urea nitrogen. Br J Nutr 31:201–105, 1974

17. Foster DL, Hellon SM, Olster DH: Internal and external determinants of the timing of puberty in the female. J Reprod Fert 75:327, 1976

18. Gill DR, Martin JR, Lake R: High, medium and low corn silage diets with and without monensin for feedlot steers. J Anim Sci 43:363, 1976

19. Goehring TB, Corah LR, Simms DD: Effect of a single zeranol implant on reproductive development of prepuberal heifers. J Anim Sci Suppl I, 61:429 (Abstr) 1985

20. Gonzales-Padilla E, Ruiz R, LeFever D, et al: Puberty in beef heifers, III. Induction of fertile estrus. J Anim Sci 40:1110, 1975

21. Gonzales-Padilla E, Wiltbank JN, Niswender GD: Puberty in beef heifers, I. Interrelationship between pituitary, hypothalamic and ovarian hormones. J Anim Sci 40:1091, 1975

22. Gonzales-Padilla E, Niswender GD, Wiltbank JN: Puberty in beef heifers, II. Effect of injections of progesterone and estradiol-17_B on serum LH, FSH and ovarian activity. J Anim Sci 40:1105, 1976

23. Hansen PH, Kamwanja LA, Hauser ER: Photoperiod influences age at puberty of heifers. J Anim Sci 57:985, 1983

24. Harrison LM, Hanse TR, Randel RD: Evidence for seasonal and nutritional modifica-

tion of ovarian and pituitary function in crossbred heifers and Brahman cows. J Anim Sci 55:649, 1982

25. Hauser ER: Seasonal effects on female reproduction in the bovine (*Bos taurus*). Theriogenology 21:150, 1984

26. Johnsson ID, Obst JM: The effects of nutrition during early rearing on the fertility and first lactation performance of beef heifers. Proc Aust Soc Ani Prod 13:460, 1980

27. Joubert DM: The influence of high and low nutritional planes on the estrous cycle and conception rates of heifers. J Agric Sci 45:164, 1954

28. Kroker GA, Cummins LJ: The effect of nutritional restriction on Hereford heifers in late pregnancy. Austr Vet J 55:467, 1979

29. Lesmeister JL, Burfening PS, Blackwell RL: Date of first calving in beef cows and subsequent calf production. J Anim Sci 36:1, 1973

30. Lusby KS, Wettemann RP, Turman EJ: Effects of early weaning calves from first-calf-heifers on calf and heifer performance. J Anim Sci 53:1193, 1981

31. Mangus WL, Brinks JS: Relationships between direct and maternal effects on growth in Herefords: I. Environmental factors during preweaning growth. J Anim Sci 32:17, 1971

32. McCartor MM, Randel RD, Carroll LH: Dietary alteration of ruminal fermentation on efficiency of growth and onset of puberty in Brangus heifers. J Anim Sci 48:488, 1979

33. Moller S: Possible fertility effects of zeranol in yearling heifers. New Zealand Vet J 32:157, 1984

34. Moseley WM, McCartor MM, Randel RD: Effects of monensin on growth and reproductive performance of beef heifers. J Anim Sci 45:961, 1977

35. Nutrient Requirement of Cattle. Washington DC, National Research Council. National Academy Press, 1984, pp 77–86

36. Plasse D, Warwick AC, Koger M: Reproductive behavior of *Bos indicus* females in a subtropical environment, IV: Length of estrous cycle, duration of estrus, time of ovulation, fertilization, and embryo survival in grade Brahman heifers. J Anim Sci 30:63, 1970

37. Poos MI, Hanson TL, Klopfenstein TJ: Monensin effects on diet digestibility, ruminal protein bypass and microbial protein synthesis. J Anim Sci 48:1516, 1979

38. Putnam DA, Elam DJ, Davis RE, et al: Dietary energy and protein effects on rumen volatile acids and ration digestibility by beef heifers. J Anim Sci 25:988, 1966

39. Ramirez VD, McCann SM: Comparison of the regulation of luteinizing hormone (LH) secretion in immature and adult rats. Endocrinology 72:452, 1963

40. Randel RD, Rhodes RC III: Effect of dietary monensin upon luteinizing hormone response to multiple GNRH challenge in prepuberal heifers. Proc 71st Ann Meeting Am Soc Anim Sci, 329 (Abstr.)

41. Randel RD: Seasonal effects on female reproductive functions in the bovine (Indian Breeds). Theriogenology 21:171, 1984

42. Raun AP, Cooley CO, Potter EL, et al: Effect of monensin on feed efficiency of cattle. J Anim Sci 39:259 (Abstr.) 1974

43. Rice LE: Coping with calving difficulties. Proceedings 2nd Annual OK Cattle Conference, Oklahoma State University 1976, p 11

44. Rice LE: Reproductive herd health management in beef cows. In Morrow (ed): Current Therapy in Theriogenology. Philadelphia, WB Saunders Co, 1980, p 534

45. Schillo KK, Dierschke DJ, Hauser ER: Regulation of luteinizing hormone secretion in prepuberal heifers: Increased threshold to negative feedback action of estradiol. J Anim Sci 54:325, 1982

46. Seidel GE Jr, Larson LL, Foote RH: Effect of age and gonadotrophin treatment on superovulation in the calf. J Anim Sci 33:617, 1971

47. Short RE, Bellows RA: Relationships among weight gains, age at puberty and reproductive performance in heifers. J Anim Sci 32:127, 1971

48. Smith MF, Burrell WC, Broadway J, et al: Estrus and pregnancy in beef heifers following use of the synchro-mate$_B$ treatment. Theriogenology 12:183, 1979

49. Spitzer JC, Wiltbank JN, LeFever DC: Increasing beef cow productivity by increasing reproductive performance. Colorado State University Experiment Station, General Series 949, 1975

50. Sprott LR: Effect of monensin and nutrition on reproductive performance in beef heifers from weaning through first postpartum period. Department Animal Science and Industry. PhD Thesis, Kansas State University, Manhattan, 1981, p 19
51. Staigmiller, RB, Short RE, Bellows RA: Induction of LH surges with 17$_B$-estradiol in prepubertal beef heifers: An age dependent response. Theriogenology 11:453, 1979
52. Stowe HD: Beta carotene and bovine reproduction. Comp Cont Ed Pract Vet, 6:S167, 1984
53. Waldhalm DG, Hall RF, DeLong WJ, et al: Restricted dietary protein in pregnant beef cows, I. The effect on length of gestation and calfhood mortality. Theriogenology 12:61, 1979
54. Wettemann RP: Body condition and reproductive performance of first-calf-heifers. Abstract presented at Southern Section of American Society of Animal Science February 1986
55. Wiltbank JN, Warwick EJ, Vernon EH, et al: Factors affecting net calf crop in beef cattle. J Anim Sci 10:409, 1961
56. Wiltbank JN, Bond J, Warwick EJ, et al: Influence of total feed and protein intake on reproductive performance in beef female through second calving. USDA Technical Bulletin 1314, 1965
57. Wiltbank JN: Wean More Pounds of Beef. Columbia, MO, National Association of Animal Breeders, 1969, p 8
58. Wiltbank JN, Kasson CW, Ingalls JE: Puberty in crossbred and straight-bred beef heifers on two levels of feed. J Anim Sci 19:602, 1969
59. Wiltbank JN: Maintenance of a high level of reproductive performance in beef cow herd. Symposium on herd health management, cow-calf, and feedlot. Vet Clin North Am 5:41, 1983

Address reprint requests to

Lawrence E. Rice, DVM, MS
Boren Veterinary Teaching Hospital
Oklahoma State University
College of Veterinary Medicine
Stillwater, OK 74078

0749–0720/91 $0.00 + .20

The Effects of Essential Trace Minerals on Reproduction in Beef Cattle

Larry R. Corah, PhD,* and Sam Ives, DVM†

The term "minor" or "trace" is used in ruminant nutrition to denote the relative amount of an element needed in the diet or by the body. There are 15 trace elements, including seven that do not commonly concern us with grazing cow herds: arsenic, chromium, fluorine, nickel, silicon, tin, and vanadium. Iron deficiency is more commonly a clinical problem with swine and poultry. Molybdenum is rarely if ever deficient and it is more commonly associated with its negative impact on copper utilization.

Deficiencies of the remaining six trace elements—copper, cobalt, iodine, selenium, zinc, and manganese—may occur in ruminants maintained on forage based diets.

The following discussion reviews the interaction of these six trace elements with reproductive function in grazing beef cattle.

COPPER

Copper (Cu) is involved in numerous body physiologic functions, such as hemoglobin formation, iron absorption and mobilization, connective tissue metabolism, and numerous enzyme functions. Copper is integral to the function of the following enzymes: polyphenyl oxidase (conversion of L-tyrosine to melanin); cytochrome oxidase (terminal oxidase in the electron transport system); ceruloplasmin or ferroxidase II (needed for iron release by reticuloendothelial cells); lysyl oxidase (formation of collagen and elastin); and superoxide dismutase (removal of toxic byproducts of various metabolic pathways).[6,12,29,46,56] The knowledge of the function of copper in these enzymes will help to

---

*Professor, Department of Animal Science, Kansas State University, Manhattan, Kansas, Member of American Society of Animal Science.
†Private Practitioner, Veterinary Clinic Inc., Mexico, Missouri

explain the clinical signs seen with copper deficiency. Once copper is absorbed, the liver acts as the storage organ (stores 40% to 70% of copper) from which the body can draw copper in times of decreased intake.

With the possible exception of phosphorus, copper is the most likely mineral to be deficient in grazing animals.[43] Copper deficiency can be a primary deficiency as a result of low copper in the total diet or a secondary deficiency resulting from altered absorption and utilization of copper. Primary deficiency usually occurs when cattle are grazing copper deficient pastures and are not supplemented with concentrate or a trace mineral mix.[34] The copper-Mo-sulfur interaction is the most important factor affecting copper utilization in secondary copper deficiencies.[34,20,48] Other factors decreasing copper absorption are dietary phytates, cadmium, zinc, silver, mercury, and iron.[46] In the rumen, sulfate is reduced to sulfide, which reacts with molybdenum to form thiomolybdates. Thiomolybdates react with copper to form copper thiomolybdate, which is insoluble and not available to the animal.[6,47,46,56] In addition, sulfide can react directly with copper to reduce available copper levels.

Clinical Signs. Reproductive disorders observed with copper deficiency in cows and heifers include decreased conception rate, infertility, anestrus, and fetal resorption.[1,3,4,6,29,40,42,45,48,59] Work at Louisiana State University[22] showed that dairy cows with higher serum copper values and higher packed cell volumes (PCV) had significantly lower days to first service, services per conception, and days to conception (56 vs 70, 1.1 vs 4.4, and 58 vs 183, respectively) than the low serum copper and PCV group.[22]

Many reported copper deficiencies appear to be secondary deficiencies complicated by molybdenum (Mo).[4,36,40,48,59] Recent research[40] suggested molybdenum's influence on reproduction was a direct effect upon the endocrine system and not one caused by decreased copper status. A control diet with 4 mg Cu/kg DM was fed ad lib (CON) or restructured (R-CON) to match the weight gain of Mo supplemented heifers. The control diet was supplemented with 5 mg Mo, or 500 or 800 mg Fe/kg DM. Onset of puberty was delayed for the Mo supplemented group by 8 to 12 weeks. Fertility was reduced to 14% and 28% in heifers and first calf heifers, respectively, given Mo compared with greater than 75% fertility in the CON and Fe groups. The LH ovulatory peak was significantly reduced in the Mo group compared with CON and Fe groups. Exogenous LH given to the Mo group to augment the LH peak did not increase conception rates. The Mo group had an increased number of animals that would not ovulate when synchronized (15 of 74) compared with 1 of 40, 2 of 37, and 0 of 40 for CON, Fe, and R-CON groups, respectively. It was concluded that Mo altered the release of LH and that it may be possible that Mo alters the secretion of ovarian steroids, particularly estrogen, or the feedback of these steroids on the hypothalamic-pituitary system, and that the whole of the latter system has to be reintegrated for resumption of normal function.[40]

In the bull calf, it has been shown that increased Mo in the diet decreased libido and induced sterility due to marked damage in interstitial and germinal epithelium and lowered spermatogenesis.[52]

Achromotrichia can be a clinical sign of copper deficiency.[4,25,29,36,46,48] Melanin is not converted from tyrosine, with a resultant lightening of the hair coat. Areas commonly affected are around the eyes and tips of the ears,[48] but lightening of the entire coat has been observed. Roughened hair coat is also seen in many copper deficient herds.[48,4] Diarrhea due to hypocuprosis or molybdenosis is also common. In severe hypocuprosis, there is a reduction in cytochrome oxidase, causing villous atrophy of the small intestine epithelial cells, reducing nutrient uptake and causing an osmotic diarrhea.[4,29,45,46] Peat scours is the common name used in areas where molybdenum is high.[47,36] Anemia in hypocupremic animals is due to decreased ceruloplasmin.[46,29,45] There is conflicting evidence as to the type of anemia associated with copper deficiency. Underwood suggested a hypochromic macrocytic anemia while Smart suggested a normchronic microcytic anemia.[46,56] Degeneration of the myocardium and aortic rupture are uncommonly reported.[45,4] Bone fractures seen in the young are increased in some herds.[36,29,45] Inability of calves to suckle at birth is an indication of neonatal ataxia.[29,45] Demyelination and/or hypomyelination, amyelination of the brainstem is the lesion observed with this manifestation of hypocuprosis. Growth rate is decreased in hypocupremic animals.[36,29,4]

Diagnosis. Diagnosis is based on integration of clinical signs, soil analysis, water analysis, content of available feed, blood analysis for Cu, liver copper content, and response to treatment.[3,29,50] Water can also be analyzed for possible sulfate contamination.[12,46,58] The NRC requirement[38] of copper for beef cattle is 10 ppm, with a range of 4 to 10 ppm, for maximum production. Ward[59] demonstrated four classifications of copper deficiency when analyzing the diet: 1) greater than or equal to 20 ppm Mo, 2) less copper with more Mo, 3) deficiency in copper without Mo, 4) normal copper and low Mo with a large protein intake (increasing sulfides). Reported reference range values for serum copper are 0.7 to 1.5 mg/mL[46] with less than 0.5 mg/ml copper considered deficient.[4] Most authors report 30 to 40 ppm[4,36,46] copper in liver (dry matter basis; DMB) as the point at which serum copper levels begin to fall and the reason why serum copper values are best used as a screening indicator of copper status.[25,43,45] Liver tissue concentrations less than 25 ppm marginal DMB are considered deficient.[29,43] Switch hair copper concentrations less than 8.3 mg/kg DM are considered marginally deficient; hair must be less than 2 months old to prevent environmental contamination. However, serum and hair copper levels do not decline until the liver is severely depleted.

When considering the amount of dietary copper, Mo, and sulfur in the diet, the ratio can be important. For optimal production, ratios of 6:1 to 10:1 Cu:Mo[12,43,59] are suggested. Below a range of 3:1, signs of molybdenosis will become evident.[4,43,47,48] Sulfur in the diet and in drinking water can decrease the copper availability.[34,43,59] Careful analysis of all parameters is necessary to make an accurate diagnosis. Grains are lower in copper than are forages.[38] Forage containing 7 to 10 μg copper/g should meet the cattles' requirements unless Mo or sulfur intake is high.

Treatment. There are many ways of treating a copper deficiency. Both oral and parenteral methods are available. Methods reported to be effective include (1) mineral mix with 0.2% to 0.5% copper sulfate,[59,30,36,4] (2) adding copper sulfate to the diet if concentrate is being fed, (3) copper oxide needles in a gelatin capsule, (4) tracerglass boluses, or (5) water treatment. The mineral mix is convenient but does not assure adequate or uniform consumption by individual herd members. Concentrate feeding has the obvious disadvantages for range cows. Copper oxide needles (20 g) placed in a gelatin capsule for oral administration with a balling-gun are an effective supplement. The needles lodge in the reticulum and abomasum where they will maintain adequate blood levels for several months.[7,30,36] Tracerglass is a phosphate-based soluble glass that has copper, cobalt, and selenium incorporated into the glass. Metering devices can be used to place copper into the water supply.[30] This can be effective if it is the only source of water. Lush pastures will decrease water intake considerably. A recent development is an "Aquatrace" pellet that is added to the stock water tank weekly to supply needed deficient elements. In work reported by MacPherson,[30] the pellets do not appear to be effective except for selenium supplementation. The other pellets, including the copper pellets, did not provide adequate supplementation of the deficient element.[30]

In severe deficiencies, parenteral application of copper is recommended. Parenteral application gives quick response and bypasses the effects of other elements in the gut.[34] Copper glycinate and copper EDTA are two common injections used.[2,4,36,59] Copper glycinate can produce abscesses at site of injection, especially when aseptic technique is not used. Copper EDTA injections have been associated with acute hepatic necrosis. Subcutaneous soluble glass has been tried and found effective. It did cause reactions to the copper at site of injection.

Dietary concentrations of 4 to 10 ppm copper have generally been considered adequate to meet requirements of beef cattle.[38] Diets with less than 3 to 5 ppm copper may result in subnormal plasma and liver copper levels.[38] The rate of dietary copper absorption is greater in young cattle than in older cattle.[43] There is evidence of breed differences in requirements and absorption, with Simmental cattle requiring twice the level of copper of Angus cattle.[43]

Toxicity

Acute toxicity may cause nausea, vomiting, salivation, abdominal pain, convulsions, paralysis, collapse, and death.[38] Levels of 200 to 800 mg/kg body weight[43] or 115 ppm[38] are considered toxic levels in cattle.

IODINE

Iodine functions in the body mainly through the thyroid hormones. Iodine is absorbed through the abomasum and small intestine easily in the ionized form. It is transported to the thyroid gland, where up to 70% of the total iodine in the body is found.[15,13] Thyroglobulin is the main storage form in the thyroid. Monoidotyrosine and diiodotyrosine are formed, which are combined to form triiodothyroxine (T_3) and thyroxin (T_4). Excess iodine is excreted mainly through the kidneys but some is lost in the feces and sweat.[15,13] Iodine as T_3 or T_4 regulates the basal metabolic rate, consumption of carbohydrates, proteins, and fats, and affects growth, development and reproductive function.[26]

Clinical Signs. Reproductive performance is decreased in hypothyroid cattle. In the female, absence of visible estrus,[8,14,17,34] infertility,[1,25] early embryonic mortality,[37,8,2] abortion,[1] dead and weakly calves,[1,15,17,53] increased incidence of retained placenta,[8,14,15,17,29] decreased conception rates,[45,14,15] uterine inertia,[17] poor mammary development in heifers at the time of calving,[17] hairless calves,[8,15] and arrested fetal development[8] have been reported. Moberg[37] showed that three of these reproductive dysfunctions could be reduced by iodine supplementation; he found a significantly higher first service conception rate in experimental herds over controls (69.1% vs 62.2%, respectively), an almost statistically significant increased incidence of retained placentas in the controls (11% vs 25%), a significantly higher incidence of irregular breeding intervals, suggesting early embryonic mortality in the control herds (20% in cows supp. vs 29% in control cows), and a significantly higher incidence of ketosis in the control herds (26% vs 58%).

A dairy herd in the United Kingdom that had low plasma protein bound iodine and pathologic changes in fetal thyroids also had a high incidence of abortions, still births, and weak calves.[42] This condition was corrected by iodine supplementation.[42]

Bulls show a decreased libido,[15,8,34,29,56] decreased semen quality,[15,56] and decreased sperm count.[17] Georgierskii states that cows and calves kept for long periods on diets moderately deficient in iodine have impaired ovarian function and the luteinizing function of the hypophysis is adversely affected.[13] The decrease in luteinizing hormone would explain the decreased libido and semen quality found in the bull.

Goiter is seen mainly in calves born to deficient cows,[29,15,13,56,8] with thyroid hypertrophy occurring in response to reduced iodine intake. Decreased growth rate and dwarfism are also noted in the young.[56,13,15,29] Part of the decreased growth may be due to the cows' reduced milk output.[29,15,8] There appears to be an increased incidence of ketosis in the hypothyroid dairy cow.[8,15]

Diagnosis. Clinical signs, mineral content of soil and plants, presence of goitrogens, size and iodine content of thyroid, protein bound iodine in the serum, and response to treatment can all be used to diagnose iodine deficiency. Minerals possibly interfering with the uptake of iodine are rubidium, arsenic, fluorine, calcium, and potassium.[43,17,8,15] Potassium appears to also cause an increase in iodine excretion in the urine.[15] Goitrogenic substances increase the iodine need in the diet by either interfering with the binding of iodine by the thyroid gland or inhibiting the selective concentration of iodine by the thyroid.[8,15] Plants such as cabbage, rape, kale, soybean meal, and dietary nitrates are goitrogenic.[13-15,29] The goiterogenic thyroid will contain less than 0.12% DM of iodine.[43] Protein bound iodine in serum will be $3-5.3$ μg/100 mL in deficient cattle.[44] Diets containing less than 0.2 ppm iodine are deficient while those with 0.2 to 2 ppm are marginal.

Treatment. Iodized salt, free choice block or loose, is recommended for all cattle regardless whether in an iodine deficient area or not.[15] If the salt will be exposed to high temperature, high humidity, or rain, the use of sodium iodide, potassium iodide, or ethylinediamine dihydroiodide is not recommended as they are volatile and easily leached out. In the case of free choice salt, insoluble iodine such as iodate at 0.01% is recommended.[8,15,34,43,56] Iodine may be added to concentrates to correct an iodine deficiency. A level of 0.5 mg/kg diet is the recommended amount.[5]

Toxicity

Iodine toxicity has occurred when dietary levels exceed 200 to 400 ppm iodine. Symptoms include anorexia, coma, death, and kidney and liver necrosis. Diets above 50 ppm can suppress growth and feed intake.

ZINC

Zinc is formed throughout the body and is utilized by various metalloenzymes or as an activator of enzymes. The enzymes are a part of nucleic acid metabolism, carbohydrate metabolism, and protein synthesis.[46,13] Ruminant absorption of zinc is relatively high when compared to monogastrics. Twenty to 40% of dietary zinc is absorbed by the abomasum and small intestine.[46,13] Calves absorb zinc more readily than do mature animals.[56] High dietary calcium or phosphorus will potentiate a zinc deficiency,[47] and copper, cadmium, iron, and Mo may also interfere with zinc metabolism. Certain proteins, particularly from seeds, increase the requirement for zinc.[46] Zinc concentrations are highest in immature plants and decline to half that level in mature forage.

Clinical Signs. Reproductive abnormalities with zinc deficiency particularly affect bulls. A decrease in testicular size is noted in growing bull calves.[41,29,9,47,56,46] Work by Pitts[41] showed that bull calves fed a zinc deficient diet from 8 to 21 weeks of age had a reduction in testicular size at 21 weeks when compared with controls. When the bull calves were put on a zinc sufficient diet at 21 weeks, their testicular size equalled that of the controls by 64 weeks. Semen quality was not affected when ejaculates were evaluated. Growth retardation and delayed onset of puberty are also noted in zinc deficient calves.[29,56] This is due in part to decreased appetite and impaired feed utilization, particularly protein synthesis.[56]

Cows appear to have a decrease in fertility and abnormal estrus behavior. Underwood states that all phases of the reproductive process may be affected, from estrus to parturition to lactation.[56]

Zinc-induced parakeratosis is common in a herd in a zinc deficient area.[46,9,56,13] In cows, the area of the dew claws and heel bulb are affected and this will eventually extend up the hock, between the legs, with a dermatosis forming around the teat base. Calves will show an inflamed nose and mouth with subcutaneous hemorrhages, unthrifty appearance, roughened hair coats, joint stiffness, swelling of hocks, delayed wound healing, and subcutaneous fluid accumulation.[9,46,13] A decrease in weight gains may be the only sign noticed in mild deficiencies.

Diagnosis. If zinc deficiency is suspected, clinical signs, soil and plant analysis, serum zinc concentrations, and treatment response information are needed. There is wide variation as to the requirement for zinc. NRC suggests 30 ppm, with a range of 20 to 40 ppm and toxic level of 500 ppm.[38] Puls[43] recommends 60–100 ppm as adequate with 75,000 ppm toxic. Underwood[56] suggests 17–32 ppm zinc in the diet. Factors affecting zinc absorption have been previously stated, with monensin effective in enhancing zinc absorption.[43] Beef cows with higher levels of milk production have higher requirements.[38] Care must be taken interpreting blood sample results, as hemolysis will increase zinc, and stress will decrease zinc concentrations in serum.[43,56,46] Most blood collection tubes and syringes contain zinc contaminated rubber; therefore, special zinc-free Vacutainers* should be used when attempting to diagnose zinc deficiency or zinc toxicity. Serum zinc concentrations less than 0.4 μg/mL serum are considered deficient.[29] Diets containing 2 to 10 ppm zinc are considered deficient while liver samples below 20 to 40 ppm are an indication of deficiency.[43]

Treatment. Zinc oxide, zinc carbonate, zinc sulfate, and zinc methionine can be used to supply zinc in the diet. They can be added to the diet if the animals are supplemented or included in trace mineralized salt mixes and fed free choice.[9,56,43] Recommendations of 0.5% to 2% zinc in salt mixtures have been made.[56,43] Powdered zinc metal (600 mg) in 0.5 mL of oily suspension injected into the neck region has also worked.[43]

Toxicity

Toxicity problems in adult ruminants are uncommon.[43] Steers have been fed diets containing 1000 ppm zinc with no reduction in performance.[38]

---

*B-D 6526, 6527; Becton-Dickinson, Rutherford, New Jersey.

SELENIUM

Although recognized in 1957 as an essential trace mineral,[46] it was often assumed that selenium (Se) deficiencies could be alleviated by supplementation with vitamin E.[57] There definitely is a relationship between Se, vitamin E, and sulfur amino acids at the cellular level.[46] Selenium functions through glutathione peroxidase, which reduces hydrogen peroxide and other organic peroxides to less harmful products. Vitamin E is an antioxidant that works at the cellular membrane level, and Se, through glutathione peroxidase, is active in the cytosol to reduce peroxides.[56]

Intestinal absorption of Se is high but can be variable depending on the chemical form of Se and other interactions with products in the diet.[46,56,13,43] Selenomethionine and selenocystine are well used by ruminants and found in many of the feeds and forages ingested by cattle.[56] Heavy metals, particularly arsenic and mercury, reduce absorption and availability of Se.[46,56] Sulfur or sulfates can also reduce availability of Se.[43]

Clinical Signs. Reproductive disorders observed in cattle are retained placenta; infertility; abortions; birth of premature, weak, or dead calves; cystic ovaries; metritis; delayed conception; erratic, weak, or silent heat periods; and poor fertilization.[46,56,43,54,34,8,42,20,16,29,57] Retention of placental membranes has been studied widely in dairy herds and it appears that Se or Se/vitamin E supplementation or injection prepartum reduces the incidence of retained placenta in Se deficient herds[20,54] but not in Se adequate herds.[16] A herd of dairy cows in Tweedsich had an abnormal number of cows retain their placentas after calving so two experiments were conducted on the herd in two consecutive years. In Experiment 1, 20 cows were treated with 15 mg Se as selenate and 680 IU of vitamin E intramuscularly 1 month prepartum. Forty-five cows were controls. The incidence of retained placenta was 0% and 42%, respectively. Experiment 2 was conducted to observe the results of vitamin E on the placental retention rate as it was believed the diet should be adequate in vitamin E. Treated animals were either given 15 mg Se as selenate and 680 IU of vitamin E intramuscularly, or 15 mg Se as selenate intramuscularly. Placental retention was classified as difficult (manual removal), delayed (greater than 6 hours to expel), or normal (less than 6 hours to expel). Controls had 63% normal, 10.5% delayed, and 26.5% difficult while retention in those receiving Se and vitamin E was 100% normal. The Se group had 71.5% normal, 21.5% delayed, and 7% difficult. There was definitely a response to vitamin E in this trial.[54]

Julien's[20] study of Ohio cows that were deficient in Se (<0.025 ppm Se in plasma) reported that supplemental Se reduced the incidence of retained placenta from 38% to 0%. Either 50 mg of Se as selenite given intramuscularly 21 days prepartum or the feeding of an equivalent average daily intake of 0.92 mg of Se as selenite during the last 60 days of the dry period was effective in this trial. Vitamin E, whether supplemental or not, had no effect on results. Kappel had similar results with a herd of dairy cows when days to first estrus, days to first service, days to conception, services per conception, or number of uterine infusions required were considered.[23]

Changes in fertility can be affected by Se status of the herd. It has been reported that beef cows on nutritionally adequate diets and injected with Se and vitamin E produced more fertilized ova when superovulated versus controls.[23] Work done by Kappel[23] and Hidiroglou[16] did not find an increase in reproductive performance in Se adequate herds when supplemental Se and vitamin E were increased. It would seem that Se/vitamin E supplementation can reduce reproductive dysfunction in a Se deficient herd but does not affect herds that ingest adequate Se.[16]

White muscle disease or nutritional myodegeneration is commonly seen in selenium deficient areas.[46,56,57,54,8,43,29] Affected animals are reluctant to move about, lose condition, become prostrate, and usually die.[56] Muscle degeneration and necrosis with increases in serum glutamic oxaloacetic transamima and lactic dehydrogenase levels in blood and tissue[57] are typical pathologic signs.

"Ill-thrift" is seen in New Zealand, occurring in Se deficient cattle of all ages. There is a subclinical growth deficit, clinical unthriftiness with rapid weight loss, and some mortality. It may or may not be associated with white muscle disease and infertility.[56] Selenium treatment improved the condition.

Diagnosis. For an accurate diagnosis, clinical signs, soil and plant analysis, blood and tissue Se levels, and response to treatment are necessary. Soil and plant analysis will determine Se intake as well as any interactions from other constituents of the diet.[46,56,13,43] Liver is by far the best tissue indicator of Se status[43] at necropsy, with 0.25 to 0.50 ppm wet weight considered adequate and levels below 0.20 ppm weight considered markedly deficient. Interpretation of serum Se levels may be difficult, in that serum levels may be extremely low (0.25 ppm) while liver levels are adequate (0.3 ppm).[43] Fetal liver values greater than 0.3 ppm wet weight are considered adequate.[43] Blood Se concentrations less than 0.5 ppm are markedly deficient, levels 0.5–0.8 ppm are considered marginal, and levels greater than 0.8 ppm are normal. NRC[38] suggests a value of .20 ppm selenium in the diet for beef cattle.

Treatment. Various methods of Se supplementation exist. Selenium or Se/vitamin E injections can be given at 3 month intervals. Allen[2] reports that when 0.05, 0.1, or 0.15 mg Se/kg body weight sodium selenate was injected into marginally deficient dairy cows, blood Se concentrations increased for up to 182 days from the higher two dosages. In beef animals with low blood Se concentrations, administration of 0.15 mg Se/kg body weight protected them for approximately 4 months.[2]

In dairy cows, oral dosing with successive 12.5 mg Na_2SeO_3 daily from 56 to 60 days prepartum, followed by weekly doses of the same amount until parturition, were effective, or at least equivalent, to a single injection of 20 mg Na_2SeO_3 both in the effect on plasma Se concentration and in reducing the incidence of retained placenta from approximately 25% to 0% in untreated cows to zero in control cows.[30]

One 30-mg pellet of 10% selenium can be placed intraruminally and last up to 1 year in adult cows.[30] Two pellets may give adequate blood levels for up to 18 months.[43] Tracerglass-C, a phosphate-based soluble-glass that has copper, cobalt, and Se incorporated in the glass structure, will continually release the elements for up to a year. Data presented by Telfer showed adequate glutathione peroxidase levels at 288 days on deficient control animals.[51] An osmotic pump intrareticular device supplies 3 mg Se/day and is effective for at least 8 months.[7a] It is becoming common practice in many areas to add Se to commercial mineral mixtures.[57] Mineral mixes should contain 25–125 ppm selenium.[43]

Toxicity

Unfortunately, selenium can be both toxic and deficient, depending on the area of the United States. Diets containing over 80 ppm are considered toxic.[43] Toxicity signs include loss of appetite, loss of tail hair, sloughing of hoofs, and death.[38] High protein diets offer some protection against high selenium intakes.

MANGANESE

Manganese (Mn) is nutritionally essential for both plants and animals. Manganese is poorly utilized from the diet, with only 14% to 18% of ingested manganese being absorbed.[13] If Mn additives are introduced into the diet, its percentage absorption decreases, but the absolute level increases.[56] Decreased Mn absorption occurs with high calcium, phosphorus, or iron levels in the diet.[47,25] Hignett[17] proposed that calcium and phosphorus intakes can determine the levels of Mn required for high conception rates. With a low Mn consumption fertility was high when calcium and phosphorus were well balanced, but when calcium was excessive relative to phosphorus or vice versa and the Mn low, fertility was depressed.[25] In the body, the highest tissue concentrations of Mn occur in the liver, kidneys, and bones.

Manganese functions as an activator of glycosyltransferases, which are necessary for mucopolysaccharide synthesis in cartilage and bone matrix. Pyruvate carboxylase is a Mn metalloprotein involved in carbohydrate metabolism. In a Mn-deficient state, magnesium replaces Mn in chicks so the actual role of pyruvate carboxylase in impaired carbohydrate metabolism of Mn deficiency is unclear.[56] Manganese has a specific lipotropic effect; it enhances the utilization of fats in the body, and counteracts fatty degeneration of the liver.[56] Furthermore, manganese has been suggested to participate in hormone synthesis in the ovary and has been shown to stimulate cholesterol synthesis; thus it indirectly influences steroid hormone synthesis.[10]

Clinical Signs. In an experiment conducted by Wilson,[60] eleven herds grazing medium to low Mn deficient pastures were used. Cows were divided alternately as they calved and half given 4 g MNSO$_4$ in the diet for 9 weeks with treatment beginning 3 weeks before first service. Results of the trial were an improvement in first service conception rates from 51% to 63% for treated cows.[60] Six of the eleven herds showed a response to Mn treatment, with a 48% first service conception rate observed for controls and 71% for manganese treated groups.[60] The main symptoms Wilson reported were anestrus and infertility, with this often being detected during rectal examination, as one or both ovaries are subnormal in size.[60] Other related signs Wilson[60] reported were calves growing poorly, "dryness," and loss of coat color. At birth the calves "knuckled over" at the fetlock. All these conditions apparently responded to Mn therapy.

Bentley and Phillips fed a group of 18 heifers a basal diet deficient in Mn (7–10 ppm) and sufficient in manganese (30 ppm) from approximately 175 lb of body weight through their second calving. A second experiment was conducted on another group of 12 heifers starting at 185 lb and continuing through either their second or third calving. The diet in Experiment 2 was divided into basal (7–10 ppm Mn), 40 ppm Mn, and 60 ppm Mn. They concluded that the Mn deficient diet caused some delay in the onset of puberty, a slightly reduced conception rate, and a greater number of calves born with weak legs and pasterns at first calving.[5]

Rojas and Dyer reported Mn deficient cows (115 mg Mn/day) required an average of four services per pregnancy; in comparison, the control group (183 mg Mn/day) required only two services.[44] Calves born to deficient dams had shorter humeri, marked reduction in humeri breaking strength, enlarged joints, stiffness, twisted legs, and general weakness.[44] No significant differences in birth weight were noticed.[44] Clinical signs continued after treatment diagnosis.

A corn silage based diet was fed to heifers and cows to provide the following trace element content: 40, 4, 45; 54, 4, 45; and 54, 9, 55 ppm of Mn, Cu, and Zn for control, Mn added, and Mn, Cu, Zn added groups, respectively. The control diet met NRC standards.[10] Days to first estrus were decreased significantly for heifers on the +Mn diet but not +Mn Cu Zn (66 v 75 and 86 days for +Mn, +Mn Cu Zn, and control respectively). Neither Mn nor Mn Cu Zn reduced the days to first estrus in cows. Adding Mn reduced days to conception for heifers when compared to the other two treatments (16 v 28 and 34 days for Mn, Mn Cu Zn, and control groups, respectively). Cows' days to conception were reduced by both the Mn or Mn Cu Zn addition (21 and 21 v 32 days for +Mn, +Mn Cu Zn, and control groups respectively). Services per conception were significantly decreased (1.1 and 1.3 vs 1.6 for Mn, Mn Cu Zn and control groups, respectively). There were no differences in conception rates between groups.[10] These data from Minnesota and the other work reported, realize the important part Mn plays in reproduction. Typical responses of females supplemented with Mn are increased ovarian activity and conception rate, and these results suggest further examination is needed in determining the Mn requirement of breeding cows.[10]

Diagnosis. Manganese concentration in the diet is the best indication of a possible Mn deficiency.[56,43] A diet is considered deficient at 1 ppm Mn or less, while 40 to 200 ppm manganese is considered adequate.[43] Blood and tissue values are not good indicators of manganese status due to extreme value variability, reflecting both individual variability and analytical technique.[56] Hair Mn bears no relationship to dietary Mn, as over 50% hair Mn is derived from the environment.[43] Evaluation of clinical signs, dietary Mn levels, and response to treatment should provide an adequate diagnosis.

Treatment. In areas where Mn deficiency is suspected, supplementation of the feed with Mn sulfate at a rate of 4 g for cows and 2 g for heifers is sufficient for either prevention or treatment of deficiency.[56] A trace mineralized salt mixture may provide adequate Mn intake but, as discussed previously, there is a wide variation in acceptance and intake of these mixtures.

Toxicity

For ruminants, Mn is among the least toxic of the required minerals. There are few documented toxicities.[38]

COBALT

Cobalt (Co) is essential in the grazing ruminant's diet, as cobalt is utilized by the rumen microflora for the production of vitamin B_{12}.[56,13] Vitamin B_{12} is absorbed by the small intestine and stored in the liver[8] and has many important functions in the body. It regulates hematopoiesis (activates the synthesis of protoporphyrin) and affects nitrogen, nucleic acid, carbohydrate, and mineral metabolism.[13] The main source of energy in ruminants (propionic, acetic, and butyric acids) cannot be utilized when the animal is in a vitamin B_{12} deficient state.[56,13] A breakdown in propionate metabolism in the metabolic pathway, where methylmalonyl-CoA is converted to succinyl CoA, a reaction catalyzed by methylmalonyl-CoA isomerase, a vitamin B_{12}-requiring enzyme, has been shown to be a primary defect in cobalt deficient sheep.[56] Vitamin B_{12} also functions as the enzyme responsible for recycling methionine, which is a part of folic acid metabolism. This provides a possible basis for the impaired nitrogen retention found in vitamin B_{12} deficient sheep.[56]

Clinical Signs. Wagner[58] reported cobalt deficiency as one of the most common causes of anestrus in New York state. Several cows within a herd may have nonfunctional ovaries and low hemoglobin values. The cows may continue to lactate and act normally otherwise. If the deficiency is severe enough, the cows will be thin, listless, and have pale mucous membranes.[58]

A herd of shorthorns with a known infertility history were divided into three groups—control, copper glycinate injections, and copper glycinate injection plus a Co bullet. The conception rates were 53%, 67%, and 93%, respectively.[1] There was obviously a Co-Cu interaction in this case. A possible explanation is that the cobalt deficiency reduces the storage of copper in the bovine liver.[43] Reproductive disorders reported by Alderman were infertility, abortion, and weak calves, and Co application to the pastures markedly improved fertility and calf viability.[1]

When cattle are grazed on Co deficient pastures, signs of deficiency are not noticed for weeks to months, depending on the age and previous history of the animals and the degree of deficiency of Co in the diet.[56] Deficiency signs occur when liver vitamin B_{12} stores are depleted. Loss of appetite is a common manifestation of the disease in ruminants.[56] If the deficiency is severe enough, poor growth and muscle wasting may occur, but it is hard to distinguish these animals from those affected by malnutrition.[56] Anemia and rough hair coat can occur, but the deficiency must be severe.

Diagnosis. Serum vitamin B_{12} levels are used most commonly to diagnose Co deficiency, as they are easy to obtain, and if taken from an adequate representative group of animals, some assessment can be made of whether or not animals are at risk.[28] Values for serum vitamin B_{12} (ng/mL) are as follows: Co deficient, 0.04 to 0.2; Co marginal, 0.25 to 0.35; and Co adequate, 0.4 to 2.5.[43] As with any suspected deficiency, clinical signs, soil and plant analysis, and response to treatment must all be assessed for an accurate diagnosis. The diet should contain at least 0.1 ppm Co to be adequate.[38] Dietary levels below 0.06 ppm are considered deficient.[43] Legumes are lower in Co than grasses.

Treatment. Cobalt bullets formed from Co oxide and finely divided iron clay can be given orally and lodge in the rumen or reticulum. Two bullets are preferred to one to prevent an impervious coating from forming on the bullet and making it unavailable.[30,56] In sheep, a steady supply of Co is maintained for more than 5 years.[56] Regurgitation of the bullets has been a problem, but use of heavier bullets has reduced the incidence.[56]

Tracerglass as described previously is another alternative that appears to be effective for up to a year.[51] Salt licks containing 120 g of Co sulfate per ton are effective if eaten, but there are problems if salt intake is poor.[8] Metering devices are available to add cobalt to the water supply.[30] Oral dosing of 20 g of Co is effective in controlling Co deficiency, but handling the animals every 14 to 28 days is required to maintain appropriate levels of Co.[30]

Toxicity

Cobalt toxicity in ruminants is rare because toxic levels are 300 times requirement levels.[38]

BIOAVAILABILITY OF TRACE MINERALS

Bioavailability is defined as the absorbability of the nutrient by the animal. Many factors influence the degree of trace mineral absorption,

Table 1. Sources and Availability of Minerals for Ruminants*

COBALT		COPPER		IODINE		MANGANESE		SELENIUM		ZINC	
SOURCE	AVAIL	SOURCE	AVAIL	SOURCE	AVAIL	SOURCE	AVAIL	SOURCE	AVAIL	SOURCE	AVAIL
$CoCo_3$	100	$CuSO_4 \cdot 5H_2O$	100	EDDI	>100	MnO	100	Na_2SeO_3	100	ZnO	100
$CoSO_4 \cdot H_2O$	100	CuO	<100	$CaIO_3 \cdot H_2O$	100	$MnSO_4 \cdot 4H_2O$	100	Na_2SeO_4	100	Zn methionine	100
Co proteinate		Cu methionate	High	KI	100	Mn proteinate		Selenomethionine	100	$ZnSO_4 \cdot H_2O$	High
$CoCl_2$	100	$CuCl_2$	>100	$Ca_5(IO_6)_2$	100	$MnCl_2$	100			$ZnCO_3$	Good
CoO	100	$Cu(NO_3)_2$	100	KIO_3	100	$MnCO_3$	100			$ZnCL_2$	High
$Co(NO_3)_2$	100	Cu_2O	<100	NaI	100	Mn ores	Low			Zn metal	High
Co bullets		CuS	Low	Poppy seeds	100					Zn ores	Poor
$CoSO_4 \cdot 7H_2O$	100	CuEDTA	High	Diiodosalicylate	<50						

*Availabilities from reviews by ER Miller (Bioavailability of minerals. 1980 Minnesota Nutrition Conference, Minneapolis, Minnesota) and WJ Miller (Bioavailability of different sources of trace minerals for livestock. University of Georgia Factsheet 82–201). Use is the number of commercial supplements or trace mineral premixes in this survey which used a specific mineral source in formulation.
Adapted from Hicks B, Owens F: Mineral supplements for feedlot cattle. In Proceedings of the Symposium on Trace Minerals in Beef Cattle Nutrition. Amarillo, Texas, Plains Nutrition Council, September 1988.

with the source of the trace mineral being one factor. An attempt to provide some information on the bioavailability of various trace mineral sources is made in Table 1.

REFERENCES

1. Alderman G: Mineral nutrition and reproduction in cattle. Vet Rec 75:1015–1018, 1963
2. Allen WM, Moore PR: Parenteral methods of trace element supplementation. Trace Elements in Animal Production and Veterinary Practice. Br Soc Anim Prod 7:87, 1983
3. Anderson DC: Dairy cattle and trace elements. Proceedings of a Course in Dairy Cattle Medicine. Massey University, 1983, p 154
4. Baldwin WK, Hamar DW, Berlach ML, et al: Copper-molybdenum imbalance in range cattle. Bov Prac 2:9, 1981
5. Bentley OG, Phillips PH: The effect of low manganese rations upon dairy cattle. J Dairy Sci 34:396, 1951
6. Bull RC: Copper. Animal Nutrition and Health, Nov–Dec:32, 1980
7. Burridge JC, Reith JWS, Berrow ML: Soil factors and treatments affecting trace elements in animal production and veterinary practice. Br Soc Anim Prod 7:77, 1983
7a. Campbell DT, Maas J, Weber DW, et al: Safety and efficacy of two sustained-release intrareticular selenium supplements and the associated placental and colostral transfer of selenium in beef cows. Am J Vet Res 51:813–817, 1990
8. Clark RG: Cobalt, selenium, iodine and sodium deficiencies in New Zealand dairy cattle. Proceedings of a Course in Dairy Cattle Medicine. Massey University, 1983, p 167
9. Cunha TJ: Zinc. Animal Nutrition and Health May:14, 1981
10. Di Costanzo A, Meiske JC, Plegge SD, et al: Influence of manganese, copper, and zinc on reproductive performance of beef cows. Nutr Rep Int 34:287, 1986
11. Fisher DD, Wilson LL, Leach RM, et al: Switch hair as an indicator of magnesium and copper status of beef cows. Am J Vet Res 46:2235, 1985
12. Gay C, Madson W: Update on copper in Washington. Washington State University Beef Research Day Report, 1986
13. Georgievskii VI, Annenkov BN, Samokhin VI: Mineral Nutrition of Animals. Butterworth & Co.
14. Harris B: Iodine needs of dairy cattle. Animal Nutrition and Health Aug–Sep:33, 1979.
15. Hemken R: Iodine. Animal Nutrition and Health Jan–Feb:12, 1981
16. Hidiroglou M, McAllister AJ, Williams CJ: Prepartum supplementation of selenium and vitamin E to dairy cows: Assessment of selenium status and reproductive performance. J Dairy Sci 70:1281, 1987
17. Hignett SL: Factors influencing herd fertility in cattle. Vet Rec 46:654, 1950
18. Ingraham RH, Kappel LC, Morgan EB, et al: Correction of subnormal fertility with copper and magnesium supplementation. J Dairy Sci 70:167, 1987
19. Julien WE, Conrad HR: Selenium and Vitamin E and incidence of retained placenta in parturient dairy cows: II. Prevention in commercial herds with prepartum treatment. J Dairy Sci 59:1960, 1976
20. Julien WE, Conrad HR: Selenium and Vitamin E and incidence of retained placenta in parturient dairy cows: II. J Dairy Sci 59:1954, 1976
21. Kalmbacher RS, Long KR, Martin FG: Seasonal mineral concentrations in diets of esophageally fistulated steers on three range areas. Journal of Range Management 37:36, 1984
22. Kappel LC, Ingraham RH, Morgan EB, et al: Plasma copper concentration and packed ALI volume and their relationships to fertility and milk production in Holstein cows. Am J Vet Res 45:346, 1984
23. Kappel LC, Ingraham RH, Morgan EB, et al: Selenium concentrations in feeds and

effects of treating pregnant Holstein cows with selenium and vitamin E on blood selenium values and reproductive performance. Am J Vet Res 45:691, 1984

24. Kappel LC, Morgan EB, Ingraham RH, et al: Effects of forage minerals on reproduction of Holsteins. Am J Vet Res 45:346, 1984
25. King JOL: Nutrition and fertility in dairy cows. Vet Rec 89:320, 1971
26. Kropp JR: Performance of first calf heifers when supplemented with amino acid chelate minerals (unpublished)
27. Lebdosoekojo S, Ammerman CB, Raun NS, et al: Mineral nutrition of beef cattle grazing native pastures on the eastern plains of Colombia. J Anim Sci 51:1249, 1980
28. Lewis G, Anderson PH: The nature of trace element problems: Delineating the field problem. Trace Elements in Animal Production and Veterinary Practice. Br Soc Anim Prod 7:11, 1983
29. Maas J: Relationship between nutrition and reproduction in beef cattle. Vet Clin North Am [Food Anim Prac] 3:633, 1987
30. MacPherson A: Oral treatment of trace element deficiencies in ruminant livestock trace element in animal production and veterinary practice. Br Soc Anim Prod 7:93, 1983
31. Manickam R, Gopalakrishnan CA, Ramanthan G, et al: Studies on the relationships between trace elements and fertility in cows. Indian J Anim Res 11:23, 1977
32. Manspeaker JE, Robl MG, Edwards GH: Chelated minerals: Their role in bovine fertility. Vet Med Sept:951, 1987
33. McClure TJ: Malnutrition and infertility of cattle in Australia and New Zealand. Aust Vet J 44:134, 1968
34. McDowell LR, Conrad JH, Ellis GL: Mineral deficiencies, imbalances and diagnosis: Part II. Feedstuffs 19:21, 1983
35. McDowell LR, Conrad JH, Ellis GL: Mineral deficiencies, imbalances and diagnosis, part II. Feedstuffs. 19:21, 1983
36. Meldrum JB, Troutt HF: A case of apparent copper deficiency in cattle. Vet Hum Toxicol 27:125, 1985
37. Moberg R: Influences of supplementary iodine, administered by evaporation on reproductive performances in cattle. Int Cong Anim Reprod 4:682, 1961
38. NRC: Sixth Revised Edition. National Academy Press, 1984
39. Owens F: The haves and the have nots. Beef May:50, 1988
40. Phillippo M, Humphries WR, Atkinson T, et al: The effect of dietary molybdenum and iron on copper status, puberty, fertility and oestrous cycles in cattle. J Agric Sci 109:321, 1987
41. Pitts WJ, Millers WJ, Fosgate OT, et al: Effect of zinc deficiencies and restricted feeding from two to five months of age on reproduction in Holstein bulls. J Dairy Sci 49:995, 1966
42. Pugh DG, Elmore RG, Hembree TR: A review of the relationship between mineral nutrition and reproduction in cattle. Bovine Practice 20:10, 1985
43. Puls R: Mineral Levels in Animal Health. Sherpa International, 1988
44. Rojas MA, Dyer IA: Manganese deficiency in the bovine. 23:600, 1964
45. Sanders DE, Sanders JA: Diagnosis and management of copper deficiency in dairy cattle. Mod Vet Prac Aug:613, 1983
46. Smart ME, Gudmundson J, Christensen DA: Trace mineral deficiencies in cattle: A review. Can Vet J 22:372, 1981
47. Stake PE: Trace element absorption factors in animals. 38th Minnesota Nutrition Conference 1977, p 137
48. Stednick JD, Tanner DQ, Leininger WC: Copper deficiency in cattle in Gunnison and Saguache counties, Colorado. Colorado State University Beef Program Report, 1985, p 104
49. Stowe HD, Thomas JW, Johnson T et al: Responses of dairy cattle to long term and short term supplementation with oral selenium and vitamin E. J Dairy Sci 71:1830, 1988
50. Suttle NF: Problems in the diagnosis and anticipation of trace element deficiencies in grazing livestock. Vet Rec 119:148, 1986
51. Telfer SB, Zervas G, Carlos G: Curing or preventing deficiencies in copper, cobalt, and selenium in cattle and sheep using tracerglass. Can J Anim Sci 64(suppl):234, 1984

52. Thomas JW, Moss S: The effect of orally administered molybdenum on growth, spermatogenesis and testes histology of young dairy bulls. J Dairy Sci 34:929, 1951
53. Thornton I: Soil-plant-animal interactions in relation to the incidence of trace element disorders in grazing livestock. Trace Elements in Animal Production and Veterinary Practice. Br Soc Anim Prod 7:39, 1983
54. Trinder N, Woodhouse CD, Renton CP: The effect of vitamin E and selenium on the incidence of retained placentae in dairy cows. Vet Rec 85:550, 1969
55. Undersander DJ, Hutcheson DP: Seasonal changes in composition of range grasses on the southern High Plains. Nutr Rep Int 30:1101, 1984
56. Underwood EJ: The Mineral Nutrition of Livestock. Commonwealth Agricultural Bureaux, 1981
57. Wagner D: Managing selenium deficient pastures. Agri-Rac 9:3, 1988
58. Wagner WC: Improving fertility in dairy cows. J Am Vet Med Assoc 140:939, 1962
59. Ward GM: Molybdenum toxicity and hypocuprosis in ruminants: A review. J Anim Sci 46:1078, 1978
60. Wilson TG: Bovine functional infertility in Devon and Cornwall: Response to manganese therapy. Vet Rec 79:562, 1966

Address reprint requests to

Larry R. Corah, PhD
Weber Hall
Kansas State University
Manhattan, KS 66506

0749–0720/91 $0.00 + .20

Some Nutritional and Genetic Considerations in the Performance Testing of Beef Bulls

William Francis Cates, BSc, DVM, PhD*

The average daily weight gain from weaning to the age of 1 year is a moderately heritable genetic characteristic in young beef bulls. Therefore, bulls that have a high rate of gain would be expected to transmit this to their offspring. Beef-cattle producers should be able to increase the productivity and profitability in their herds by including this attribute as one of the criteria in the selection of herd sires.

Record of Performance (ROP) Bull Testing Stations provide breeders with an opportunity to compare their bulls with others under uniform management conditions. This reduces the variations that would occur if animals were tested in small groups on their home premises. When the test conditions are uniform, the difference in rate of gain between bulls of the same breed and approximately the same age should represent their genetic capability for this trait. While consigning bulls to performance test stations will increase costs for the owner, the reliability of the test results will be far greater. Another advantage of larger stations is that more professional expertise can be made available to carefully monitor the program and to provide special services. This should include research studies that will have direct application for the producer who wants to improve the productivity of his herd. The only limitation on research that may be done would be to ensure that the performance test itself would not be compromised.

While the rate of gain is important, it has not been found to be the most profitable trait in beef cattle. In commercial beef operations, reproductive traits have been identified as being at least five times as important economically as growth and milk producing ability.[21] With prevailing prices, it was also observed that gain in the feedlot was about

---

*Professor, Herd Medicine and Theriogenology, University of Saskatchewan, Western College of Veterinary Medicine, Saskatoon, Saskatchewan, Canada

twice as important as quality of product. If high gaining bulls are to be of any real value to the beef industry, they must have good reproductive capacity. Every performance test program should include all the assessments of reproductive potential that can be done on bulls of this age. The time, effort, and expense involved can be better justified if as many profitable traits as possible can be identified.

High gaining bulls finishing a performance test should always be subjected to careful examination for overall physical soundness. Any unsoundness, such as poor foot and leg conformation, can limit the useful lifespan of a bull, and some of these longevity-limiting conditions could be passed on to offspring. There are cases of this in dairy cattle; for example, a cow with good milking ability can become crippled so early in life that her lifetime milk production is greatly reduced because of bad feet or legs. This same problem occurs in beef cattle; instead of producing 8 or 10 calves a cow may produce only 5 or 6 because of her limited lifespan.

THE PERFORMANCE TESTING PROGRAM

As there are very few uniform guidelines that apply to all test stations, a wide range of management and feeding practices may exist. This is especially true concerning energy-intake levels. The bulls' age at the start of the test and the length of the test period may also vary between stations. Bulls entering a test program are generally required to have been born within a specified time span: usually within 90 days. While animals usually start on a test at weaning, age at end of test could range from 12 to 20 months[10] because performance tests in the past have varied considerably in length. A more common practice is to have a 28-day adjustment period, followed by a 140-day test period. There is a trend now to shorten the test period to 112 days while maintaining the 28-day adjustment period. This approach is less costly and is believed to measure growth rate as accurately as the longer test periods.

Bulls starting a performance test at the Saskatoon ROP Test Station must be between 196 to 285 days of age when they enter the station. They are fed an adjustment ration for 28 days and are then put on a test ration that was formulated to contain 67% total digestible nutrients (TDN) on a dry matter basis, for 112 days. Consequently, these bulls will range in age from approximately 11 to 14 months at the end of the test, and their average age will usually be somewhere between 12 and one half and 13 months.

A starting weight is established (Glossary) for the bulls by weighing them on two successive days and taking the average. They are weighed every 28 days during the test. The final weight is established at the end of the test by again taking the average of weights on two successive days.

Scrotal circumference measurements are taken on all bulls (that have a normal scrotum and normal scrotal contents) as soon as the final weights have been obtained. All the bulls that index high enough to qualify for the station sale are examined for physical soundness. Special emphasis is placed on the examination of the feet and legs. The pelvic reproductive organs and the penis and prepuce are then examined on bulls that pass these preceding evaluations.

The bull test results, including all performance data, various indices (see Glossary), feed conversion, and ration description are published in a pamphlet form. An index is used to compare a bull on average daily gain and weight per day of age to his contemporaries within that breed. Contemporaries are animals of the same sex and similar ages (not more than a 90-day spread in this case) that are managed together so that each animal has an equal chance to demonstrate its performance ability. It is calculated (see Glossary) by dividing a bull's individual record by the contemporary average and multiplying by 100. If the result of this calculation is 100, the animal is considered average for his group. Similarly, if it is 105, the animal is considered to be 5% above and if it is 95 the animal is considered to be 5% below the group average. Finally, a combined index is calculated for average daily gain and weight per day of age. The bulls are also ranked according to their combined index (combined rating) and their average daily gain (average daily gain rating). Some stations may index across breeds. When this is done, the British breeds are usually considered to be 100, the Limousin 103, the Charolais and Simmental 118, and the Maine-Anjou 124.

At the Saskatoon ROP Test Station, the actual scrotal circumference is obtained at the end of the test, it is adjusted (see Glossary) for age, and both are reported in test results. Since no bull at this station is sold if it falls more than 2 cm below the breed average for age, the required scrotal circumference for each bull is calculated and listed in the published results of the test. There is a breed-adjusted scrotal circumference index calculated and bulls are ranked as to age-adjusted scrotal circumference measurement. Backfat measurements are also provided in the published bull test results. With the information provided this way, the best single attribute or the best combination of attributes can be readily identified.

PROBLEMS ASSOCIATED WITH ROP TEST PROGRAMS

There are varying opinions as to the optimal energy level to feed in ROP stations, the kinds of evaluations that should be done, and the kinds of research studies that can be done in conjunction with the performance test. There is also concern about the apparent lack of genetic progress in many station contributors' herds.

An important problem in measuring performance in bulls is the wide range of rations used. The TDN levels used for growing bulls have varied from about 60% to nearly 80%. It is not likely that these different energy levels are all equally good and if so this should be clearly established. Alternatively, it would seem important to identify the optimal level of energy necessary to correctly rank bulls for their rate of growth and to determine whether different breed types require different energy levels. It must also be established that the selected energy level will not cause harm to the bull's overall health, physical soundness, or reproductive capacity. While it could be argued that few adverse effects have been observed in bulls during the performance test period, little creditable research has been done to eliminate the possibility. More specific research is still needed to establish safe energy intake limits to prevent impaired spermatogenesis or subclinical laminitis.

In the past, performance testing of bulls has consisted almost entirely of measuring rate of gain. While this was the original purpose of the program, there are other valuable traits that should be important to cattle raisers. One of these is reproductive capacity; therefore it is important to establish that a performance-tested bull's reproductive system is developing normally. In addition, the high correlation between testes size in bulls and reproductive traits in females[20] argues for extra attention being paid to scrotal circumference measurement as a selection criteria for maternal traits. The performance-testing program should be an important part of the development and use of any new evaluation procedures identifying productive and reproductive attributes in bulls.

There is an unexploited opportunity in most test stations to identify some undesirable conditions of possible genetic origin. Most test-station patrons contribute bulls regularly over a number of years, allowing repeated sampling of animals from individual herds. Over the course of time, a research investigator may be able to identify heritable conditions that a cattle raiser might want to eliminate from the herd. One area that needs considerable improvement in many purebred beef cattle herds is the selection of animals for foot and leg conformation. This would provide both improved function and increased longevity. The heritability of some foot defects, such as bilateral claw conditions, could be studied by examining bulls at the end of performance testing to locate the herds of origin. An example of one of these is "bent" or "corkscrew" claw, where both lateral claws of the hind feet are affected. Occasionally, both medial claws of the front feet will also be affected in the same animal. This condition can be identified at the end of the test, as it often begins to become evident on animals of about 1 year of age.

For breed associations that would like to reduce the incidence of chromosomal anomalies, screening bulls in a performance-test station may be an economical way of locating affected herds. Once the herd of origin is located, related animals can be examined individually. For example, the impact of a 1 : 29 Robertsonian translocation on one such herd was studied, after it was located by identifying the condition at the Saskatoon ROP Test Station.[17] Rapid improvement could be made in purebred beef cattle if breed associations and test station contributors would work together to take advantage of the assembled animals to identify and reduce the incidence of genetic and chromosomal abnormalities.

Another problem for ROP programs can be the station contributors' perception and use of them. Apparently, many view ROP stations as a merchandising device and not as a method for the selection of genetically superior individuals. In an analysis of 22 years of data at the Saskatoon ROP Test Station,[11] it was found that only the Angus breed had shown any significant improvement in rate of gain over that period of time. It has also been observed that only about 35% of the bulls finishing the test will pass all the various selection criteria to be eligible for the bull sale that follows the test. Of the bulls not qualifying for sale, 10% to 12% will be sent directly to slaughter from the station. As most of these have been shown to earn highest carcass grade, marketing at this time should result in about the greatest economic return for the least investment. However, many more bulls are taken out of the station by the owners and are presumably sold as breeding animals. These observations may indicate that many contributors are just using the test station as a method of selling their bulls and not as a means of collecting information for breed improvement. This should be of concern to breed associations, because it tends to limit genetic progress.

OVERNUTRITION

For more than 70 years, it has been known that overfeeding breeding animals interferes with reproductive capacity. In 1909, a reproductive impairment of male animals that was manifest primarily by an absence of sexual interest was described.[22] From clinical observations, two specific reasons for this problem were identified. They were overfeeding and the lack of exercise, which generally went along with the practice of overfeeding. It was observed that some male animals seemed to withstand overfeeding better than others, but that bulls of the beef breeds were especially susceptible. It was also observed that younger animals were less likely to be affected by overfeeding and lack of exercise, but when these animals were allowed to carry too much fat for too long, there was an increasingly greater risk of damage to their breeding capacity. It was concluded that the more prolonged the overfeeding, the greater the likelihood of permanent impairment. It was found that many animals of good genetic value were temporarily or permanently damaged by fitting for the show ring. Things have changed very little.

In a more recent study, the effect of two levels of dietary energy fed from weaning time to 21 months of age on the breeding ability of beef bulls was investigated.[9,10] Bulls raised on the primarily forage diet spent twice as much time in grazing and nongrazing activity as the concentrate fed bulls. In the forage fed group, only about 5% of the feet needed trimming, while 70% of the feet in the concentrate fed group had to be trimmed. In mating trials, 100% of the forage fed bulls completed copulation compared to only 10% of the concentrate fed bulls. In addition, the sexual response time was much faster in the forage fed bulls. Although semen quality of the concentrate fed bulls was better early in the trial, the best quality semen was found in the forage fed bulls by the end of the trial.

In another feeding trial, young Angus and Simmental bulls were fed either a low or a high energy diet over a 140 day feed test.[16] The low energy intake group was limit-fed to gain about 2 lb/day on a 70% TDN ration. The other group was fed the same ration free choice. In this study, the limit-fed bulls also had significantly better libido than those fed the higher energy.

Overfeeding of high-energy rations can also be expected to reduce a bull's breeding capacity through interference with testicular thermoregulation. High ambient temperature, febrile disease conditions, and scrotal insulation can all cause dramatic changes in spermatogenic activity. Exposing bulls to experimental chamber temperatures of 86°F and 100°F for 5 weeks and 2 weeks respectively, caused impaired seminal quality without loss of sex drive.[2] Two of the four bulls used produced ejaculates that were practically devoid of sperm for at least 2 months after the exposure. In another trial, bulls of *Bos taurus* and *Bos indicus* breeds were found to develop some impairment of seminal quality with as little as 12 hours exposure to an ambient temperature of 104°F.[18] There was an increase in the number of abnormal cell types and a decrease in motility and the number of live cells. The peak occurrence of abnormal cells was between 28 and 42 days after exposure, and it coincided with the highest number of dead cells. The degree of impairment was noticeably greater in the *Bos taurus* breeds than in the more heat tolerant *Bos indicus* breeds.

A report of the effects of febrile disease in the human male should be of some interest in any discussion of impaired spermatogenesis.[15] Three medical students, with known normal semen quality, in samples previously contributed for a research project, coincidently acquired a febrile disease. Two had chickenpox and one staphylococcal pneumonia. In the chickenpox patients, the fevers did not exceed 103°F and lasted less than a week. The patient with pneumonia had a fever of 99.5°F to 104°F for about 3 weeks, and he had the greatest seminal quality impairment. However, all had serious seminal quality changes that did not return to normal until about 2 months after these patients left the hospital.

Williams[23] reviewed Lagerlof's work and described how Lagerlof had used scrotal insulation in bulls to induce varying degrees of testicular degeneration. He had devised an enveloping sack of rubber fabric with a cotton lining that could cover the scrotum. With 4 or 5 days of insulation, large numbers of abnormal cells would appear in the semen. Although there was some decrease in motility, there was no great drop in numbers, and recovery occurred in 4 to 6 weeks. When the scrotum was insulated for 11 to 16 days, degeneration was severe. Most of the sperm cells became abnormal in shape, and there was a great reduction in cell numbers to the point where no cells were found for about 4 months. This was followed by a regeneration process that appeared to last about 3 months.

One of the most convincing reports on the detrimental effects of overfeeding was a study in which 34 Hereford bulls were put on a feeding trial from 3 to 24 months of age.[19] Bulls were fed to gain about 1.75 kg/day on the high plane of nutrition and 1 kg/day on the low plane diet. Semen was collected from animals in both groups at 42, 52, 76, 104, and 130 weeks of age. Bulls were killed at intervals of 12, 24, 52, 76, 104, and 130 weeks of age and their reproductive organs were examined. The age at which the first sperm cells appeared in the ejaculate was not reduced by the high nutrition. However, there was a noticeable increase in the number of abnormal cells appearing in the semen by 52 weeks of age in the high plane group, and by 76 weeks of age there was a significant difference between groups. Furthermore, these sperm-cell abnormalities were similar to those seen in a short duration heat stress experiment previously reported.[18] As the abnormalities increased, sperm-cell motility also declined. When the nutritional planes were reversed at 104 weeks of age the trend toward abnormalities did not stop. From 52 weeks of age on, there was a greater amount of fat covering the dorsal pole of the testicle and in the spermatic cord of the bulls on the high level of feed. Reversing the energy levels later in the experiment did not reduce this accumulation of fat to any great extent. On histological sections, more fat could also be seen surrounding the vessels of the pampiniform plexus on the heavily fed bulls.

When subjected to breeding soundness evaluation, highly fitted 2-year-old bulls have been reported to have unusually low satisfactory rates.[1,3] When these bulls were examined about 75 to 90 days after sale time, 36% to 43% were classified as satisfactory potential breeders. When the same bulls were reexamined about 5 to 6 months after sale time, a range of 68% to 71% were classified as satisfactory potential breeders. The primary reason for not being classified as satisfactory on the first examination was reduced semen quality. A community pasture manager with 20 years of experience reported that these bulls will consistently lose 250 pounds or more after purchase.[8] He estimated that their breeding effectiveness, the first year in the pasture, was only 25% of what it would be if they were in good breeding condition.

Feeding trials at the Agriculture Canada Research Station at Lethbridge, Alberta indicate that young Hereford and Angus bulls of 12, 15, and 24 months of age are all susceptible to the high-energy intake induced damage to reproductive capacity.[4,5,6] The effect of high (80% concentrate and 20% forage) energy intake was compared with that of medium (100% forage) energy intake. Semen quality and daily sperm cell production were reduced in the bulls on the high-energy intake. The epididymal sperm reserves were also reduced by as much as 75% in some cases. The bulls on the high-energy diet had the greatest backfat thickness at all ages. The bulls on the high-energy diet had a greater scrotal circumference at 12 months of age, but this difference disappeared by the time both groups reached 15 months. In another study, Coulter and Kozub examined the fertility of bulls used for multiple-sire breeding under range conditions.[7] They observed that continental breed bulls with less backfat sired more calves, whereas detrimental effects were observed in those with as little as 2 mm of backfat. It would appear that more research is justified on the relationship of backfat and fertility in bulls, since it may provide an effective monitoring system to prevent excessive fattening of bulls.

POST-PERFORMANCE TEST EXAMINATION

Puberty has been reported to occur in young bulls of the beef breeds when they reach about 9 to 10 and one half months of age.[12] The same study indicated that, regardless of breed, puberty occurred in these bulls when their scrotal circumference reached about 28 cm. After reaching puberty, normally developing beef bulls all appear to require approximately 14 to 16 weeks for a series of seminal quality changes before the ejaculate can be considered adequate for breeding purposes.[13] In this latter study, it was observed that scrotal circumference, sperm-cell density, percentage of morphologically normal sperm cells, progressive motility, and seminal protein concentration all increased during this transitional period. During the same period of time the percentage of proximal protoplasmic droplets decreased.

These two studies would indicate that young bulls must be allowed to go through this transitional period, and as a result they should not be expected to pass accepted semen quality criteria until they complete this maturation process. Therefore, bulls should not be subjected to culling based on inadequate semen quality until they are at least 14 and one half months of age. We believe that bulls should be required to pass minimum satisfactory seminal quality criteria by the time they have reached a full 15 months of age. If performance-tested bulls are subjected to a semen quality evaluation when their average age is just under 13 months and their age range may be from 11.5 to 14.5 months, less than half of them are likely to be classified as satisfactory potential breeders. The results of 7 years of semen quality evaluations of performance-tested bulls at the Saskatoon ROP Test Station are the basis for this observation (Table 1). Many ROP test stations have instituted semen quality evaluations and have apparently used some undefined "adjustment" factors to allow a higher percentage of bulls to be classified as satisfactory. This practice can not be condoned, because the present state of knowledge does not appear to be adequate to confidently predict whether bulls with substandard semen quality at this age will be satisfactory at 14 and one half to 15 months of age. While it would be desirable to do a complete breeding soundness evaluation on bulls that have just completed a performance test, it may be expecting too much biologically. However, owners should be encouraged to have this examination done when or slightly before a bull reaches 15 months of age. Selection and/or culling for testes size at the end of the performance test is advocated and should ensure as much as any single examination that seminal quality at 15 months of age will be satisfactory. Culling at this age would also apply some selection pressure against late puberty. If heifers are expected to conceive at 15 months, it is also

Table 1. *Number of Bulls with Satisfactory Semen Quality*
after Performance Testing

YEAR	NUMBER OF BULLS EVALUATED	AVERAGE AGE (DAYS)	% BULLS SATISFACTORY
1973	97	386	34
1974	79	385	34
1975	105	383	36
1976	104	388	38
1977	130	384	41
1978	—	—	—
1979	75	388	48
1980	37	371	32

reasonable to expect young bulls to be minimum satisfactory breeders at the same age. Requiring both males and females to be reproductively functional by 15 months of age would seem to be a sound management practice for purebred cattle raisers, especially if they expect to fulfill the requirements of commercial cattle producers, who want to breed heifers early in life.

Another advantage of culling just as early as the bull's reproductive development permits is that the cost of production of these animals is still relatively low in comparison to their potential slaughter value. The sooner the culls are identified, the more likely the opportunity to profit from their disposal. The production efficiency of the beef industry would be improved if more bulls were culled for both low gaining ability and low reproductive potential just as soon as these characteristics can be identified.

While it may be best from a reproductive developmental point of view to examine bulls at 15 months of age, it is unlikely that test-station contributors will be persuaded to eliminate the performance-test bull sale in favor of slightly later sales. Many contributors are aware that some of the bulls are too young for a meaningful breeding soundness evaluation, which would include semen evaluation. They are also aware that testicular size is important for good semen quality. However, they often do not appreciate the importance of a thorough physical examination. Fortunately, there are a number of very useful examination procedures that can be performed on young bulls at this age. If performed carefully, a physical and specific reproductive examination will probably eliminate well over half of the bulls that would be culled at 15 months of age when semen evaluation can also be included.

Performance-tested bulls should be culled for any unsoundness, especially those that are known to be heritable. Although breeders generally underestimate the value of identifying these defects as part of a breeding soundness evaluation, veterinarians that examine test-station bulls should look for and promote the culling of as many conformation defects as possible.

After the general physical examination, the scrotum and its contents should be carefully examined. This examination and the scrotal circumference measurement must take place in a reasonably warm environment, otherwise the scrotum and testicles are drawn too close to the body for proper evaluation. There are three essential parts to this examination. The first is to clearly identify the scrotal shape. The second is to accurately palpate the scrotum and all the anatomical parts within it. The third and final step is to be able to correctly measure the scrotal circumference. This should not be done if steps one and two reveal abnormalities. The normal shaped scrotum has a distinct neck (Fig. 1). The length of the scrotal neck will increase some as the bull matures, and bulls finishing a performance test should already have a clearly evident scrotal neck (Fig. 2). The scrotum is part of the bull's testicular thermoregulatory system, and its shape will change to fulfill that function. When the ambient temperature is low, the testicles and scrotum are pulled closer to the animal's body, and the scrotal neck may not be visible. When the ambient temperature rises, the testicles are lowered and the neck of the scrotum is clearly visible in a normal bull. Some bulls may have a congenitally short scrotum (Fig. 3) and it can be readily recognized by visual inspection. Others may have an accumulation of fat (Fig. 4) in the neck of the scrotum, which can also be recognized by visual inspection and by palpation of the fatty tissue in and around the spermatic cord and over the dorsal pole of the testicle. Some bulls may have a combination of these two abnormalities (Fig. 5).

Careful palpation is very important. Palpation may reveal parts of the epididymis to be underdeveloped, or absent, or even epididymitis. The testicles should be palpated to determine whether they are of normal consistency and of about equal size. Similarly, the scrotal neck and scrotal skin should be thoroughly examined.

Accurate scrotal circumference measurement requires that the bull's testicles be well down in the scrotum and that scrotal wrinkles are smoothed out. If not, the measurement is almost invariably too high. A scrotal circumference measurement may be meaningless in some situations. Good examples of this are the abnormalities shown in Figures 3, 4, and 5. Another would be in the case of a horizontal testicle. The scrotal circumference measurement is only of value when the scrotum and its contents are completely normal.

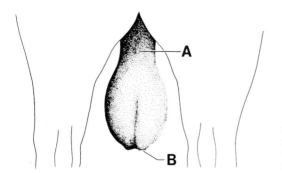

Figure 1. A, The normal shaped scrotum has a distinct neck. B, The outline of the cauda epididymis generally is visible on the ventral aspect.

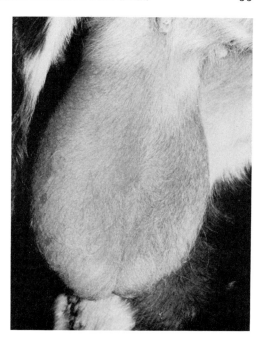

Figure 2. Right craniolateral view of the neck of the scrotum of a 1-year-old Hereford bull.

Guidelines for scrotal circumference measurement can be obtained from published[14] sources or developed within a station. The best source is within each individual station as this would eliminate difference in management and measurement technique. This would require at least four measurements taken on all bulls at approximately equally spaced intervals throughout the test period. Table 2 was developed from measurements obtained at the Saskatoon ROP station. Four mea-

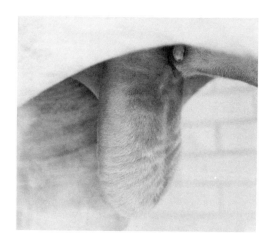

Figure 3. Right lateral view of congenital short scrotum on a young Charolais bull.

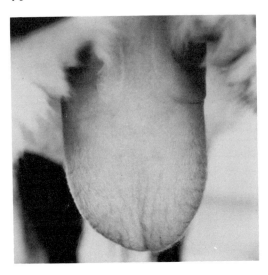

Figure 4. Caudal view of accumulation of fat in the neck of the scrotum of a young Hereford bull.

surements were taken during the test period, for 3 consecutive years. Data were broken down into 10-day age intervals so that contributors could visualize where their bull's scrotal circumference measurement was in comparison to the breed average at that age. In the Saskatoon ROP Test Station Sale, bulls are not eligible if they are more than 2 cm below the breed average (adjusted for day of age), and no sale candidate can have less than a 30-cm scrotal circumference measurement.

The pelvic reproductive organs and the penis and prepuce can be examined most efficiently if two examiners work together. One can perform the pelvic examination while the other examines the penis and

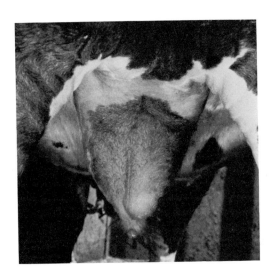

Figure 5. Caudal view of congenital short scrotum and fat accumulation around the top of the testicles in a young Hereford bull.

Table 2. *Mean Scrotal Circumference (CM) of Performance-tested Bulls Compared by Age and Breed*

AGE (DAYS)	ANGUS	CHAROLAIS	GALLOWAY	HEREFORD	MAINE ANJOU	SIMMENTAL	SHORTHORN
210	21.5*	20.5	20.1	21.0	20.5	22.4	21.0
220	22.5	21.5	21.0	22.0	21.5	23.4	21.9
230	23.5	22.4	21.9	22.9	22.4	24.5	22.8
240	24.5	23.4	22.8	23.8	23.4	25.5	23.7
250	25.4	24.3	23.7	24.6	24.3	26.4	24.5
260	26.3	25.1	24.5	25.4	25.1	27.3	25.3
270	27.1	25.9	25.2	26.1	25.9	28.2	26.1
280	27.9	26.7	26.0	26.9	26.7	29.1	26.8
290	28.7	27.5	26.6	27.5	27.5	29.9	27.5
300	29.4	28.2	27.3	28.1	28.2	30.6	28.1
310	30.1	28.9	27.9	28.7	28.9	31.4	28.7
320	30.7	29.5	28.5	29.3	29.6	32.1	29.2
330	31.3	30.1	29.0	29.8	30.2	32.7	29.8
340	31.9	30.7	29.5	30.2	30.8	33.3	30.2
350	32.4	31.2	30.0	30.6	31.3	33.9	30.6
360	32.9	31.7	30.4	31.0	31.8	34.5	31.0
370	33.4	32.2	30.8	31.3	32.3	35.0	31.4
380	33.8	32.6	31.2	31.6	32.7	35.4	31.7
390	34.2[c]	33.0[b]	31.5[a]	31.9[a]	33.2[b]	35.9[d]	31.9[a]

*Standard error of the estimate averaged over all breeds = ± 2.14 cm
Unlike letters (a b c d) are significantly different (p < .01).

prepuce. Gentle rectal examination followed by massage of the pelvic urethra often stimulates a bull to relax and partially protrude his penis. The British breeds respond very well to this technique and may even completely protrude the penis and prepuce by massage alone. However, the examination can often be expedited by grasping the tip of the penis as soon as it protrudes from the preputial orifice. A gauze sponge held in the hand will provide a secure grip on the tip of the penis. Before grasping the penis, the examiner's other hand should be used to deflect the preputial hairs and any part of the prepuce that may otherwise prevent a firm grasp of the glans penis. Gentle sustained traction while the pelvic organs are being massaged will generally expose the entire penis and prepuce for inspection. An electroejaculator should be held in reserve for those cases in which this technique fails (it can also be used with the few bulls that kick at the examiner's hand). If this part of the examination is left until last, then only those bulls that pass all the other sale selection criteria will need to be examined. This would seldom be greater than about 35% to 40% of the population that was present at the final weigh off.

The most common findings in bulls of this age during the penile-preputial examination are incomplete penile-preputial separation (Fig. 6), hair rings (Fig. 7), persistent penile frenula, and fibropapillomas. Incomplete penile-preputial separation is observed more in the polled breeds than in the horned breeds. It is not a serious problem, but it may serve as a site for hair ring formation. These unseparated areas can be

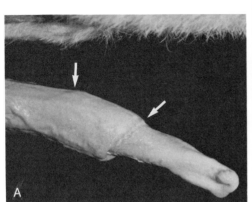
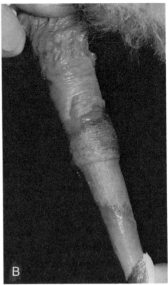

Figure 6. A, Incomplete penile-preputial separation in a 1-year-old polled Hereford bull (*between arrows*). B, After manual separation of the penile-preputial tissue.

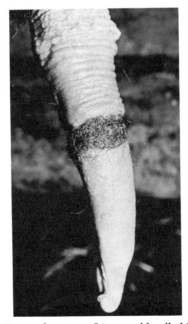

Figure 7. Hair ring on the penis of 1-year-old polled Hereford bull.

easily and quickly broken down and covered with a medicated ointment as the examinations are in progress. However, it is best done while the bull is being stimulated with the electroejaculator. Otherwise, the bull is likely to kick the examiner because of the momentary pain that this separation causes. Hair rings can be easily removed during the examination procedure. Hair rings can cause serious penile injury, including urethral fistula and amputation of the tip of the penis. Persistent penile frenula can be easily diagnosed and surgically corrected if the owner so desires. However, there is evidence from observations at this station of its heritability. Fibropapillomas may occur on the penis, prepuce, or both. They can be removed by cryosurgery or surgery. Although this may have to be repeated once or twice, corrective procedures at this time will insure that the animal is ready for breeding at 15 months of age. One condition that may be difficult to diagnose during this part of the examination is congenital short penis. The penis of almost all the bulls this age can be extended sufficiently to permit proper examination. However, a few animals seem to be able to resist attempts to fully extend the penis by traction. There are also some younger animals in a performance test group that simply need more time to complete penile development.

SUMMARY

Performance testing started after it was recognized that growth traits were heritable. In the early years of performance testing there was a tendency to feed higher levels of energy for longer periods of time. More recently, the trend has been to feed lower levels of energy for shorter periods. There are still differences in opinion as to the appropriate level of energy to use. Although it is important that the level of energy fed is adequate to correctly establish a bull's ability to gain, it is essential to know that it will pose no risk of impaired spermatogenesis or cause any degree of laminitis.

Clinical observations and research on overfeeding clearly show that both libido and spermatogenesis can be impaired by excess energy intake. The damage in 2-year-old bulls can be very extensive and in some animals it may not be reversible. The scant amount of research in yearling bulls indicates that there is considerable potential danger from overfeeding energy as well.

Test stations are under used in regard to performing research that would help identify heritable defects that would interfere with the productive and reproductive efficiency of beef cattle.

The first performance testing programs emphasized average daily gain from weaning to 1 year of age, so "performance" has traditionally meant rate of gain to most cattle raisers. The term "performance" is now starting to acquire a broader and more inclusive definition. For many breeders, it now includes weight per day of age, which is in part a maternal trait, and some kind of male evaluation for reproductive potential that can also be extrapolated to the female side. One of the first breakthroughs in this regard was to recognize the heritability of testicular size, and that testicular size could be fairly accurately determined by scrotal circumference measurement. It was also found that there was a favorable relationship between larger testicle size and the ability to produce high quality semen. As a result, it became a common practice to include scrotal circumference measurements in the published bull test results. However, many test station patrons were, and still are, content to consider the scrotal circumference measurement alone as an evaluation of a bull's breeding potential.

Unfortunately, less than half of the bulls finishing a performance test at ages ranging from 11 to 14 months will be able to produce semen of completely acceptable quality. However, the development of their testicles and other reproductive organs is far enough advanced so that many of the animals with the best and poorest breeding potential can be recognized. A thorough general physical examination as well as a careful examination of the reproductive organs by a competent clinician familiar with the developmental changes that are occuring in bulls of this age is necessary to identify a young bull's future breeding potential.

REFERENCES

1. Barth AD, Oko RJ: Abnormal Morphology of Bovine Spermatozoa. Ames, Iowa State University Press, 1989, p 143
2. Casady RB, Meyers RM, Legates JE: The effect of exposure to high ambient temperature on spermatogenesis in the dairy bull. J Dairy Sci 18:14, 1953
3. Cates WF: Observations on scrotal circumference and its relationship to classification of bulls. Proceedings of and Annual Meeting of the Society for Theriogenology, Cheyenne, 1975, p 1
4. Coulter GH, Kozub GC: Testicular development, epididymal sperm reserves and semen quality in two-year-old Hereford and Angus bulls: Effect of two levels of dietary energy. J Anim Sci 59:432, 1984
5. Coulter GH, Carruthers TD, Amann RP, et al: Testicular development, daily sperm production and epididymal sperm reserves in 15-month-old Angus and Hereford bulls: Effects of bull strain plus dietary energy. J Anim Sci 64:254, 1987
6. Coulter GH, Bailey DRC: Epididymal sperm reserves in 12-month-old Angus and Hereford bulls: Effects of bull strain plus dietary energy. Anim Repro Sci 16:169, 1988
7. Coulter GH, Kozub GC: Efficacy of methods used to test fertility of beef bulls used for multiple-sire breeding under range conditions. J Anim Sci 67:1757, 1989
8. Griffin DG: The economics of bull management in community pastures. Paper presented at mid-winter conference of Saskatchewan Vet Med Assn Saskatoon, 27 Jan 1989
9. Hentges JF Jr, Neal FC, Capote FA, et al: Effect of nutrition on potential reproductive potency of bulls. J Anim Sci 23:307, 1964
10. Hentges JF Jr: Level of feeding and bull performance. In Cunha T, Warnick A, Koger M (eds): Factors Affecting Calf Crop. Gainesville, University of Florida Press, 1967, p 102
11. Koots KR, Cohen RDH, Nicholson HH: Yearly trends in the performance of bulls entered at the Saskatoon ROP bull test station. Can J Anim Sci 68:965, 1988
12. Lunstra DD, Ford JJ, Echternkamp SE: Puberty in beef bulls: hormone concentrations, growth, testicular development, sperm production and sexual aggressiveness in bulls of different breeds. J Anim Sci 46:1054, 1978
13. Lunstra DD, Echternkamp SE: Puberty in beef bulls: Acrosome morphology and semen quality in bulls of different breeds. J Anim Sci 55:638, 1982

14. Lunstra DD, Gregory KE, Cundiff LV: Heritability estimates and adjustment factors for the effects of bull age and age of dam on yearling testicular size in breeds of bulls. Theriogenology 30:127, 1988
15. MacLeod J: Effect of chickenpox and of pneumonia on semen quality. Fertil Steril 2:523, 1951
16. Morrow RE, Elmore RG, Brooks AL, et al: Growth and reproductive development of beef bulls tested on two levels of energy. J Anim Sci 53(suppl 1):188, 1981
17. Schmutz SN, Moker J: Impact of a 1:29 Robertsonian translocation on a herd of purebred beef cattle. Can J Anim Sci, in press
18. Skinner JD, Louw GN: Heat stress and spermatogenesis in *Bos indicus* and *Bos taurus* cattle. J Appl Physiol 21:1784, 1966
19. Skinner JD: Nutrition and fertility in pedigree bulls. *In* Gilmore D, Cook B (eds): Environmental Factors in Mammalian Reproduction. London, Macmillan, 1981, p 160
20. Smith BA, Brinks JS, Richardson GV: Relationships of sire scrotal circumference to offspring reproduction and growth. J Anim Sci 67:2881, 1989
21. Trenkle A, Willham RL: Beef production efficiency. Science 198:1009, 1977
22. Williams WL: Veterinary Obstetrics Including the Diseases of Breeding Animals and of the Newborn. Ithaca, NY, Published by the author, 1909, p 138
23. Williams WL: Researches concerning the morphologic changes in the spermatozoa and in the testicles of sterile or subnormally fertile bulls (a review). Cornell Vet 24:361, 1934

GLOSSARY

TERMS AND DEFINITIONS

Actual Scrotal Circumference: Measured at final weigh off.

ADG: Average daily gain.

ADG on Test (calculated using the equation): (Weight at end of test − starting weight)/112 days = ADG on test.

Adjusted Scrotal Index: The age-adjusted circumference relative to the other bulls of the same breed on test, calculated as follows: (Age adjusted circumference of individual/average age adjusted circumference of breed) × 100 = adjusted scrotal index.

Adjusted 200 Day Weight (calculated using the equation): Adjusted ADG from birth to start of test × 200 days + birth weight = adjusted 200 day weight. Correction factors are used to adjust calves from 2 to 4-year-old dams to level of performance equivalent to calves from mature dams. The figure is obtained from herd test data.

Adjusted 365 Day Weight (calculated using the equation): (End of test weight at station/age in days) × 365 = adjusted 365 day weight.

Breed ADG Index: The gain of each individual calf relative to the average daily gain of all bulls for that breed at the station, expressed as a percent using the following equation: (ADG of individual/age ADG of breed) × 100 = breed ADG index.

Fat Depth: Obtained by ultrasonic measurement from a position between the 12th and 13th ribs and is expressed as a total depth in mm (1 in = 25.4 mm; 1 mm = 0.04 in).

Final Weight: Average of weights taken on 2 successive days at the end of the 112-day feeding period.

Required Scrotal Circumference: Minimum scrotal circumference necessary for eligibility for the special ROP bull sale, adjusted for the age and breed of the bull based on cumulated data obtained at this station. No bull with a scrotal circumference less than 30 cm is eligible for the sale irrespective of age or breed.

Start of Test Ranking: The ranking of the individual calf at start of test relative to all calves of the same sex in the contemporary group on the herd test based on adjusted 200 day weight.

Starting Weight: Average of weights taken on 2 successive days following a 28-day adjustment period at the station.

Weight per day of age index (WDAI): (WDAI of individual/average WDAI of breed) × 100 = WDA station index.

Address reprint requests to

William Francis Cates, BSc, DVM, PhD
2118 Haultain Avenue
Saskatoon, Saskatchewan
Canada S7J1P6

0749–0720/91 $0.00 + .20

Grazing Management as it Affects Nutrition, Animal Production and Economics of Beef Production

S.D. Parsons, PhD,* and C.D. Allison, PhD†

The use and management of rangeland has been largely neglected in the development of the ranching industry. It is our intention to (1) show the close relationship that exists between economics, animal performance, grazing management, and supplementation; (2) illustrate how manipulation of one affects the outcome of another; and (3) outline some practical considerations on grazing management and supplementation.

Traditionally, practical animal nutrition has been considered to be the determination of a ration based on the animal's requirements on the one hand and the nutritive value of available feedstuffs on the other. In practice, nutrition of the grazing animal commonly revolves around what, and when, to supplement. Interestingly, texts on ruminant nutrition simply ignore the role of grazing in general, and grazing management in particular. Equally, the needs of livestock have been neglected in the design and development of most grazing systems.[8]

So, despite the fact that production of beef and sheep is primarily dependent upon grazing, we face the rather odd situation where the nutritional fate of the grazing animal has been largely neglected by both the animal and range scientists. As the philosopher, James Watt, is purported to have said, the truth lies somewhere in the chinks between departments. It is a truth that has been sought somewhat haphazardly by producers and feed sellers alike. Each has sought solutions to real problems of maintaining or increasing animal performance. But again, largely through ignorance, the role of grazing management has been ignored.

Such neglect has occurred despite the fact that economically ef-

*President, Ranch Management Consultants Inc., Albuquerque, New Mexico
†Professor of Range Science, New Mexico State University, Las Cruces, New Mexico

fective beef production is highly dependent upon grazing management that must consider the needs of the animal and the forage plant simultaneously. Sound grazing management should result in a healthy sward while simultaneously improving individual animal performance and enabling an increase in stocking rate.

ECONOMICS

Because it is our assumption that the ultimate goal of the livestock producer is economic and profitable production, economics must provide the framework for our considerations. Fortunately, only a small part of the rather complex economics of a ranching business need concern us here. Increased production has been the major goal of agricultural scientists, while economics has been largely ignored by them.

If we pursued the dream of increased production to its limits, every cow in the herd would produce twin calves, each weighing 600 pounds or more at weaning. Apart from its novelty, this herd may or may not be an attractive economic proposition. For instance, consider only one cow in the herd. The income she produces is offset by the costs of producing that yield. The costs directly associated with this one cow are interest on the capital invested in the cow, the supplementary feed cost, and veterinary and medicine expenses. These costs vary in direct proportion to the number of cows in the herd and are known as direct costs. The difference between the income and direct costs is known as gross margin. Gross margin is the financial contribution the cow makes toward overhead costs. Thus one goal in ranch economics is to increase the gross margin produced per head. This is achieved either by increasing income or by decreasing direct costs.

If the herd consisted of only one cow, producing even an exceptional gross margin, the commercial ranching operation would show a loss. This is true simply because one cow could not produce enough income to cover the land, labor, vehicle, administrative, and other expenses that make up the overhead costs. So a second economic goal would be to have more cows, each producing a positive gross margin.

The third alternative for increasing profit is to reduce overhead expenses by reducing land-related, labor-related, and administrative overheads. In practice, a rancher losing money generally cuts expenditure by not replacing capital equipment or by taking a smaller draw from the business. To maintain living standards in the face of unprofitability many ranchers in the United States borrow against their land or subsidize the ranch income from nonranch activities. Clearly, living on capital is not a viable long-term alternative so it is necessary to examine ways of improving profitability. Specifically, in the extensive livestock business there are only three things that can be done to improve profit[10]: (1) Improve gross margin per head; (2) increase number of head; (3) decrease overhead costs.

In this article we are primarily concerned with improving gross margin per head. Gross margin of the livestock enterprise is the main concern of the animal scientist or animal advisor. Though some of the advisor's actions might influence the overhead costs, or the number of head, in the main his activities impinge on gross margin.

ANIMAL PERFORMANCE, NUTRITION AND GROSS MARGIN

Generally, gross margin of the grazing animal increases in direct proportion to production level — for any given direct cost outlay. The better the steer gains or the better the cow herd reproduces, the better the gross margin, but there are additional factors that affect gross margin.

Gross margin of the steer operation is greatly influenced by market price, both at time of purchase and at time of sale, and to a lesser extent by production considerations. By contrast, gross margin in the cow/calf operation is greatly influenced by production levels and to a lesser extent by market price. For this reason production technique, nutrition, and grazing management assume an important role in the economics of the breeding herd. It would be true to say that the single most important factor affecting cow/calf gross margin is reproduction. The cow that does not produce a calf does not produce an income. But the direct costs of maintaining a barren cow remain essentially unchanged. Therefore the gross margin contribution from such a cow is negative. Another way of expressing this is to say that the barren cow depreciates in value.

Because the gross margin of the breeding cow is most dependent upon production levels and the nutritive value of grazing, the breeding cow will be used as the example animal in this article.

Reproduction and Gross Margin

Wiltbank[4] has identified six factors critical in insuring high reproductive performance. These may be grouped as three nutritionally related variables, namely, body condition score at calving, cows gaining weight immediately prior to breeding, and well grown heifers; and three husbandry related variables, namely, a 60-day breeding season, bulls evaluated for breeding soundness, and 48 hour calf removal. The length of the breeding season also has nutritionally related considerations, in that a short breeding season permits greater uniformity within the herd for grazing management and supplementation purposes. It is clear that high reproductive performance is highly dependent upon nutrition.

Reproduction and Nutrition

The relationship between reproduction and nutrition has long been known and researched. Richards et al[14] showed that body condition score at calving and weight changes immediately prior to breeding were the two factors that should receive most attention in order to improve conception rates. These are both factors well within control of management, but they are often expensively achieved, especially where cows are overwintered on hay, silage, and similar conserved feeds. To improve gross margin it is essential that attention be focused on lower cost nutrition.

For extensive animal production, which for all practical purposes covers beef production from nondairy herds as well as sheep and goat production, the major source of nutrition is grazing. There may well be isolated incidences where beef cows and ewes receive most of their nutrients from crop residue or confinement feedlots, but these should be considered outside the mainstream and beyond the normal economic parameters for profitability. Thus, we may summarize by saying:

$$\text{Gross margin} = \text{f(animal performance)}$$
$$\text{Animal Performance} = \text{f(nutrition)}$$
$$\text{Nutrition} = \text{f(grazing)}$$

GRAZING MANAGEMENT AND NUTRITION

Surprisingly, animal scientists and ranchers have paid little attention to the impact of grazing management on providing nutritional needs of cattle. They seem to have simply assumed that the grass is there, that it will grow, and that it will provide nutrients as long as it is of the right species. As rangelands have deteriorated, the typical rancher has treated the symptoms while lamenting the fact. Seldom do ranchers concern themselves with the causes, nor indeed do they seem to consider their typical grazing practices to be one of the major causes for rangeland deterioration.

Despite the fact that grass species of economic importance evolved under the influence of heavy grazing,[9] it is modern grazing management that has caused, and is still causing, rangeland degradation. The grazing regimen that existed prior to our pervasive influence was different from that which is practiced by most ranchers today.

Grazing and Rangeland Deterioration

Once defoliated by grazing or burning, the typical bunch grass sacrifices reserve energy materials stored in roots and the basal parts of the plants in order to put out new leaf.[17] Repetitive defoliation of the individual plant before it has had an opportunity to restore its root reserves means the demise of that individual plant. This phenomenon is known as overgrazing. Overgrazing is said to occur because of frequency of bite and severity of bite.

Overgrazing was largely avoided under natural conditions by the migratory habits of large herbivore herds. But with homesteading, control of vital water points,[16] and the sedentary habits of modern people, that graze-rest-graze pattern was broken and replaced by extended periods of continuous grazing, which are enormously detrimental to the health of the plant. Resulting range deterioration was mistakenly believed to be caused by overstocking.

Overgrazing takes place individual plant by individual plant, and not over a range as a whole. Thus, it is possible to have severe overgrazing, albeit over a limited percentage of the area, when one horse is turned loose for extended periods in a large pasture. The fallacy is that overgrazing can be avoided by reducing stocking rate. However, a lower stocking rate designed to control overgrazing simply means that fewer plants in the pasture will be overgrazed and more plants will be undergrazed. Because undergrazing, and the consequent plant moribundity, are just as detrimental to range health as overgrazing, reduction in the stocking rate does not necessarily lead to improvement in range health. A brief discussion of the physiology of plant growth will serve to explain the apparent contradiction that a range can be simultaneously overgrazed but understocked.[1]

Photosynthesis and Plant Growth — the Basis of Sound Nutrition

Plants are remarkable natural factories upon which all life depends. Through photosynthesis the leaf converts light, water and carbon dioxide into sugar. Through further processing, and with the addition of phosphorous, nitrogen, sulfur, and other minerals, the sugar is converted to starch, fats, and proteins which are then consumed by other forms of life. All the technology that we use in agriculture is simply designed to improve the efficiency with which we harvest sunlight energy transformed by plants.

Part of the energy trapped by the leaf is used in manufacturing the protein, cellulose, and lignin needed to build the plant. Energy is also converted to reserves of starch, fats, and oils, which are stored in the roots to enable life to continue during dormant phases and to provide initial growth once the leaf has been removed. Starch, oils, fats, and sugar are also stored in the seeds to provide the initial source of energy required at the time of germination until the new plant grows enough leaf material to begin to synthesize its own energy from light, water, and carbon dioxide.

Tiller Production

In addition to the leaves produced by each plant, new growth takes place from the base of the plant in the form of new tillers. Once the tiller produces a seedhead it becomes dormant and dies, but before a tiller dies it sends out one or more new tillers that each eventually develop their own root system and become established as independent plants within a colony of plants that we know as a grass tuft. These plants in turn produce new tillers and thus the healthy grass tuft grows bigger as it gets older. Each tiller in turn produces new leaves, so in the healthy sward there is an increase in the number of leaves, as well as the number of tillers, and hence an increase in the size of the factory able to convert sunlight energy to a form useful for humans and other animals.

Rate of Plant Growth and Feed Availability

Not considering the individual plant, but the plant community as a whole, new herbage growth increases rapidly at first and then progressively less rapidly as competition for light increases. Climate, available soil nutrients, and soil moisture, as well as plant species, determine the rate of plant growth. Apart from ensuring that a leafy pasture is maintained through correct grazing management, little can be done by management to influence the rate of plant growth in a natural rangeland. Therefore management attention should focus on maintaining the sward in a condition in which it is able to grow at its fastest rate.

A grass community that has been grazed too severely would have insufficient leaf material to trap sunlight energy, so growth would be slow. Conversely and ironically, a plant community with too many leaves will also reduce the amount of sunlight energy trapped by the plant. Slow growth in the overgrown community occurs for a variety of reasons. Older leaves do not photosynthesize as efficiently as younger leaves and as the plant grows, these older leaves tend to shade the younger more efficient leaves. To avoid both too little plant material and too old a plant, representing the extremes of slow growth, it is necessary to keep growth in the steep part of the sigmoid, or S shaped, growth curve (Figure 1).

Phase I represents slow growth, which occurs when a large portion of leaf, the plant "factory," has been removed. Phase II represents efficient production; the period of most rapid growth when there are sufficient leaves to intercept the maximum amount of light and provide the necessary energy for plant growth. Phase III represents the period when growth slows due to excessive shading and less efficient photosynthesis of older leaves. During Phase III, the death rate of plant tissue

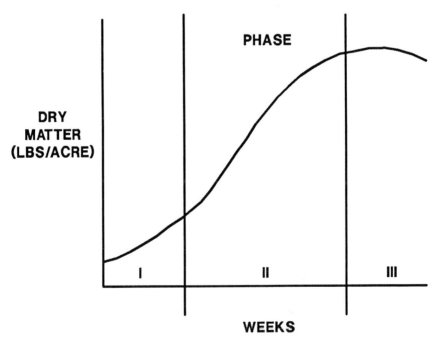

Figure 1. Sigmoid growth curve.

starts to exceed the growth rate and the proportion of dead, low quality feed becomes high. So, from an energy production perspective, both Phases I and III are energy inefficient phases and should be avoided.

Climatic conditions also affect the number and rate of emergence of leaves from the individual tillers. In spring when temperatures are low, even if moisture is adequate, the rate of growth is likely to be slow. As the season progresses and temperatures rise, so the rate of growth increases if there is adequate moisture. Toward autumn when temperatures fall and daylight hours shorten, growth slows. This expected pattern of changing growth rates would be further modified by availability of soil moisture.

To maintain grass growth in the steep Phase II portion of growth it is necessary to observe three requirements: (1) The pasture should not be grazed too short. (2) Prolonged periods in Phase III detract from the efficiency of photosynthesis through shading and senescence and should be avoided. Bear in mind that these requirements apply to individual plants as well as to the pasture as a whole. (3) Because of varying rates of growth, the period between grazings must vary according to the rate of growth to keep the plant growing in Phase II. When growth is fast, the rest periods must be shorter. When growth is slow, the rest periods must be longer.

Plant Growth and Plant Health

The factors discussed previously are important in understanding why plants die from overgrazing or undergrazing and why plants die during drought. First, consider the dangers of underuse. Visualizing an ungrazed tuft, it is fairly apparent that the leaves of the individual tillers in the middle of the clump will be shaded by surrounding tillers. Thus, they do not trap sunlight energy efficiently. Consequently, they translocate little energy to their roots and are unable to send up new tillers the following year. The tillers that are not replaced die. By contrast, the tillers on the outer edges of the clump survive because they trap sufficient energy and are able to replace themselves.[6] This phenomenon is often observed as plants with dead centers growing throughout the range.

In the case of overgrazing, all the tillers in the clump are likely to be equally afflicted and all of them would die. Overgrazing occurs when the plant is defoliated so frequently that to maintain vital life processes, the plant depletes root energy reserves.

Seeding versus Vegetative Growth

Vegetative growth is more important than generally recognized. Though ranchers tend to be very concerned about producing sufficient seed, probably more than 90% of new perennial plant growth occurs through vegetative propagation. For this reason, any activity, such as over-rest, that results in lowered tiller production will cause a decrease in pasture productivity.

ANIMAL REQUIREMENTS AND GRASS MANAGEMENT

There is more involved in grazing management than simply producing the maximum amount of grass growth within any one year,
however. The reason the rancher produces grass is primarily to produce livestock and livestock products. Ranchers are in the business of
converting sunlight energy to a product demanded by the consumer.
Obviously, the requirements of the animal must be taken into account
in any grazing system.

Plane of Nutrition as Related to Phase of Grass Growth

Not only are Phases I and III energy inefficient zones for grass
production, they are also inefficient zones from an animal nutrition stan
point. In Phase I, animals are likely to perform poorly, will lose weight
and exhibit poor reproductive performance due to a lack of feed quantity. In Phase III, by contrast, there is an adequate amount of feed, but
animals absorb fewer nutrients because of poor feed quality.

Most ranchers understand and accept those extremes when confronted with pastures that exhibit a uniform sward in either Phases I or
III. However, they probably do not recognize that animals on a continuously grazed pasture are confronted by those extremes most of the
time. This occurs and is perpetuated by the grazing behavior of the
animal. In most lightly stocked, continuously grazed pastures, one finds
overgrazed and underused grasses side by side. The problem is exacerbated by low stock density and is known as low density grazing.

Typically, animals will return to a previously grazed, less mature
plant rather than to an older, lignified, mature plant. Thus, in the
unmanaged but confined pasture situation, where animal migration has
been prevented, one finds plants that are overgrazed (Phase I) and
plants that are completely ungrazed (Phase III) side by side. Much has
been said and written about area selective grazing, but in essence it is a
situation that develops and is perpetuated by too low a stock density
(number of animals per acre at any moment in time). Thus it could be
more correctly called "low density grazing".[15]

When confronted with low density grazing the grazing manager
periodically defoliates the underused material by mowing or burning.
The symptoms are treated but the cause is ignored. Whereas mowing is
not ecologically harmful, it is expensive, and burning can be both
expensive and ecologically harmful when repeated frequently. The
consequence of repeated fire is the gradual change of plant species,
deterioration of the water cycle and reduction in stocking rates because
of reduced energy flow.

Though it may be possible to maintain animal performance, with
continuous grazing this is generally only achieved at the expense of the
natural resource. There are consequent effects on the two other economic parameters, namely, number of units that can be stocked and
overhead expense. Low density grazing can be avoided by increasing
stock density and by allowing plants that have been defoliated an
adequate time to recover before they are again grazed.

Meeting the Animal's Nutritional Requirements

Perhaps the most common, and most frequently overlooked, problem in grazing animal nutrition is getting the animals to consume sufficient nutrient energy. If the animal was able to consume more energy, performance would improve. Both quantity and quality of feed affect intake. In Phase I, short feed results in the animal being unable to ingest sufficient nutrients to satisfy requirements. In Phase III, the feed quality limits energy intake.

While it is reasonably obvious why an absence of feed should limit energy intake it may be less apparent why animals should consume insufficient energy when there is an abundance of mature grass. As the plant matures, the cell walls thicken and become infused with lignin. Lignin renders the major energy components of the plant, cellulose and hemicellulose, less digestible by the micro-organisms within the rumen. As the digestibility decreases, so the rate of passage of ruminal material decreases, and consequently there is decreased feed intake. The net result is that although the total energy component of the pasture has probably increased, that which is available for micro-organism breakdown and ultimately for animal nutrition decreases.

There is, therefore, an optimum time to graze grass plants so that the maximum amount of high quality feed is produced per acre while avoiding poor feed quality.

When grass is harvested while it is still young, the feed quality is high although the yield is low. As the grass matures, the yield increases but the quality decreases. Fortunately, if the grass plant is used before it reaches Phase III, the degree of lignification will be small and daily intake will be greater. Thus, in broad terms, what is good for the plant is also good for the animal. The sward should be managed so that growth remains in Phase II for as long as possible.

Grazing Intensity and Animal Performance

There is more to providing sufficient intake than simply deciding when a grass plant should be grazed. As far as grazing management is concerned, additional factors that affect intake are: (1) the feed available to the animal each day—the feed allowance; (2) the amount of residual material left by the animals; and (3) the percentage of the available feed that is used.[13]

In general terms, the optimum grazing intensity of a paddock, within certain limits, is dependent upon the desired animal performance. The higher the level of animal performance required, the less the paddock should be defoliated. As the paddock is defoliated, the animal is forced to eat more dead leaf relative to green leaf. Consequently, rate of digestion decreases and total nutrient intake declines, leading to poorer performance. Thus, to achieve maximum animal performance, paddocks should be grazed lightly.

As the amount of feed available per animal per day is increased, one can expect individual animal performance to increase (Fig. 2a). To

PDCTN
/HEAD

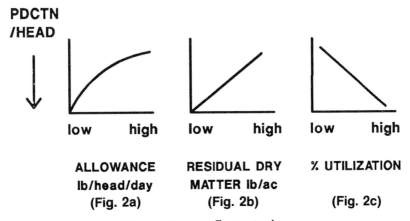

| low   high | low   high | low   high |

ALLOWANCE	**RESIDUAL DRY**	**% UTILIZATION**
lb/head/day	**MATTER lb/ac**	
(Fig. 2a)	**(Fig. 2b)**	**(Fig. 2c)**

Figure 2. Factors affecting intake.

increase daily allowance, one would either decrease the stocking rate or move the animals more rapidly to fresh pasture. Grazing management then becomes a balancing act. When the grazing period is shortened the rest period also decreases. The danger of too short a rest is that there might have been inadequate plant recovery by the time the animals return. Fortunately, a reasonably well-informed manager cognizant of the principles can rapidly gain the experience needed to maintain the correct balance.

Closely related to feed allowance is the amount of residual dry matter left by the animals once they have been moved from the paddock. The more feed left, the greater the animal performance during that particular grazing (Fig. 2b). Thus, if the animal is forced to scrape the bottom of the barrel we should expect poorer performance; but, if the animal can be more selective in what it eats, we can expect better performance. As the percentage of the available feed consumed increases, animal performance can be expected to decrease (Fig. 2c).[13]

GRAZING MANAGEMENT TO PROMOTE IMPROVED NUTRITION WHILE IMPROVING PASTURE GROWTH

Ideally, once a plant has been defoliated it should have adequate time to recover before again being grazed. The recovery period would approximate the time interval of Phase II (see Fig. 1), and would vary depending upon the growth rate, which would in turn be influenced by temperature and moisture conditions. To allow an adequate period for recovery and regrowth, animals need to be removed from the pasture, but because they must be housed somewhere during this recovery period, a large pasture would be subdivided into individual paddocks, each of which is treated as an individual entity within the block of rangeland allocated to the herd.

It may be conceivable to divide a pasture in two, resting one half while grazing the other. The practical limitation of such a system is that the length of the grazing period in the grazed paddock equals the length of the recovery period in the rested paddock. If the graze period is optimally short from the animal's perspective, the rest period would be too short to allow adequate regrowth. Conversely, if the recovery period was attuned to the requirements of the plant, the graze period would be so long that animal performance would suffer. Therefore, several paddocks are necessary to ensure an adequate rest period. Pasture scientists have suggested that 8–10 paddocks are adequate for this purpose.[5] While a lower number of paddocks might be adequate when considering the plant only, field experience shows that so few paddocks do not result in adequate animal performance.

For bunch grasses growing under range conditions, the desirable rest period is likely to be greater than 50 days and could be as long as 90 days. Thus, with 10 paddocks, nine of which are resting, the graze period will be at least 6 days for each paddock. With a longer rest period or fewer paddocks, the graze period would increase in duration. The longer the grazing period, the lower the plane of nutrition for the animal.[2,3] This phenomenon is fairly obvious when observing rotationally grazing animals. During the first day in a new paddock animals have access to the greatest amount of feed of the highest quality. Having selected on the first day, both the quantity and quality of feed available will be lower on the second, and so on through the grazing period (see Fig. 3).

The duration of the rest period and the duration of the graze period are inextricably tied. Since the rest period is dependent upon growth rate and is therefore beyond the control of management, the duration of the graze period can only be reduced by increasing the

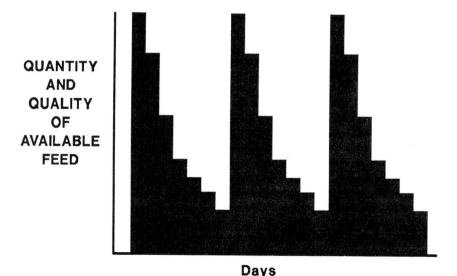

Days

Figure 3. Decreasing nutritional plane with increasing duration of grazing period.

number of paddocks. There is no single ideal number of paddocks because the duration of the recovery period, as well as the animal's requirements, will vary considerably during the season and from year to year. However, as a general observation, we may conclude that a grazing period of 3 days or less is desirable. Thus, if animals are grazing a pasture that requires a recovery period of more than 50 days, more than 18 paddocks per herd are required in order to maintain a high plane of nutrition for the animals.

Under intensive grazing circumstances where portable fences can be used for strip grazing, the duration of the graze period can be more easily determined and controlled, but under extensive range conditions the number of paddocks tends to be fixed. Under these circumstances combining herds and thus altering the number of paddocks per herd provides the greatest opportunity for varying duration of graze period for an individual herd. Combining herds to increase number of paddocks while lengthening the rest period to accommodate slower growth during drought, for instance, has become common practice among those who practice controlled grazing under extensive conditions.

Fitting Animal Requirements to Pasture Growth

Even under the most ideal conditions, the grass does not grow at a uniform rate year round. For that reason the animal requirements should be matched to pasture growth. Ignoring market considerations, the ideal would be to fit peak animal nutritional requirements (e.g., lactation and rebreeding) to peak pasture production. For the past several decades, however, the reverse has been true. There has been a tendency in the United States to ignore the natural cycle. The popular perception is that by calving earlier, weaning weights will be heavier, and income will be higher. Shortfall in feed availability is made up by supplement. If supplementation is inadequate, a drop in conception rates is likely. In either event, there are economic ramifications that should be considered. Experience with many ranchers in several regions suggests delaying the breeding season and reducing supplement cost can frequently improve the gross margin.

Because grass growth is seasonal and animals require feed year round, it is necessary to accumulate surplus feed during the growing season and to budget use of accumulated feed during nongrowing periods. Feed can be accumulated by pasture deferment but that practice is likely to lead to excessively mature Phase III grass, especially in the higher rainfall areas where grass growth tends to be faster. Feed of a higher quality can be accumulated through rotational grazing where excess growth is accumulated in every paddock. Feed quality is more likely to be maintained when grass growth is arrested through periodic grazing (defoliation) throughout the growing season.

Thus, the desirable practice is to periodically graze each paddock while allowing excess feed to accumulate during the growing season. By continuing the rotation through dormancy this accumulated feed is budgeted until growth resumes. It is a fairly simple matter at the end of growth to estimate the amount of feed available. This control of "standing hay," ensures that the animals' requirements can be met, and that a minimum of feed is wasted through trampling and fouling.

Fluctuating Stocking Rates During Drought

Annual fluctuations in rainfall and grass growth pose an additional problem with which the grass farmer must contend. Many ranchers avoid the problem of a fluctuating carrying capacity (amount of feed available), by adopting a "safe" stocking rate. Though this is a simple management strategy, it is neither biologically nor economically efficient. Feed accumulated during years of abundance simply becomes moribund. Apart from losses through highly lignified feed, the weakened state of Phase III grass frequently leads to advancing plant succession and its related problem of brush encroachment.

Matching stocking rate to amount of feed available from one year to another minimizes the accumulation of old gray grass over a period of time, and therefore reduces the need and necessity to artificially defoliate plants by burning or mowing. Of course, a new set of problems arises if animal numbers are to be varied from year to year. However, through judicious enterprise selection and other drought management practices, a strategy can be developed that is both biologically and economically advantageous.

Three Cycles in Grazing Management

In summary, we can say that there are essentially three biologic cycles that dictate grazing management practices: (1) In the short term, the sigmoid pattern of growth requires that plant defoliation be followed by periods of recovery. In practice, rotationally grazing of several paddocks affords good animal performance, a healthy sward and increased stocking rates. (2) Annual growth patterns are such that feed needs to be accumulated during the growing season and budgeted through dormancy. Fitting animal requirements to forage production and careful budgeting ensure high animal production per area of land. (3) Between years, fluctuation in available feed requires adjustment of stocking rates to fit carrying capacity, while minimizing problems that occur with underuse.

THE ROLE OF SUPPLEMENTATION

With the high economic demands placed on optimum animal performance, it is only in the exceptional situation that pastures need not be supplemented. Supplementation with minerals to make up for forage deficiencies is usually essential. In addition, it is often economically advisable to supplement with energy and/or protein. In the context in which the word supplement is used here, hay should be considered as a substitute for nonavailable pasture, rather than as a supplement.

Supplementation should be seen as making up deficiencies that exist in the available forage, with the aim of increasing forage intake and hence animal performance. Therefore, the type of supplement to use will depend upon the state of the forage. The field of supplementation is vast. However, a brief examination of the energy and protein requirements will serve as a useful background in understanding which supplement should be used under different circumstances.

Supplementation with Energy

Range and pasture livestock frequently have an energy intake lower than animal requirements when high animal performances are expected. During such periods animals lose weight because they are drawing on previously accumulated fat reserves as a source of energy. If such reserves are inadequate or the dietary energy shortage is prolonged, production will suffer. Energy supplementation therefore becomes an alternative option.

However, energy supplementation using energy rich foods such as grains has both economic and physiologic limitations. If it was economically feasible to feed unlimited amounts of highly concentrated energy, grazing as a source of nutrients would be unnecessary. Only when the beef to grain price ratio is high, does some grain feeding become economically feasible, and even then, there are physiologic limits to how much grain it is advisable to feed.

Cellulolytic bacteria, which break down the major energy producing components of grass in the rumen, function best at a pH of 6.5 or above. If starch-rich grains are fed as a supplement, the relatively rapid breakdown of starch to organic acids results in a drop in ruminal pH and the replacement of cellulolytic bacteria with amylolytic bacteria, which are starch users. This is frequently witnessed as a decrease in grass and other forage intake, resulting in the observation that "the animals are on welfare." However, this is an involuntary physiologic reaction that can be avoided by limiting the starch intake to approximately 0.4% of body weight.[7] Beyond that level of starch intake, substitution of starch for cellulose will occur at an increasing rate.

Feeding oil-rich energy sources such as cotton seeds, or sugar-rich energy sources such as molasses, does not have the same substitution effect as the starch-rich energy sources. Generally, energy intake is likely to decline as the protein content of the grass decreases and as the lignin content increases. Supplementation of such forage with protein results in an increased ruminal micro-organism population. The consequent increased rate of digestion and increased feed intake results in an increase in energy intake. Protein supplementation for this purpose has become standard practice in many grazing situations.

Protein Supplementation

The major source of protein for the grazing ruminant is microbial protein. The abundant micro-organisms occupying the rumen use non-protein-nitrogen, or degradable protein, as a source of ammonia from which they synthesize protein for their own requirements. When the microbes die and pass from the rumen they are washed into the omasum, abomasum, and lower intestines, where the microbial protein is readily digested. The amino acid component of microbial protein meets the animal's requirements almost perfectly.

If the animal is on an energy-deficient diet, the microbial population declines. While the animal is able to meet energy requirements by drawing on fat reserves to make up dietary deficiencies, it will now be protein deficient because of the reduced microbial population. This protein deficiency can be corrected through adding undegradable protein to the diet. Undegradable protein bypasses the rumen and is directly available to the animal. The value of different sources of undegradable protein to the ruminant depends on its amino-acid content. Fishmeal and various meat meal supplements would be examples of high quality undegradable protein. Cottonseed meal is a more commonly used source for range cattle. It should be noted that the degradability of protein depends, among other factors, upon how long the protein remains in the rumen and how long it is exposed to microbial activity.

Undegradable protein is also required when the animal's requirements exceed the supply of microbial protein, even when the diet is not energy deficient. This may occur, for instance, during peak lactation.

Protein Supplementation to Increase Energy Intake

Unless there is an absolute absence of forage, an alternative strategy for increasing energy availability is to ensure adequate supply of degradable protein in the diet. Typically, as the grass matures and becomes lignified, the protein content of the pasture decreases. Research[12] suggests that at a crude protein level in the forage of less than 7%, the micro-organism population declines because protein is the limiting factor. By feeding a degradable protein or non-protein nitrogen supplement to the animal, the microbial population can be increased, resulting in increased digestion of the forage material, and therefore, indirectly, an increase in energy intake.

Type of Supplement to Use Under Different Pasture Conditions

Since supplementation involves correcting nutrient deficiencies in forage, the first step in supplementation is the identification of the forage characteristics. For purposes of demonstration, we have elected to show (Table 1) supplementation policies that might be adopted with four broad pasture categories, interacting with four different physiologic stages of development in the cow herd. For each physiologic state we have assumed that the cow is either thin (Body Condition Score ≤4) or in adequate condition (BCS ≥5). The range of alternative supplements have been limited to the broad categories of:

DP = Degradable Protein; BPP = By-pass Protein; E = Energy;
None = No Supplement

We should emphasize that the selected array of supplements represent only one scenario, and is not offered as a general recommendation.

Table 1. *What and When to Supplement**

| | | GRASS STATUS | | | |
| | | QUANT: PLENTY
QUAL: POOR | LITTLE
POOR | LITTLE
GOOD | PLENTY
GOOD |
PERIOD	BCS				
Late lact	<4	DP	Wean/destock Energy/BPP	Wean/destock Energy	None
	>5	DP	Wean/destock Energy/BPP	Wean/destock Energy	None
Post wean	<4	DP	Energy/BPP	Energy	None
	>5	DP	Energy/BPP	Energy	None
Lactating	<4	BPP Energy(?)	Energy/BPP	Energy	None
	>5	BPP	Energy/BPP	Energy	None
Flushing	<4	BPP/Energy Fast move	Energy/BPP	BPP/Energy	Fast move
	>5	BPP/Energy Fast move	Energy/BPP	BPP/Energy	Fast move

*CHOICES: DP = Degradable Protein   BPP = By-pass Protein
            E = Energy   None = No supplement

Note: This is one possible scenario and portrays what we might do if faced with the above situations. It is NOT a recommendation. Note in particular:

Flushing cows in good condition with energy is an insurance policy while energy is cheap. Drop energy when energy cost per cow exceeds 10% (?) of calf value. Bear in mind that a drop in open cow value may justify a higher energy feed cost. Daily carbohydrate supplementation should not exceed 0.4% of the animal's body weight.

NPN In animal science circles, opinions differ as to the value of non-protein nitrogen. At best it can be used when there is an abundance of energy with a relatively low protein content. When the animal's nutritional demands increase (e.g., lactation), response to NPN tends to be disappointing, because high quality BPP is required to make up for deficiencies in supply of microbial protein.

SUMMARY

Until recently, the nutritional fate of the grazing animal has been largely ignored by both animal and range scientists despite the economic dependence of the extensive livestock industry on nutrition from grass.

Of the three factors that can be manipulated to improve profit gross margin per animal, is one that is directly affected by nutrition and, hence, grazing management. The relationship between economics and grazing management may be summarized as: Gross margin = f(Animal Performance); Animal Performance = f(nutrition); Nutrition = f(grazing).

Economical beef production must consider the needs of the animal and the forage plant at the same time. The health of the sward must be maintained while improving individual animal performance and simultaneously increasing stocking rate. Generally, plants that have been defoliated require a period of recovery before again being grazed. A sward is kept in a vigorous state by preventing repetitive defoliation at the one extreme, and avoiding excessive shading (mature growth) of photosynthetic material at the other. This state is best achieved where livestock grazing is controlled. For any individual paddock, periods of grazing are followed by periods that allow adequate physiologic recovery of the plants.

A grazing regimen that keeps the plant in a healthy state is fortuitously also well suited to the nutritional requirements of the animal. Animals on overgrazed pastures are likely to suffer from inadequate feed intake because of deficiencies in feed quantity. Conversely, on over-rested pastures, intake deficiency results from paucity in feed quality. On most unmanaged ranges, overgrazed and over-rested plants are likely to be found side by side. By controlling duration of the rest period as well as duration of the grazing period through pasture subdivision, requirements of both the plant and the animal can be met.

With artificially high economic demands placed on animal production, some form of supplementation is required in most modern livestock situations. Whereas energy is frequently the nutrient limiting production it is seldom economically feasible to supplement the grazing animal directly with energy.

Protein supplementation to increase forage intake, and thus indirectly energy intake, has become standard practice in many grazing situations. When there is adequate forage with a low crude protein content ($\leq 7\%$), microbially degradable protein is the preferred choice. However, when the animals are in an energy deficient state, either through a shortage of available forage or because their requirements exceed energy intake levels, by-pass protein is required.

REFERENCES

1. Acocks JPH: Veld Types of South Africa, ed 2 (Memoirs of the Botanical Survey of South Africa No. 40). Pretoria, Department of Agricultural Technical Services.
2. Allison CD: Factors affecting forage intake by range ruminants: A review. Journal Range Management 38:305, 1985
3. Allison CD, Kothman MM: Effect of level of stocking pressure on forage intake and diet quality of range cattle. American Society Animal Science (Western Section) 30:174, 1979
4. Anderson RS, Fillmore HL, Wiltbank JN: Improving reproductive efficiency in range cattle: An application of the O'Connor management system. Theriogenology 26:2, 1986
5. Booysen P deV, Klug JR, York BS: Number of camps for rotational grazing of veld. Grassland Society South Africa 9:145, 1974
6. Dankwerts JE, Aucamp AJ: The rate of leaf emergence and decay as criteria for optimising the grazing rotation in semi-arid grassveld. Grassland Society South Africa 2:1985
7. Horn GW, McCollum FT: Energy supplementation of grazing ruminants. In Proceedings, Grazing Livestock Nutrition Conference, University of Wyoming, 1987, p 125
8. Kothmann MM: Nutrition of livestock grazing on range and pasture lands. In Church DC (ed): Digestive Physiology and Nutrition of Ruminants ed 2 (vol 3 — Practical Nutrition). Corvallis, O&B Books, 1980, p 56

9. McNaughton SJ: Serengeti migratory wildebeest: Facilitation of energy flow by grazing. Science 191:92, 1976

10. Parsons SD: The three secrets for improving profit. In Putting Profit into Ranching. Albuquerque, Ranch Management Consultants, 1986, p10

11. Parsons SD: The Ranching for Profit School—unpublished material. Albuquerque, Ranch Management Consultants

12. Petersen MK: Nitrogen supplementation of Grazing Livestock. In Proceedings, Grazing Livestock Nutrition Conference, University of Wyoming, 1987, p 115

13. Rattray PV, Clark DA: Factors affecting the intake of pasture. NZ Agricultural Science 18:141, 1984

14. Richards MW, Spitzer JC, Warner MB: Effect of varying levels of postpartum nutrition and body condition at calving on subsequent reproductive performance in beef cattle. J Anim Sci 62:300, 1986

15. Savory CAR, Parsons SD: The Savory Grazing Method. In Beef Cattle Science Handbook (International Stockman's School, Tucson) Agriservices Foundation, 1980, p 216

16. Treadwell EF: The Cattle King. Santa Cruz, Western Tanager Press, 1981

17. Waller SS, Moser LE, Reece PE: Understanding Grass Growth: The Key to Profitable Livestock Production. Kansas City, Trabon Printing Co, 1985

ACKNOWLEDGMENTS

We are indebted to Dr RH Diven, Agriconcepts, Tucson, AZ for much of the background material employed in our discussion on nutrition.

Address reprint requests to

S.D. Parsons, PhD
Ranch Management Consultants Inc.
7719 Rio Grande Blvd NW
Albuquerque, NM 87107

0749–0720/91 $0.00 + .20

Nutritional and Managerial Considerations for Range Beef Cattle Production

Harley A. Turner, PhD* and Timothy DelCurto, PhD†

Rangeland, which covers over 1 billion acres (400 million ha), excluding Alaska, makes up the largest classification of land area in the continental United States. This represents 54% of the land area and consists of grasslands, shrublands, and open forest. This land mass under current management practices is estimated to supply forage for over 200 million animal unit months. This supplies over one third of the total forage required by the nation's beef herd in addition to forage for other domestic and big-game species. Rangelands contribute to the food supply of people in only one way and that is by providing feed for grazing animals. The majority of these rangelands lie in the 17 western states. In addition there are approximately 1 million acres (40 million ha) of native meadow hay in the western United States.

These rangelands and native meadows are extremely heterogeneous in nature and represent the most variable commodity that is encountered in livestock nutrition and management. Soil type and depth, annual and seasonal precipitation, temperatures, altitude, topography, ecological sites and management of these lands all contribute to their variability. Much of the data presented here were collected on the Eastern Oregon Agricultural Research Center, located in southeastern Oregon. This rangeland and meadowland is closely related to much of the ranges and meadows in the western United States. These data and general principles can be extrapolated and applied to grazing animals on forages anywhere in the world.

---

*Associate Professor, Department of Animal Science, Oregon State University, Eastern Oregon Agricultural Research Center, Burns, Oregon
†Assistant Professor, Department of Animal Science, Oregon State University, Eastern Oregon Agricultural Research Center, Burns, Oregon

Livestock operators can usually tell you the nutritive value of grains, supplements, hay, or other feedstuffs they purchase, but few have a clear understanding of the value of forages they graze and how they change over time. This discussion will identify the nature of range feed, including nutritive value of forages throughout the year, nutrient needs of the livestock and the relationship of these nutrient needs to the nutrients the various classes of cattle can get from the forage base. Discussions will include managerial manipulations that strive for optimum range livestock production and supplemental feed strategies, options beyond economic supplementation, time of calving, time of weaning, producing slaughter animals on range, and other strategies for improving efficiency of range operations. Parasite control, implanting, feed additives, routine herd health practices, and many other factors involved with good animal management are important for optimum production but outside the scope of this article. Obviously, with all of these alternatives we need to practice good "range management" to maintain range condition and consider the effects on wildlife. This discussion will not include range management techniques, such as removing brush, fertilizing, grazing systems, etc., for increasing or improving range forages, or the effects of the management schemes on wildlife.

DESCRIPTION OF THE AREA WHERE THE BASIC RESEARCH WAS CONDUCTED

Grazing regions of the western United States have been divided into three distinct units based on seasonal precipitation patterns.[15] The Great Basin pattern lies between the Rocky Mountains and the Sierra Nevada and Cascade Mountains and is characterized by primarily winter and spring precipitation and moisture-deficient summers. The Southwestern pattern, including Arizona, southern Utah and Nevada, and parts of New Mexico, is biseasonal and is characterized by winter precipitation followed by spring drought and summer precipitation followed by fall drought. The Plains pattern occurs in the area bounded on the west by the Rocky Mountains and on the east by the Appalachian Mountains. Precipitation in this area is greatest in the spring and summer and then tapers off in the fall and winter.

Common ecological units within the Great Basin pattern are the sagebrush-bunchgrass of the lower elevations, where much of the data that will be presented have been collected, and coniferous forest communities in the mountains. There are approximately 20 million acres of sagebrush-bunchgrass rangeland in eastern Oregon alone. This region also contains extensive riparian and flood meadow areas.[30] The northern intermountain region alone contains nearly 1 million acres of native flood meadow bordering local streams and lakes.[7] The Eastern Oregon Agricultural Research Center, Squaw Butte Range, is typical of much of the sagebrush steppe of the Great Basin, and the hay meadows are typical of native meadows throughout the region.

The Squaw Butte Range is in the Payette section of the Columbia Plateau at an elevation of 4600 feet (1400 m). The soils are mostly sandy loams of basaltic origin underlain with a calcium carbonate layer varying from 2 to 4 feet (0.6 to 1.2 m) below the surface.[11]

The climate is characterized by cold winters, hot summers, and low precipitation levels, arriving mainly during the winter. Average annual precipitation is 11.7 inches (29.7 cm). About 60% occurs as snow during the fall and winter and only 25% as rain during the growing season in the spring and early summer.[13] The combinations of late spring and early fall frosts, and limited amounts of precipitation during the warmer months result in short grazing seasons and permit only one growth cycle, resulting in all grass forage species maturing at about the same time with little difference in nutritive value between species.

Shrubs form a major component of desert range vegetation. Woody vegetation is primarily Wyoming big sagebrush (*Artemisia tridentata* subsp. *wyomingensis*), low sagebrush (*Artemisia arbuscula*), and juniper (*Juniperus occidentalis*). Other shrubs found in the region include several other sagebrush species (*Artemisia tridentata* spp.), bitterbrush (*Purshia tridentata*), green rabbitbrush (*Chrysthamnus vascidiflorus*), and gray rabbitbrush (*Chrysthamnus nauseous*). Except for bitterbrush, the shrub species of the basin are not palatable to cattle.

Herbaceous vegetation consists of cool-season grasses, primarily of native species bluebunch wheatgrass (*Agropyron spicatum*), Idaho fescue (*Festuca idahoensis*), sandberg bluegrass (*Poa sandbergii*), squirreltail (*Sitanion hystrix*), thurbers needlegrass (*Stipa thurberiana*), and several other species of stipas. Introduced grass species include crested wheatgrass (*Agropyron desertorum*) and cheatgrass (*Bromus tectorum*).

Elevation of the Harney Basin, which encompasses the native flood meadows, is 4100 feet. This is a wide alluvial plain typical of native flood meadows. Soils of the area are generally silt loams and are mildly calcareous and slightly alkaline. The area is irrigated by wild flooding in the spring for a period from 6 to 12 weeks, usually starting in April. Active growth ceases within 2 to 3 weeks after recession of flooding.

Vegetation consists of as many as 100 species; however, over half of the biomass is made up of rushes (*Juncus* spp.) and sedges (*Carex* spp.).[7] The principal sedge is rusty sedge (*Carex subjunca*) and the dominant rush is baltic rush (*Juncus balticus*). The remaining 25% consists of grass and shrub species. The most abundant grasses are Nevada bluegrass (*Poa nevadensis*), meadow barley (*Hordeum brachyantherum*), meadow foxtail (*Alopercurus pratense*), and beardless wildrye (*Elymus triticoides*). The principle clover species is annual whitetip clover (*Trifolium variegatum*).

TYPICAL GAINS OF CATTLE THROUGHOUT THE GRAZING SEASON ON RANGE

Livestock weight gains on range diminish dramatically as the grazing season progresses and plants mature. With the precipitation pattern allowing only one growth cycle on forages in the Great Basin, there is only one period of high nutrient value and rapid gain during the year. This occurs in late spring and early summer and essentially dictates a situation in which, without forage or livestock management manipulation, there is a period of 3 months of high forage quality and animal performance and 9 months of poor quality feeds and poor livestock production.

Typical gains of suckling calves and yearlings on range are presented in Figure 1.[18] Gains peak between May 15 and June 10 and exceed 2 pounds (0.9 kg) per day during this time and drop off rapidly over time. Figure 2 presents typical gains of fall- and spring-calving cows, with parturition occurring during October to November and March to April, respectively.[16] The same pattern is displayed, with extremely high weight gain early in the grazing season and eventual weight loss by late summer and early fall. Most of the data were collected on crested wheatgrass seeding, but gain response to grazing is essentially identical on native species. For management reasons, crested wheatgrass seedings need to be fenced off and managed separately from native ranges, primarily because of differences in preference. Native flood meadows provide for somewhat higher gains, but the general trend is the same.[8]

The gain patterns presented in Figures 1 and 2 are simplistic and represent a composite over many years. There are many factors that affect these responses. Previous winter nutrition and management, quality of cattle, yearly climate patterns, condition of animals, etc., will modify the actual gain within a given time frame. Cattle grazed at lower elevations will shift the gain charts to the left and higher elevation vice versa, but the trend remains the same. Management schemes to allevi-

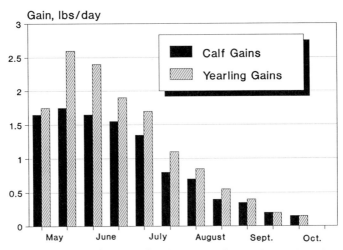

Figure 1. Typical weight gains of suckling spring-born calves and yearlings on sagebrush-bunchgrass range.

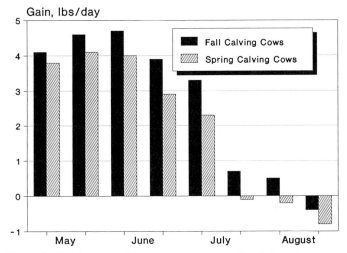

Figure 2. Weight gains of lactating cows on sagebrush-bunchgrass range.

ate poor production over much of the year will be dealt with in subsequent sections.

NUTRITIVE VALUE OF RANGE FORAGES THROUGHOUT THE GRAZING SEASON

The gain data presented in the previous section are a direct reflection of the nutrient value of the range forages. These values are dependent on elevation, yearly climatic factors, and diversity of the forage base. As with the gain data, the general trend of forage quality throughout the grazing season will be presented and represents a composite over many years.

Concentration of certain chemical constituents of range forages are shown in Figure 3.[18] The critical nutrients, protein, energy, and phosphorus all decline as the grasses mature and cell wall constituents increase. The precipitation pattern permits only one growth cycle, resulting in all grass species, native or introduced, maturing at about the same time with little difference in quality between species. Supplementing minerals and vitamins will not substantially improve performance. However, if grazing is in a deficient area, then these minerals need to be supplied. Mineral content of plants varies considerably from one area to another. Other than phosphorus, minerals that can be deficient or, in some cases, excesses can occur, are magnesium, potassium, copper, zinc, selenium, and cobalt. Mineral nutrition problems are very localized and need to be evaluated on that basis. Vitamins A and E are the only vitamins of concern. Vitamin E deficiency is not commonly recognized and vitamin A deficiency is only a problem if on dry bleached feed over a period of 6 months or more.

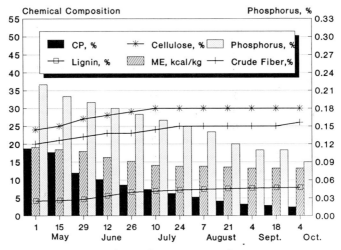

Figure 3. Chemical compositions of range grasses.

In addition to the reduction of nutrient content of the forage, the declining nutritive value to livestock is compounded by declining availability of the nutrients as shown by digestibility values in Figure 4.[18] This slows rate of passage and consequently total forage intake, which leads to poor livestock performance.

Browse, woody-stemmed perennials, and forbs, usually hollow-stemmed annuals, including most weeds, also make up an important component of range feed. Browse is generally higher in protein and

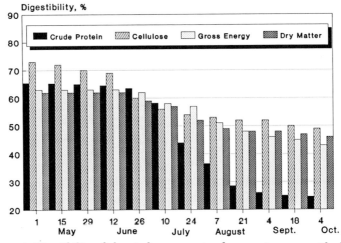

Figure 4. Digestibility of chemical components of grasses in range cattle diets.

lower in energy than grasses, with forbs exhibiting both seasonal and yearly variation, making them unpredictable with regard to availability and quality (Fig. 5). Browse and forbs are much more important in wildlife and sheep diets than in those of cattle, with cattle diets typically containing little to none of these forages. However, under certain conditions of availability and quality of grasses, as compared to the browse and forbs, they can become an important component of the diet.

NUTRITIVE REQUIREMENTS AS RELATED TO ANIMAL CAPABILITY TO OBTAIN NUTRIENTS FROM THE FORAGES

Nutrient requirements of various classes of livestock at different stages and levels of production can be fairly accurately determined from guidelines.[17] This information, in conjunction with the nutrient content and digestibility data presented in the previous section and determining the voluntary intake of grazing animals allows us to estimate the relationship between the animal's needs and what it can get from the forages. Energy expended for travel will increase requirements for range animals somewhat over small pasture or confinement feeding, but this can be calculated. Otherwise requirements are the same. Gathering data to make these needed evaluations involves laborious and expensive techniques such as chemical analyses of forages, digestibility determination either in vitro or in vivo, or fecal output for intake estimates and often employs rumen and esophageal fistulated animals, internal markers, or a wide array of other techniques described in various publications.[5,6,14] The recent development of boluses

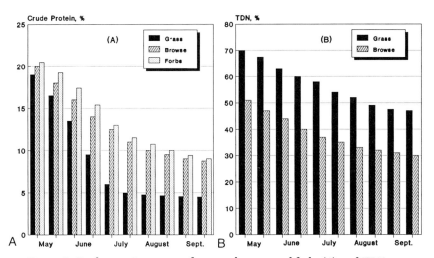

Figure 5. Crude protein content of grasses, browse, and forbs (A), and TDN content of grasses and browse (B) at various dates during the grazing season.

containing external indicators such as chromic oxide for estimating
fecal output will help make gathering of these data more practical. Data
of this nature that have been collected in a research unit or other
rangelands can be applied to many other situations.

Figure 6 presents the digestible nitrogen and metabolizable energy yearling steers can obtain from range forage and the requirements
to gain 2.2 (1 kg) or 1.1 pounds (0.5 kg) per head per day. Protein for
either level of gain is becoming limited by late June to early July
whereas energy becomes limiting by late June on the higher level and
mid July on the lower level.

Digestible nitrogen and metabolizable energy that mature cows
can obtain from range forage are presented in Figure 7. The protein
deficiencies occur at about the same time as with the growing animals
for lactating cows and a little later for gestating cows. Phosphorus
deficiencies occur at about the same time as protein for all classes of
animals. The lactating cow is short of energy by late July, with the
gestating cow capable of meeting her energy requirements throughout
the grazing season.

PRESCRIPTION SUPPLEMENTAL LEVELS TO
FILL VOID BETWEEN ANIMAL'S REQUIREMENTS
AND NUTRIENT INTAKE

Supplemental feed is employed when nutrients from the forage
base become insufficient or inadequate for the level of production
desired. Due to economic considerations, supplementation under western range conditions is usually centered around feeding a minimum
amount of concentrates to supply the deficient nutrients. Substituting

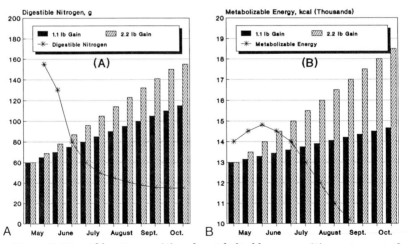

Figure 6. Digestible nitrogen (A) and metabolizable energy (B) requirements for
550-lb yearling steers and the amount of each derived from range forage.

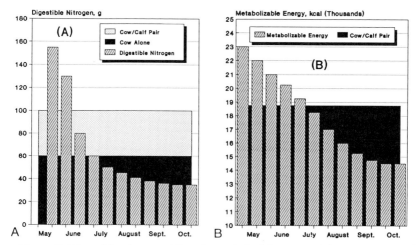

Figure 7. Digestible nitrogen (A) and metabolizable energy (B) requirements of lactating cows and the amount of each derived from range forage.

supplements for forage is, under most conditions, a costly practice. Forage availability should be adequate to provide maximum intake to negate substituting and also of high enough quality to at least provide maintenance and some gain for growing animals to make the supplement program profitable. In general, the higher the quality of forage, the more efficient and profitable the supplements. Obviously there are situations in which low quality forages must be supplemented to maintain animals.

A typical prescription supplement schedule for yearlings on range is presented in Figure 8.[33] This schedule is derived from the data

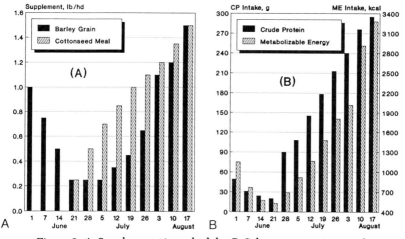

Figure 8. A, Supplementation schedule. B, Subsequent nutrient intake.

presented in previous figures and is designed to provide for 2 pounds
(0.9 kg) daily gain on yearling steers. Increased supplemental levels
above those shown have not proved to be economically sound, primarily because of increased costs, decreased forage intake and subsequent
diminishing return from the supplement. Supplemental nitrogen is not
necessary between turnout date in early May to mid June; however, the
barley produces the amounts indicated and is needed for energy.

Previous figures would indicate that supplements are not needed
during May and early June to maintain 2 pounds (0.9 kg) or more daily
gains on yearling steers. However, if small amounts of nutrients are
provided during this time, extremely efficient and profitable gains can
be realized and these gains are not negated by compensatory gains later
in the season. Figure 9 presents a composite of data where steers were
supplemented from turnout in early May as opposed to starting in mid
June. Increases of 0.4 pounds (0.2 kg) during this period were realized
over those not receiving a supplement and this gain did not affect
subsequent gains throughout the summer. Responses from energy supplementation in early spring, despite forage nutrient values being very
high, may be attributed to the relatively high moisture content of the
forage, which tends to limit dry matter consumption, an imbalance of
protein and energy, slowing of rapid passage which decreases digestion
and absorption by the host animal, or providing nutrients while adaptation to a new feedstuff via shifting of microbial populations occurs.
Most of the protein of immature lush plants is in the form of nonprotein
nitrogen and the supplemental energy source may be providing carbon
chains for use of this form of nitrogen or the nitrogen contained in the
concentrate may be providing by-pass protein. Data indicate that, because of decreasing forage quality, it is impractical to supplement for
economic production beyond the middle of August.[33] Beyond this

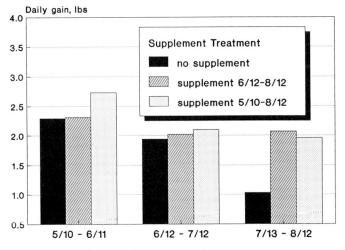

Figure 9. Daily weight gain of yearlings on different supplement treatments.

point, an increased supplement level inhibits forage intake and substitution rather than supplementing nutrients occurs.

These supplements were hand fed on a daily basis with adequate trough space to allow all animals to eat at the same time. For training of animals to the supplement and not reducing grazing time and subsequent forage intake, time of supplementation and setting up of a routine time and method to establish optimum grazing behavior also improves performance.[1] The gain response is under continuous grazing and high pasture use. By grazing half or less of the available forage, typical gains have been 2.6 to 3.2 pounds (1.2 – 1.5 kg) per day.[9] The cow herd can then follow the yearlings and use the remaining forage.

Gains on summer range vary considerably, depending on forage quality, quality of cattle, previous winter gain, management grazing systems and many other factors. Over the years, yearlings on Squaw Butte have had average gains of 1.2 to 1.8 pounds (0.5 – 0.8 kg) per day during the summer without supplements and 2 to 3 pounds (0.9 – 1.4 kg) with daily supplements. In the foregoing examples, supplemental protein was provided from cottonseed meal and energy from rolled barley. However, as long as protein and energy are provided, many different feedstuffs can be used with similar results. Nonprotein nitrogen sources, such as urea and biuret, under proper conditions, have resulted in gains approaching or equaling those with cottonseed meal, as long as the energy provided by feeding cottonseed meal was replaced by barley or other energy sources.[22] Nonprotein nitrogen is not effective with low quality forages unless additional energy is provided. However, care should be taken when urea is fed because of palatability and toxicity problems.[3,4] Urea supplements should be thoroughly mixed and precautions taken to insure that individual animals do not get more than their share. The concentration of urea in the diet is critical. Biuret, a condensation product of urea, essentially two urea molecules hooked together, releases nitrogen more slowly and is less toxic.

Creep feeding on summer range has been marginally effective. Under certain conditions it will pay but often does not. Likewise, supplementation of the cow herd during the traditional grazing period has not been practical or profitable under range conditions. Even in situations in which cows lose weight on range, they recoup losses when moved to meadow aftermath (forage), higher elevation range, rakebunch hay, or other fall feed prior to severe weather conditions of winter.

In general, unless in an area where specific minerals or vitamins are known to be deficient, minor nutrients are adequate. However, a good phosphorus source should be available to animals at all times, regardless of the management program. Two-compartment salt boxes with plain or trace mineral salt on one side and a 50 – 50 mix of salt and a phosphorus source on the other side have worked well. Intake of the phosphorus is low when forage phosphorus levels are high and high when forage phosphorus levels are low. Care must be taken, though, to monitor intake to provide enough phosphorus, but not allow excess consumption, because phosphorus is an expensive supplement.

The supplement programs described to this point have involved daily feeding of animals. They are not always practical or possible, particularly on the large expanses of western rangeland. For one reason or another, many producers cannot or will not feed a supplement unless it can be fed free choice at infrequent intervals. Supplemental programs based on free choice with controlled consumption of the supplement are desirable. Many vehicles for feeding supplement ad lib have been tried, including blocks, pellets, salt-limiting mixes, liquid feeds, etc., but none has been totally satisfactory in terms of controlling intake at the desired levels. Supplementation at the proper level enhances intake up to mid August, but additional feed decreases forage intake.[25]

Every other day and every fourth day energy supplement regimens have been tested against daily supplementation with gain reduced by one-fourth to one-half pounds (0.1–0.2 kg) per day on the alternative feeding. Late July and August gains were reduced by as much as 1 pound (0.5 kg) per head per day as compared to daily feeding.[33] These data indicate that a method of feeding supplements must be devised so that animals receive their supplements daily. Up to weekly supplementation of adequate amounts of protein, phosphorus and many other minerals and vitamin A has generally been shown to be sufficient. However, energy needs to be supplied daily for the most efficient conversion by the animal.

Salt has been used to control intake of supplements since the early 1930s with varying success. Salt levels have to be continually adjusted and in some cases exceed 50% to adequately control intake. Daily intake of salt has exceeded 2.5 pounds (1.1 kg) per day without ill effects,[26] but the use of salt to control intake seems to consistently reduce daily gains as compared to hand feeding.[33] Also, salt consumption is hard to predict with any great accuracy. It varies from year to year, day to day, pasture to pasture, animal to animal, etc., and depends on forage quality, quantity, type, maturity, and other factors such as previous salt consumption and weather. Salt content of the feed and water also have an effect. Adjustments on these types of supplement programs have to be made frequently, and it is very difficult to get a consistent daily intake of supplement at the levels desired. Although salt does work in some situations, it certainly is not the answer to controlling intake.

Feeding molasses as a supplement to cattle has been practiced since 1850, and urea with molasses since about 1950. Liquid feeds offer many benefits, including improved feed palatability and masking of undesirable flavors, consistent distribution of urea, high phosphorus availability, less waste, convenience, accessibility, and for mixing of top dressings, improved feed penetration, improved feed texture, and reduced dust and wind loss. Liquid feeds also serve as a vehicle for feeding medicaments, vitamins, minerals, antibiotics, and other feed additives. Liquid supplements are easily mechanized, with materials being handled by pumps from tanks, which allows rapid dissemination with little hand labor.

Problems connected with liquid feeds include controlling the consumption level on a herd basis, uniform consumption by individual animals, difficulty in maintaining uniformity of product, equipment cost, and weather changes, particularly cold weather, which can disrupt intake patterns. Overconsumption of urea-molasses products caused by lack of feed, ice or snow covered feed, insufficient water, letting cattle have access to liquid feed prior to feeding hay, etc., can be a major problem and cause digestive disturbances, diarrhea, inefficient animal performance, and possibly death. Calcium can be a problem ingredient, particularly in feedlots, because it is not soluble and is difficult to suspend in liquids. Urea is often used because amino acids and/or natural proteins are difficult to suspend. High levels of phosphoric acid or salt, used for intake control, may result in corrosion of metals, particularly in conjunction with water condensation, and subsequent dilution. Corrosion of galvanized metals can result in zinc toxicity.

Total energy intake can also be a problem with liquid feeds. Molasses is a good source of energy (about 88% of the energy value of barley); however, most liquid feeds contain only 50% to 70% molasses. This lower energy restricts urea use, particularly in high roughage situations, and leads to poor animal performance. In supplement schedules that call for 2 to 3 pounds (0.9 – 1.4 kg) of barley, it would require 3 to 7 pounds (1.4 – 3.0 kg) of liquid supplement to be isocaloric. In general, when a supplement exceeds 3 pounds, roughage intake is reduced. Also, liquid supplements become very expensive at these levels. Fats, both animal and vegetable, and alcohols, both ethyl and propylene glycol, have been added to liquid supplements as a way to increase energy in liquid supplements. The price of these additions is often prohibitive to wide scale use.

Properly used with the right class of animals, liquid supplements can be as effective as any other supplement type as long as needed nutrients are provided. Some managerial and nutritional problems must be worked out, particularly continual availability of forage, regular feeding, intake control, and energy level, before their optimum value is reached. Liquid supplements are not always the best buy in terms of nutrients or cost and any supplement containing urea should be used with caution.

Blocks of various types offer many of the same advantages and disadvantages as liquid feeds. Blocks can serve as a vehicle for nonprotein nitrogen, medicaments, antibiotics, vitamins, minerals and other feed additives in addition to masking undesirable flavors, cutting waste, reducing dust, and providing a certain amount of convenience. As with other supplementation methods, with the exception of hand feeding, controlling intake, both on a group basis and between individual animals, is the biggest problem with blocks. Intake control measures in blocks are primarily through the ingredients and/or the physical characteristics of the block. As with liquid feeds, results from range studies using blocks have not been encouraging.[33] Blocks can be an effective supplement method when properly produced and used. However, as with all the other free choice supplement methods, intake is still a major problem and more work needs to be done on this.

Daily hand feeding of supplements is still the preferred method, where possible. Daily gains have always been reduced with any of the convenience supplement schemes. However, this does not fit into all management schemes or situations. Cost, ease of handling, mixing, and feeding facilities all have to be considered along with the manager's abilities. Mechanics and supplementation cost have to be determined in each individual situation. Salt control, blocks, liquids, pellets, etc., all offer viable alternatives to hand feeding in specific instances.

The relative advantages of each kind of supplement need to be evaluated to determine where it fits into the livestock program. Final costs of production are more important than out-of-pocket costs. Consider the feeds available and the nutrients required by the animals and compare the available supplements that will supply the proper nutrients at the best price. The cheapest supplement may not be the most profitable to feed in terms of animal performance per unit of cost. Safety, nutrient adequacy, and management must be considered along with cost before the decision is made to feed one type or another.

OPTIONS BEYOND ECONOMICAL SUPPLEMENT LEVELS

Data indicate that because of decreasing forage quality it is impractical to supplement for economic production of market animals beyond the middle of August under the range conditions at Squaw Butte. Beyond this point an increased supplement level inhibits forage intake and a substituting of expensive concentrates for relatively cheaper forage occurs.

Sell Market Animals or Move to Better Feed

By removal of salable yearlings from range early, the remaining feed can be used for maintenance of the breeding herd. Along with early weaning, which will be discussed in the next section, additional condition can be put on the cows before the winter.

A viable option is to put yearlings on better feed. This may be meadow aftermath from the haying operation on irrigated meadows, rake-bunched hay, irrigated pastures, higher elevation ranges, etc. However, when cattle are moved to a new feed source it takes a 2 to 4 week adjustment period before efficient gains are realized. Thus, it is important that the feeding period prior to sale of these animals is long enough to warrant moving them as opposed to early sale off range.

Time of Weaning

Traditionally, calves in the Great Basin region have been weaned at about 7 months of age, during late October or the first part of November. However, as shown in previous figures, gains of these calves are very poor by late August. By removing these calves early, they can be put on better feed with the cows remaining on range. Dry cows do well on range feed during the fall and without the suckling calf will come into the winter in better condition. The condition of cows coming into the winter is important, as the total nutrients required to get the cow through the winter and bred back in the spring are reduced as condition going into the winter is increased.

Figure 10 presents some early weaning data from the Squaw Butte herd. Early-weaned calves were removed from their dams on September 12 and put on meadow aftermath and regrowth plus supplemented with 2 pounds (0.9 kg) of barley and 1 pound (0.5 kg) of cottonseed meal. Late-weaned calves remained on range with their dams until October 12 and then were managed with the early-weaned calves. On November 12 all calves were fed meadow hay and received 2 pounds (0.9 kg) of barley and 1 pound (0.5 kg) of cottonseed meal throughout the winter.

Early-weaned calves outgained late-weaned calves by 20 pounds (9 kg) from September 12 to October 12, despite going through the stress of weaning and adjusting to new feed. During the next period of time, from October 12 to November 12, the early-weaned calves outgained late-weaned calves by 31 pounds (14 kg) and were now 51 pounds (23 kg) heavier. Late-weaned calves compensated somewhat over the remainder of the winter, but were still 24 pounds (11 kg) lighter on April 12.[20]

These results would likely favor early-weaning more if calves were weaned somewhat earlier for the early-weaned group and closer to the traditional mid-November date for the late-weaned calves. The advantage of early weaning depends on the quality and expense of feed available for the early-weaned calves and the options available for the late-weaned calf, such as moving the cow-calf pair to higher elevation range or to better feed, such as irrigated pasture or rake-bunched hay. In many cases early weaning does provide a management tool for increasing productive efficiency off rangelands.

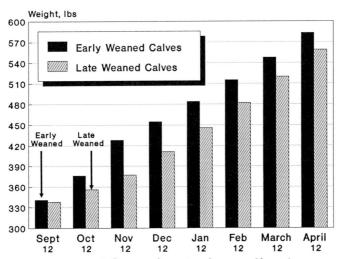

Figure 10. Influence of weaning date on calf weight.

Chemical Curing of Range Forages

Manipulating the forage chemically presents another option for combating poor quality as plants mature. An example of this potential for providing higher quality late-season forage entails growth arrestation of plants while they are high in nutritive value, through application of paraquat (1,1'-dimethyl-4, 4' bipyridinium ion), a bipyridylium herbicide. Crested wheatgrass was treated in mid to late June when the plants were in early anthesis. The chemical was foliar applied at various rates and concentrations with ×77 surfactant employed.[29] A description of treatments and ramifications with various grasses, weather conditions, concentration levels, mode of action, residues, and other information has been reported.[28]

As shown in Figure 11, late-season daily gains of yearlings are increased by over 0.5 pound (0.2 kg) per head per day on chemically cured forage. Chemically cured forage retained higher levels of phosphorus, potassium, lignin, ash, and protein (Fig. 12) and reduced levels of calcium and ether extract, with cellulose being similar. The values in Figure 12 represent change in forage quality due to both maturity and selective grazing. The relative decline of phosphorus between naturally and chemically cured forage closely followed that of protein.[29] Forage intake was increased by about 1 pound (0.5 kg) per head per day on treated forage. The increased quality of forages not only improves daily gains and allows growing animals to be grazed later into the season but also represents a substantial savings in the amount of supplementation needed and improves the efficiency of supplements provided. The addition of 1 pound (0.5 kg) of supplement (barley and cottonseed meal) provided an additional gain of 0.4 pounds (0.2 kg) per head per day.

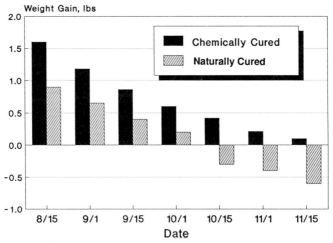

Figure 11. Daily weight gain of yearlings on naturally and chemically cured range forage.

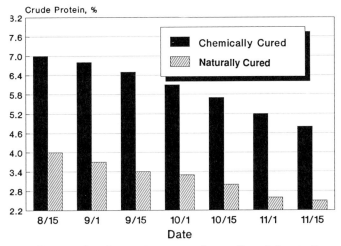

Figure 12. Percent of crude protein content of naturally and chemically cured range forage.

Chemically cured forage appears to have a great deal of potential on perennial grass stands on rangelands. The question with chemicals is whether the potential market is great enough for companies to produce them for this purpose and whether they can be cleared for this use. Paraquat is cleared for other uses in the United States and use on grasses in other countries. Paraquat was used as an example here and, of course, other materials may provide similar results.

Producing Slaughter Animals on Range

Following the supplement schedule described earlier, steers in mid-August are carrying a great deal of condition. It was postulated that by leaving these cattle on range and gradually increasing the concentrate level to a full feed, using the range as a roughage source, steers could be brought to a suitable slaughter grade in about 90 days. There are many alternatives that can be employed. The relationships involved in beef production and marketing need to be considered. Production and growth rate need to be considered from birth through the entire growing phase, with feed requirements, efficiency, and economics all being accounted for in reaching an acceptable goal for slaughtering these steers by mid-November. Beyond this time, requirements accelerate considerably due to cold weather, and animals probably should be removed from range prior to that time. Management considerations to provide for continuous growth need to be employed from birth to slaughter to insure that these animals reach an acceptable slaughter weight.

A typical supplement schedule to bring steers to full feed is presented in Figure 13. The level of concentrate was increased daily as long as the feed was cleaned up each day and held constant or de-

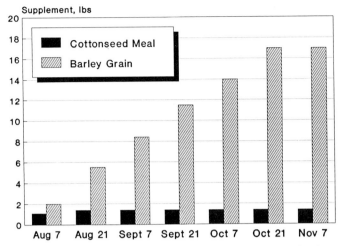

Figure 13. Daily supplement intake of yearling steers during the finishing period.

creased if feed was left. When concentrate levels reached 8 pounds (3.6 kg), the ration was fed twice daily. When full feed, approximately 1.75% of body weight, was reached in mid to late September, feed was presented free choice.

This range regimen (Treatment 1) is compared to four other treatments in Figure 14. Treatment 2 represents feedlot steers to mid November; treatment 3, range to mid-November and then feedlot to early January; treatment 4, feedlot to early January; and treatment 5, irrigated pasture to mid-September then feedlot to early January. All animals were on the prescribed supplement schedule to mid-August.

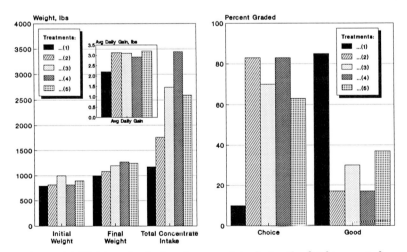

Figure 14. Weight gain, feed, and carcass data during the finishing period.

Steers slaughtered off range weighed less, gained less, and graded lower than steers on the various feedlot systems. However, their total concentrate intake was 34% to 76% of that of the feedlot steers and returned more per dollar invested in feed. Adding yardage, interest on investment, equipment, and environmental preservation costs give the range-fattened steers an advantageous position. Detailed data on treatments, feeding regimens, carcass, and economic evaluation have been reported.[32] Economic evaluations are valid only for a given market and need to be calculated for the price structure or time-frame that exists.

Some consumer preference studies have shown the consumer would buy more of the USDA good grade if it were available.[10] Taste panel work in these trials was somewhat inconclusive. However, these trials and others show that although taste panels detect differences between forage, forage plus limited grain, and feedlot beef, differences were small and all were rated in the favorable zone of the hedonic scale. It has also been concluded that it is important to feed British breeds to slaughter weights of 1,000 to 1,050 pounds (454–476 kg) on limited feed to insure scoring in the acceptable zone.[27]

There are many other alternative systems and management schemes of producing slaughter cattle, including use of irrigated pasture or improved pastures in conjunction with the range feed. A short feeding period at the end of a fairly high grain supplement while still on pasture may be desirable to change color and taste of fat and still provide a substantial savings of grain.

One of the most exciting possibilities in terms of producing an acceptable carcass with a small amount of grain is by using the chemical curing of grasses for late-season grazing as previously described. Acceptable carcasses from range could be produced with as little as 10% of the grain intake of normal feedlot regimens.[32] Many other alternatives, including incorporating straw and other waste products into the systems, calving in the fall and finishing these calves on range, various winter feeding regimens, and different rations have been studied.[10,12,20,24,36]

There are a number of inherent advantages to fattening steers on range or pastures. Because of the low density of cattle in comparison to feedlots, range feeding, in many situations, does not contribute to water and air pollution problems. Less confined conditions also provide for drier, healthier feeding conditions and eliminate the need for manure removal. Range feeding also has less expense in permanent feedbunks and handling equipment. Hauling expense, overhead costs of middlemen and selling expenses may also be less because of retained ownership and keeping the cattle at the same location.

Other factors need to be considered before range finishing can become a large scale industry. One is carrying capacity of available ranges. The previously reported study was conducted on crested wheatgrass ranges with a carrying capacity of about 2.5 acres (1 ha) per animal unit month (AUM). On ranges with a carrying capacity of more than 5 acres (2 ha) per AUM, the distance cattle have to travel for feed could have an adverse effect on rate of gain. Average carrying capacity of semiarid ranges is about 10 acres (4 ha) per AUM. Thus, opportunities are somewhat limited.

Another consideration is that these ranges are, in general, best suited for cow-calf production. It seems unlikely that production of slaughter animals off range would, or should, increase to the extent that it would adversely affect the number of brood cows that can be carried. Also, limited supplies of grain are produced in these arid regions. Slaughter beef production should probably be limited to higher quality ranges and areas in which grains are readily available.

The possibility that production of slaughter grade cattle from range or grass will replace production from the feedlot is remote. On the contrary, it provides another marketing channel for cattle producers and another choice of meat for consumers. We will undoubtedly always produce feedlot beef in this country. A market will probably always exist for highly finished beef for certain clientele, such as restaurants, hotels, and caterers and for a portion of the population that simply prefers beef with a high degree of finish. However, a tremendous market also exists for those who want a leaner cut of beef, prefer the taste of short fed animals, or would like to buy a cheaper grade of beef. Consumption of imported beef is an indication of preference for this type of product, and we should be competing stronger for a share of this market. One reason these countries can undersell us is that they depend heavily on forages rather than more expensive concentrates for production. However, low land and labor costs also are considerations.

Data suggest that range or pasture supplemented steers can be adequately finished by any one of several systems, depending on many factors including a market for the grade of cattle produced. The overall beef system used ultimately responds to the market place and to profitability.

Time of Calving

Time of breeding and subsequent calving is another management tool for getting optimum production out of a given forage situation. Again, it is important to inventory the forage resource with respect to quality and relate this to nutritional needs of the animals on a year-round basis. Availability of outside feed sources such as hay, grain, irrigated pasture, etc., also need to be considered, along with management preferences and capabilities.

On most desert range operations, parturition occurs during March and April. Problems encountered at this time include poor calving weather, long breeding seasons, and light weaning weights. Problems such as infectious diarrheal and respiratory diseases are compounded by calving on wet muddy flood meadows during the spring before cattle are allowed on the range. Wind is also prevalent at this time of year, and wind-chill can adversely affect calf morbidity and mortality.

By calving during the fall (October and November), a calf is produced that is big enough to efficiently use the early high-quality forage available in the spring; with the cow still producing some milk, make rapid gains during this period. This program allows calves to stay on the cow longer and continue to make economical gains. Spring-born calves are not big enough during late April to mid June to effectively take advantage of the high quality forage. By the time they are mature enough to use range feed, quality has declined substantially in both protein and energy content. The spring-born calf cannot get much from the forage at this time and the cow's milk production has declined due to the decreased forage quality. Fall calving, while increasing the cost of wintering the lactating cow versus a dry cow, provides a bigger calf to use high quality range feed and increased weaning weights. Wintering cows and creep feeding calves will be dealt with in a subsequent section on winter feeding.

Weaning weights of fall-born calves at Squaw Butte have exceeded that of spring-born calves by 150 to 200 pounds (68–91 kg), with over 1,100 calves over 5 years included in the data (Fig. 15). Most of the fall-born calves were creep fed 20–100 pounds (9–45 kg) of feed. Due to confinement on winter feed grounds, creep feeding of the fall-born calf is more practical than on ranges with spring-born calves. Most of the weight advantage is due to higher gains early in the spring on range, creep feeding, and the additional length of time on the cow. Weaning the spring-born calves later does not appreciably increase their weaning weight, since little gain is made by these calves beyond the first of September, under the existing forage conditions.[18,35]

Conception rates and weaning percentages were also slightly higher in fall-born cows (P > .05). Conception rates and weaning percentages represent all cows exposed to breeding. Cows that were

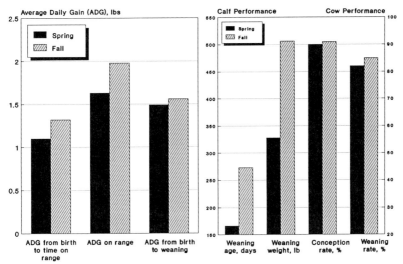

Figure 15. Performance data of spring- and fall-born calves and cows averaged over 5 years.

culled because of pregnancy test results, advanced age, cancer eye, or other reasons prior to weaning were tabulated as not weaning a calf.

Winter management of these fall-calving cow-calf pairs is more conducive for intensive management and nutrition practices to improve efficiency of both production and reproduction. Clinical cases of calf-hood diseases, such as scours, and respiratory problems are minimal in fall-born calves, requiring treatment of less than 1%, whereas 10% required treatment in the spring-born calves. Weather conditions are favorable and meadows are bare and dry during October and early November. This same morbidity rate occurred at weaning time with spring-born calves that required considerably more treatment. With cows congregated on hay meadows, the identification and treatment of problems and diseases are also facilitated with the fall calving.

Concentration of the fall-calving cows on winter feedgrounds also facilitates breeding programs. Artificial insemination programs are much easier to accommodate and, with natural breeding, fewer bulls are needed. The advantages of confinement breeding have proved to be beneficial in shortening the breeding season and the calving interval. The data from Squaw Butte do not indicate much of an advantage in conception rates over a 60-day breeding season. However, compared to most range operations, the station cows are on relatively small range pastures, not exceeding 2000 acres (810 ha), and stockwater is hauled, which means animals are more concentrated. The difference in conception and weaning rates would likely be much higher in favor of fall calving on most range operations.

Fall calving offers many advantages, particularly on desert range operations where higher elevation ranges or improved feed resources are not available for cow-calf pairs in late summer and fall. However, a major deterrent to fall calving is the policy of public agencies in charge of public grazing of counting a calf over 6 months of age as a full animal unit on rangelands. This in effect halves the size of the cow herd. This makes it nearly impossible to incorporate fall calving where public rangelands represent a majority of the summer feed. With over 80% of the desert rangelands administered by the Bureau of Land Management or Forest Service, this represents a large deterrent to fall calving. These policies exist despite data showing that the fall-calving cow-calf pair consumes only 25% more forage than the spring-calving pair.[16] In addition, the older calf and cow spread out over the range better, improving distribution and reducing overgrazing in riparian areas, waterholes, meadows, etc. Despite problems with public rangelands, time of calving does provide viable alternatives for many range operations. Producing slaughter grade animals off range from fall-calving cows is discussed in other publications.[9,32]

WINTER FEEDING PROGRAMS

Winter nutritional needs are dependent on managerial goals and subsequent range grazing programs throughout the following grazing season. Winter supplementation programs are simpler and more easily adopted. Harvested hay provides a nutritionally constant feed source and therefore a stable supplement that does not change over time. Also, cattle are in more confined areas, making supplementation easier.

The following discussion will assume hay is being harvested at the proper time, which provides hay with crude protein ranging from 7% to 9%. Date of harvest or maturity of plants at harvest probably contributes more to quality of hay than any other single factor. The earlier hay is harvested the more available nutrients are for production. However, due to spring flooding conditions in many areas, meadows can seldom be cut prior to late June or early July. These dates happen to correspond to near maximal levels of protein and dry matter production on the meadows. Protein and energy content of meadow hay harvested at various dates and digestibility of various nutrients are presented in Figure 16.[21]

Growing Animals

Much of the roughage used for wintering calves and yearlings in most of the west is native meadow hay. Factors contributing to its low quality for growing animals are relatively low levels of crude protein, low digestibility, and high crude fiber values. Young animals simply cannot consume adequate quantities for acceptable performance. Weaner calves on hay alone do little more than maintain themselves and, in some cases, may lose weight.

Many studies reporting the effect of winter gain on summer gains have been conducted with the idea of obtaining inexpensive gains on grass and selling long yearlings as feeders in the fall. High rates of winter gain together with the increased number of days on feed have a

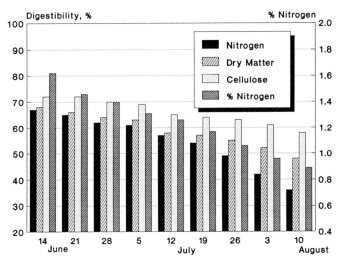

Figure 16. Apparent digestibility of nitrogen, dry matter, cellulose, and nitrogen content of hay harvested at different dates.

significant negative effect on subsequent summer gain. However, calves restricted to limited winter gains for long time periods (100 days or longer) are considerably lighter at the end of the summer grazing period. In short-grass years when growing stock must be sold in the spring to maintain the cow herd, there is a considerable economic loss from the restricted winter feeding program. Total digestible nutrients required during the winter per pound of gain accumulated during both the winter and summer periods reach a minimum when animals gain 1.2 pounds (0.5 kg) per day during the winter, with the greatest return over feed costs occurring at about 1.6 pounds (0.7 kg).[2] Steers should be fed to gain 1.5 to 1.8 pounds (0.7 – 0.8 kg) per day when feed cost-cattle price relationships appear favorable and 1.0 to 1.4 pounds (0.5 – 0.6 kg) per day under less favorable conditions. Calves can gain up to 1.6 pounds (0.7 kg) per day in the winter without substantially affecting summer gain as long as the animals are supplemented during the summer to gain at a maximum rate. Without supplementation, the summer gains are drastically reduced with increased winter gain levels. The size of the calf entering the winter period also affects the economics of the optimum winter gain. Other management goals, such as producing range-slaughter animals and target weights for optimum development of replacement heifers also need to be considered for determining desired winter gains.

Supplemental protein and energy must be fed along with native meadow hay to provide economical gains for wintering weaner calves and yearling cattle. Protein is critical here or in any feeding regimen because if protein is deficient and microbial protein needs are not met, then microbial numbers are decreased, digestion of forage is reduced, rate of passage is slowed, and consequently intake is reduced. Energy and other nutrients are shorted as well, due to reduced dry matter intake. A combined supplement of 1 pound (0.5 kg) of cottonseed meal plus 2 pounds (0.9 kg) of barley, or their equivalent, with a full feed of good meadow hay provides a well-balanced growing ration for weaner calves. Figure 17 represents a typical gain response and cost per pound of gain with and without supplements. Feed values used were $50, $100, $200/ton for hay, barley, and cottonseed meal, respectively. Supplements were fed on a daily basis. Gains on hay alone have varied from 0 to 0.6 pounds (0.3 kg) per day, depending on the hay quality. Supplemented calves have gained 0.9 to 1.7 pounds per day (0.4 – 0.8 kg) depending on the quality of hay and calves. Supplementing above this level will reduce hay intake and often increases cost per pound of gain. A phosphorus source should be available on a free-choice basis.

Under carefully controlled conditions, nonprotein nitrogen products such as urea and biuret can be used in place of cottonseed meal as a protein source. Gains will approach those of cottonseed meal as long as the energy lost from the removal of the cottonseed meal is replaced by barley or another energy feed. In a properly balanced and well-mixed ration, urea can increase efficiency and lower cost of production. Increased frequency of feeding will increase performance with urea supplement. However, under less controlled conditions, palatability and

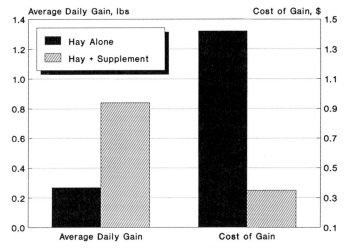

Figure 17. Winter daily weight gain and cost of weight gain for weaner calves with and without supplement.

toxicity problems can arise when urea is fed. Results from urea with low energy, high roughage, or limited feeding programs can be disappointing. Biuret is more palatable and acceptable to the animal and is less toxic, making it a more desirable source of nitrogen under these circumstances. Increased efficiency can often be realized by supplying the supplemental nitrogen with both a natural and nonprotein source.[23]

Condensing meadow hay bulk through different processing methods offers some opportunity for greater consumption and, consequently, an improvement in calf performance. Chopping or wafering hay does not seem to offer much improvement. Pelleted hay can increase intake by 25% or more and roughly double gains over long hay.[19,39] The main disadvantage of processed hays is added costs of grinding and pelleting, along with transportation costs to and from the feed mill, or the cost of equipment to do it in place. Supplements, in most cases, are probably a cheaper way of improving performance.

High quality alfalfa hay alone often will provide adequate winter gains on growing animals. Average to poor quality alfalfa does require an energy supplement. Poor to average quality alfalfa hay does not provide more energy than average quality meadow hay. Whereas chopping did not improve performance with meadow hay, calves on chopped alfalfa consumed more and gained considerably more than those on long hay.[19]

Alfalfa also can be used effectively as a protein supplement for meadow hay. Two to three pounds of alfalfa will provide as much protein as a pound of cottonseed meal and, when fed with an energy level similar to the standard supplement, will give similar gain responses.

Mature Cows

Older animals with the capacity for more feed can usually meet their requirements from meadow hay provided adequate amounts are available. In many livestock operations, supplements are used primarily in the winter for maintenance. In general, mature pregnant cows on a full feed of meadow hay or limited alfalfa do not need additional nutrients. However, lactating cows, first-calf heifers, and replacement heifers do, on occasion, need supplemental nutrients. The overall objective of most wintering programs is to get cows through the winter as economically as possible in condition to calve, milk well, and rebreed in the spring.

Grass straw, a by-product of the grass seed industry, may provide beef producers with a cheap source of roughage for maintenance purposes and help grass producers recover the cost of removing the straw. Cows have been successfully wintered on grass-straw-alfalfa mixes and on grass straw plus 0.7 pounds (0.3 kg) of cottonseed meal and 1.3 pounds (0.6 kg) of grain. Depending on straw quality and cattle condition going into the winter, ratios of 4:1 to 1:1 of grass straw to alfalfa will adequately maintain pregnant cows. Lactating cows require about a 1:2 ratio.

Harvesting and feeding hay is the most expensive practice of a range cattle operation. It costs approximately $30 per ton to produce hay and feed it out. Wintering cows on rake-bunched hay has proved to be a viable alternative. With this system, hay is cut, then raked into small piles, 80 to 120 pounds (35 to 54 kg), and left in the field. Cows are then strip grazed, by using New Zealand type electric fences, throughout the winter. Figure 18 shows the weight gain change of these cattle as compared to traditionally hand-fed cows on harvested feed. Cows grazing rake-bunched hay came out of the winter in better condition than controls and did not receive any supplements or supplemental hay. Conception rates, calving interval, weaning weights, and attrition rates have been equal between control and treatment groups.[31]

Cattle have been wintered on rake-bunched hay now for 10 years and in only 1 year was emergency hay fed. In that year, the bunches were smaller and the high ground was grazed first, leaving the low areas where snow was as deep as 3 feet and a very unusual ice rain put a layer of ice on top of this, making it impossible for cows to find the hay. With higher, more compact bunches being used now and using low ground early, this can be avoided.

The rake bunches appear to emit heat, possibly due to fermentation, and to some extent tend to remain reasonably open, or at least visible, through the snow. They discolor and are not attractive, but have a sweet smell similar to haylage. During the one year when supplemental hay was required, cows would leave the feed ground early and search for rake-bunches, showing a definite preference for them. Bunches have been successfully grazed through long periods of 24-inch snow cover and under 12 inches of water toward spring.

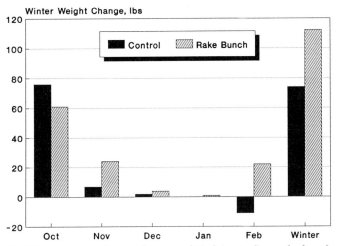

Figure 18. Winter weight change of cows on baled (control) or rake-bunched hay.

Weekly fence movements seem to be near optimum, creating very little waste, in fact less than with traditional feeding.

One of the keys to the increased performance of cows on rake-bunched hay and reductions of waste occurs in the spring when the weather warms and the meadows become wet and muddy. Cows on the rake-bunched hay continue to graze aggressively through this period, whereas the traditionally fed cattle tended to brawl and follow the feed wagon, tramping hay into the ground. They would then leave the feed ground and attempt to graze emerging spring grasses.

The cost of wintering cattle on rake-bunched hay has been $30 to $40 less per head than the traditional feeding of harvested hay. The bunches appear to have little effect on subsequent production and composition of forages produced by the native flood meadows.

Feeding the ionophore, monensin, a biologically active compound produced by *Streptomyces cinnamonensis*, has proved effective in either putting additional weight on cows over the winter or keeping the weight constant and reducing hay intake.[37,38] Cows fed a full feed of meadow hay plus 200 mg of monensin had daily gains of 0.2 pounds (0.1 kg) higher than cows fed meadow hay alone.[34] In studies where cow weights were kept equal between control cows receiving meadow hay and cows receiving meadow hay plus monensin, hay savings of up to 13% were realized. This represents another management tool for improving productive efficiency of range cattle operations. Monensin feeding has also partially alleviated the negative reproductive performance of replacement heifers receiving implants.[34] The use of monensin with very low quality forages can seriously affect weight gains and body condition scores in pregnant cattle.

One of the major nutritional concerns of calving in the fall is the nutrient requirements during the winter. During cold weather, energy must be provided for maintenance as well as for lactation and conception. An early assumption was that lactating cows on meadow hay and their calves would need additional energy and possibly protein to meet maintenance, productive, and reproductive requirements. For 3 years cows were supplemented at two energy levels with three protein sources, which included cottonseed meal, biuret, and urea. Calves were creeped at two levels, free choice and half of free choice. Calf gains were similar from cows on the two energy levels and pounds of calf weaned actually favored the cows on low energy due to a 4% higher mortality rate in calves from high energy cows. Most of these calf losses were due to respiratory problems, pneumonia, and scours. Cows fed biuret performed considerably lower than those fed the other protein sources. The higher creep level added 11 pounds (5 kg) to the weaning weight and 19 pounds (9 kg) of calf production per cow.[35] Due to these results, the last 7 years of the study, the previous high energy cow supplement was eliminated and the previously low energy ration was compared to hay alone and compared to free-choice creep feeding to no creep and all the interactions. Biuret was retained as a protein source and compared to cottonseed meal. This provided two energy levels and two protein sources.[35]

The addition of protein alone (biuret) to meadow hay did not improve performance. Cows on hay alone produced 16 pounds (7 kg) more calf per cow. On the high energy level cottonseed meal and biuret cows produced with a slight advantage of 9 pounds (0.4 kg) over those receiving cottonseed meal alone. Figure 19 shows summary data from these trials. When calves were not creep fed, all supplements fed to cows produced a negative response in pounds of calf produced per cow. Supplementation of cows produced negative effects in most cases and would not be feasible. However, creep feeding efficiency was increased when cows were supplemented with additional energy. Throughout these trials there was a slight negative effect on cow production and reproduction when calves were creep fed and cows were not supplemented. The larger calf may exert more aggressive nursing behavior, increasing milk flow and nutrient requirements of the cow.

Creep feeding year around as opposed to either summer or winter was compared to no creep for 1 year. Results show that creeping both winter and on range to be inefficient. Either creep in the winter or summer alone provided more efficient gains. It would be more convenient and feasible to creep on the winter feedgrounds than on summer range. Details of creep feeding results have been reported.[35]

The data indicate feeding good quality meadow hay alone may be the most profitable way to winter fall-calving cows and their calves. During times of high cattle prices in relation to feed costs, it may be profitable to supplement the hay with both protein and energy and to also creep feed the calves. Winter creeping of calves without supplementing cows may also pay when price conditions are favorable. Supplementing cows without creeping the calves did not pay under any conditions in these trials. These results are somewhat surprising; how-

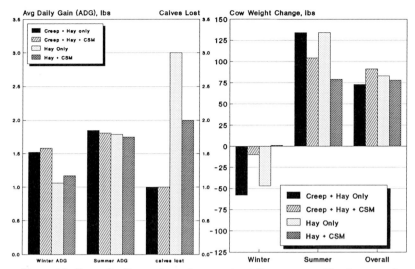

Figure 19. Creep feeding and supplementation influences on calf and cow performance during the winter and subsequent summer feeding period.

ever, some of the treatments may have altered hay intake. These conclusions are valid with good quality meadow hay or better forage, but results would be different with poor quality hay. Heavier milking cows would have higher nutrient requirements and may also change results somewhat.

One other management consideration that may be beneficial for many range operations is early turnout of the mature cows. This requires saving feed on range from the previous growing season for use early in the spring of the next year. The current year's growth on range is not adequate to maintain cattle until early to mid May, so old feed must be used or harvested feed hauled to range to maintain cattle at an adequate level. By turning out March 1 and calving on range, many of the health problems connected with calving on the wet muddy meadows are negated. Cattle can spread out more on range and the brush and juniper provide excellent thermal cover for young calves. This also facilitates the rake-bunch treatment by getting them off the meadows prior to spring flooding.

SUMMARY

A number of nutritional and managerial schemes have been presented to help optimize range livestock production. Forage quality, animal requirements, and the animals' ability to meet their requirements from the forage is presented. After determining the nutritional value of the forages and animal requirements, prescription supplementation produces very efficient additional gains. Management alternatives to compensate for poor quality forage on range in late summer and early fall, such as selling market animals, moving to better feed, chemical curing of forages, time of calving, time of weaning, and using the range as a feedlot are discussed. Winter feeding programs using native flood meadow hay as a base were also presented for both growing animals and mature cows. Included were discussions on using rake-bunched hay, an ionophore, and feeding strategies for wintering cows. Material presented illustrates a philosophy of range nutrition with methods and procedures that are adaptable to grazing systems in all parts of the world. It should be noted, however, some data need to be extrapolated to fit local conditions.

REFERENCES

1. Adams DC, Kartchner RJ: Effects of time of supplementation on daily gain, forage intake and behavior of yearling steers grazing fall range. Proc West Sec Am Soc Anim Sci 34:158, 1983
2. Castle EN, Wallace JD, Bogart R: Optimum Feeding Rates for Wintering Weaner Calves. Tech Bul 56 Ore St U, 1961, p 20
3. Chapupa W: Problems in feeding urea to ruminants. J Anim Sci 27:207, 1968
4. Clanton DC: Non-protein nitrogen in range supplements. J Anim Sci 47:765, 1978
5. Cochran RC, Adams DC, Wallace JD, et al: Predicting digestibility of different diets with internal markers: Evaluation of four potential markers. J Anim Sci 63:1476, 1986
6. Cochran RC, Vanzant ES, DelCurto T: Evaluation of internal markers isolated by alkaline hydrogen peroxide incubation and acid detergent lignin extraction. J Anim Sci 66:3245, 1988
7. Cooper CS: The effect of source, rate and time of nitrogen application upon the yields, vegetative composition and crude protein content of native flood-meadow hay in eastern Oregon. Agron J 48:543, 1956
8. Cooper CS, Wheeler RR, Sawyer WA: Meadow grazing-1: A comparison of gains of calves and yearlings when summering on native flood meadows and sagebrush-bunchgrass range. J Range Manage 10:172, 1957
9. Daugherty DA, Britton CM, Turner HA: Grazing management of crested wheatgrass range for yearling steers. J Range Manage 35:347, 1982
10. Daugherty DA, Turner HA, Church DC, et al: Range vs feedlot finishing. II. Performance and carcass quality comparison of feedlot and limited grain finishing of fall-born steers. Proc West Sec Am Soc Anim Sci 31:143, 1980
11. Eckert RE Jr: Vegetation-soil relationships on some Artemisia types in northern Harney and Lake Counties, Oregon. PhD Diss Ore St U, 1957, p 208
12. Ellis WC: Determinants of grazed forage intake and digestibility. J Dairy Sci 61:1828, 1978
13. Gomm FB: Climate and agriculture of Malheur-Harney basin, Oregon. Spec Rep 530 Ore St U, 1979, 23 p
14. Harris LE, Lofgreen GP, Kercher CJ, et al: Techniques of Research in Range Nutrition. Utah Agricultural Experiment Station Bulletin, 1967
15. Humphrey RR: Climate as a factor. In Range Ecology. New York, The Ronald Press Co, 1962, p 6
16. Kartchner RJ, Rittenhouse LR, Raleigh RJ: Forage and animal management implications of spring and fall calving. J Anim Sci 48:425, 1979
17. National Research Council: Nutrient Requirements of Beef Cattle. Washington, DC, National Academy Press, 1984, p 90
18. Raleigh RJ: Symposium on pasture methods for maximum production in beef cattle: Manipulation of both livestock and forage management to give optimum production. J Anim Sci 30:108, 1970

19. Raleigh RJ, Turner HA: A comparison of long vs chopped alfalfa or meadow hay for wintering weaner calves. *In* Research in Beef Cattle Nutrition and Management. Spec Rep 380 Ore St U, 1973, p 1
20. Raleigh RJ, Turner HA, Phillips RL: Weaning and post-weaning management of spring born calves. *In* Research in Beef Cattle Nutrition and Management. Special Reports 288 Oregon State University, 1970, p 5
21. Raleigh RJ, Rumburg CB, Wallace JD: Digestibility of native flood meadow hay at different stages of growth. Proc West Sec Am Soc Anim Sci 15:LVI-1, 1964
22. Raleigh RJ, Turner HA: Biuret and urea in range cattle supplements. Proc West Sec Am Soc Anim Sci 19:301, 1968
23. Raleigh RJ, Turner HA: Nonprotein nitrogen for wintering calves. *In* Research in Beef Cattle Nutrition and Management. Special Reports 270 Oregon State University, 1969, p 3
24. Raleigh RJ, Turner HA: Irrigated pastures as a complement to range. *In* Research in Beef Cattle Nutrition and Management. Special Reports 574 Oregon State University, 1980, p 18
25. Raleigh RJ, Wallace JD: Effect of supplementation on intake of grazing animals. Proc West Sec Am Soc Anim Sci 14:XXXVII-1, 1963
26. Riggs JK, Colby RW, Sells LV: The effect of self feeding salt cottonseed meal mixtures to beef cows. J Anim Sci 12:379, 1953
27. Schupp A, Binder T, McKnight W, et al: Acceptance of beef finished on range or with limited grain. Station Bulletin 714 Louisiana State University, 1979
28. Sneva FA: Chemical curing of range grasses with paraquat. J Range Manage 20:389, 1967
29. Sneva FA, Raleigh RJ, Turner HA: Paraquat-cured herbage for late season grazing. J Anim Sci 36:107, 1973
30. Stoddard LA, Smith AD, Box TW: Grazing areas of the world. *In* Vaux HJ (ed): Range Management. New York, McGraw-Hill, 1975, p 25
31. Turner HA, Angell RF: Systems for reducing dependency on harvested forage for wintering cows. Proc West Sec Am Soc Anim Sci 38:197, 1987
32. Turner HA, Raleigh RJ: Production of slaughter steers from forages in the arid west. J Anim Sci 44:901, 1977
33. Turner HA, Raleigh RJ: Supplementation considerations for beef cattle. Special Report 489 Oregon State University, 1977, p 15
34. Turner HA, Raleigh RJ: The effect of zeranol and monensin on reproductive performance of spring-born replacement heifers. Proc West Sec Am Soc Anim Sci 35:138, 1984
35. Turner HA, Raleigh RJ: Winter nutrition of fall-calving cows and calves. Sta Bul 665 Ore St U, 1985, p 24
36. Turner HA, Whittington DL, Raleigh RJ: Marketing steers directly off grass. *In* Research in Beef Cattle Nutrition and Management. Spec Rep 480, 1977, p 1
37. Turner HA, Raleigh RJ, Young DC: Effect of monensin on feed efficiency for maintaining gestating mature cows wintered on meadow hay. J Anim Sci 44:338, 1977
38. Turner HA, Young DC, Raleigh RJ, et al: Effect of various levels of monensin on efficiency and production of beef cows. J Anim Sci 50:385, 1980
39. Wallace JD, Raleigh RJ, Sawyer WA: Utilization of chopped, wafered, and pelleted native meadow hay by weaned Hereford calves. J Anim Sci 20:778, 1961

Address reprint requests to

Harley A. Turner
Eastern Oregon Agricultural Research Center
HC71, 4.51 Highway 205
Burns, OR 97720

0749-0720/91 $0.00 + .20

Polyether Ionophores — Effect on Rumen Function in Feedlot Cattle

Larry R. Corah, PhD*

Feed costs represent from 75% to 80% of the cost of producing beef. For the cattle industry to continue to produce excellent quality, competitively priced beef, cost of production is of paramount economic importance. Thus, additives that can improve feed efficiency and/or rate of gain have economic merit.

Polyether antibiotics have been used for a number of years in the poultry industry as coccidiostats. However, in the early 1970s, biological screening of these compounds showed potential efficacy in cattle diets. Monensin sodium was the first ionophore cleared by the Food and Drug Administration for use in feedlot cattle. This occurred in 1976, and its clearance for stocker cattle occurred in 1978. In 1982, lasalocid sodium was cleared for use in feedlot diets.

The clearance of polyether antibiotics was a significant scientific advancement for the field of ruminant nutrition.[14] There are at least 76 known polyether ionophores. Ionophores have the conventional polyether ring, but will vary in their chemical composition and even to a slight extent, in their biological activity. The first cleared ionophore, Monensin sodium, had an empirical formula of $C_{36}H_{61}O_{11}Na$ with a molecular weight of 692. Lasalocid sodium has an empirical formula of $C_{34}H_{53}O_2Na$ with a molecular weight of 612.8.[10]

BIOLOGICAL AND ECONOMIC EFFICIENCY

Initial research conducted with ionophores focused mainly on their application in the feedlot industry. Predominant benefits of ionophores in stocker and feedlot diets can include:[1] (1) improved feed efficiency; (2) improved rate of gain in stockers and a slight improvement in

---

*Professor, Department of Animal Science, Kansas State University, Manhattan, Kansas; Member of American Society of Animal Science

average daily gain in feedlot cattle; (3) decreased feed intake which may enhance the carrying capacity of cattle on a given quantity of forage; (4) a potential protein sparing effect, thus, possibly lower protein requirements, or at least more efficient use of the dietary protein content; (5) increased digestibility of low quality forages; (6) some reduction in the incidence of coccidiosis in cattle; (7) a decrease in the incidence of lactic acidosis; (8) some reduction in the incidence of feedlot bloat; (9) partial intake regulation in self feeding supplement systems; (10) some reduction in the incidence of pulmonary emphysema. To illustrate, the effect of ionophores on feedlot performance, Table 1, summarizes a number of research trials and illustrates the efficacy of the two cleared ionophores, monensin sodium (Rumensin), and lasalocid sodium (Bovatec).[13]

MODE OF ACTION

An ionophore is a compound that makes cations lipid soluble.[14] In the preliminary clearance of monensin sodium, the predominant mode of action discussed and assumed to be the factor influencing the biological efficiency was the alteration of the ruminal volatile fatty acid ratios. Specifically, the proportion of propionate was increased and the portion of acetate and butyrate decreased. In the typical ingestion of feed stuffs, the cellulose portion of roughages is broken down in the rumen by cellulase enzymes with the product being glucose. As the starch from grain is digested by rumen amylase enzymes, the starch molecules are converted into glucose sub units. In the rumen, the glucose is further quickly converted to pyruvate and volatile fatty acids (VFAs), which become the major dietary energy sources in ruminants. The relative proportion of these VFAs will vary based on the type of diet. In a predominantly roughage diet, VFA molar percentages are commonly 65% acetic, 20% propionic, and 12% butyric. In contrast, in feedlot diets where 70% or more grain is fed, the molar percentages VFA are 40% acetate, 37% propionate, with the remainder being butyrate and other VFAs that occur in a lesser percentage.[10]

The conversion to propionate is more efficient in the ruminant than the conversion to either acetate or butyrate. Glucose breaks down into two propionate molecules which can enter the tricarboxylic acid cycle. In contrast, if glucose breaks into two molecules of acetate, there

Table 1. *Summary of Ionophore Trials with Feedlot Cattle (1979, 1980, 1981)*

| | NO. OF TRIALS | PERCENT DIFFERENCE VERSUS NEGATIVE CONTROL | | |
		GAIN	INTAKE	F/G
Rumensin	53	+2.5	−5.1	+7.2
Bovatec	17	+6.4	−4.6	+9.9

(From Wagner D: Ionophore comparisons for cattle. The Bovine Practitioner 19:151, 1982; with permission.)

are also two molecules of CO_2 gas produced, which is a wasteful by-product in the conversion process. In the metabolism of butyrate, methane is formed.[10]

EFFECT ON RUMEN METABOLISM

One of the main effects of ionophores is to alter the rumen microflora to favor propionate production. A further effect on the rumen is that methane production is reduced when ionophores are included in the diet. Two factors result in the metabolizable energy value of feed stuffs being increased. First, there is an increase in the dry matter digestibility of the diet and an increase in hydrogen retention with proprionic acid production.[5]

Although enhancement of animal performance through improved retention of carbon and energy in the rumen diet is a logical partial explanation, scientists have suggested that other factors are obviously involved in the benefit derived from ionophore inclusion in the diet.

EFFECT ON NITROGEN METABOLISM

Shortly after the elucidation of the VFA influence, scientists indicated that ionophores may have a protein sparing effect. Ruminal studies have indicated that the presence of an ionophore causes a reduction in ammonia production, resulting in an increased protein flow from the rumen to the lower gut.[1]

This early research speculated that the impact of the ionophore on the rumen could be due to a resulting depression of available proteolytic and deaminative enzymes, or possibly a direct effect on both protease and deaminase activity.[1]

Recent research has given a clearer understanding of how the ionophores may improve nitrogen utilization. Work by Newbold and associates[9] has shown that ionophores inhibit the growth of gram-positive bacteria[4] and that ionophores cause a change in the composition of the rumen microbial flora. It has been further shown that ionophore inclusions will influence the metabolic activities of the surviving resistant rumen microbial species, particularly their influence on ion gradients across the bacterial cell wall membrane and on other energy-dependent processes. Bergen and coworkers[1] concluded that the underlying mode of action of ionophores is on transmembrane ion fluxes and the dissipation of cations and protein ingredients. They conclude that this action destroys primary membrane transport of cells, thereby interfering with cellular solute uptake coupled to primary transport systems. Their interpretation was that cells respond to this metabolic insult by maintaining primary transport by expending metabolic energy.

From the affect on cellular activity, the increased flow of nonammonia nitrogen from the rumen observed when ionophores are included in the diet is apparently attributed to lowered proteolytic, peptidolytic, and deaminase activity of the ruminal microorganisms. The probable effect of ionophores on amino acid deamination appears to be twofold. One is the elimination of gram-positive deaminating bacteria. The other is the interference in amino acid breakdown in surviving species arising from the mechanism whereby the bacteria adapt to grow in the presence of the ionophore.[9]

EFFECT ON MINERAL METABOLISM

Recent research has indicated that the feeding of ionophores will:[12] (1) increase the apparent absorption of sodium, magnesium, and phosphorus; (2) increase the retention of magnesium and phosphorus; (3) alter the soluble concentration of certain minerals in ruminal fluids of steers fed high energy diets.

As previously explained, ionophores impact ion exchange at the cellular level and, thus, it would appear logical that some impact on mineral metabolism would be apparent.

Of interest, however, is the recent evidence that increasing the dietary level of sodium and potassium may decrease the response of cattle to ionophores.[11] Although not fully determined, this research evidence indicates that excess dietary potassium and sodium levels will alter the level of VFA production, possibly alter the acetate : proprionate ratio, and may depress microbial activity in the rumen. This is particularly significant when high levels of salt are used to limit grain or protein supplements in a self feeding system.

Other Beneficial Effects

The rumen and serum lactate levels of cattle are decreased as they are transferred from either high forage diets to high grain diets, or from irregular intake of daily concentrates to high grain diets, resulting in a buildup of lactic acid, which can cause lactic acidosis.[8] Nagaraja demonstrated that inclusion of ionophores in the diet resulted in higher rumen pH values and lower lactate concentrations. In this study, the control cattle exhibited classic signs of acidosis such as lower blood pH and increased blood lactate, while the ionophore treated cattle exhibited none of the acidosis signs.

The incidence of coccidiosis in the cattle industry is fairly widespread. A number of specifically cleared coccidiostats are available and commonly used in the cattle industry. However, the fact that ionophores are antibiotics and initially cleared as a coccidiostat for use in the poultry industry would give a strong indication that they would show some coccidiostat efficacy in cattle. Research conducted by monitoring the incidence of clinical infections of coccidia in cattle has shown that at normal stocker and feedlot doses, ionophores are effective in at least partial control of coccidiosis.[5]

Since the inclusion of ionophores in feedlot diets, numerous feedlot operators have reported that the incidence of feedlot bloat has decreased. In research work done by Hartley and coworkers,[7] they showed that 300 mg of monensin sodium reduced the severity of bloat and attributed this result to its ability to inhibit the growth of the bloat causing strains of *Steptococcus bovis*. This work with feedlot cattle has been recently substantiated in stocker cattle grazing wheat pasture in which monensin reduced the incidence of wheat pasture frothy bloat. Branine and coworkers[3] postulated that this was possibly due to maintaining a ruminal pH above that required for maximal foam stability and strength. This relates to the fact that an optimal pH is required for ruminal foam formation.[2] Not to be overlooked in the beneficial effect of ionophores on preventing feedlot bloat, is the fact that its inclusion in the diet tends to create a more uniform feed intake, which is very advantageous to a favorable rumen environment.

An added benefit of ionophore inclusion in the diet is its efficacy in the reduction of the incidence of face and horn fly. Work by Harold and coworkers clearly indicates that enough monensin is apparently passed on to the fecal material to result in an increased incidence of larvae mortality, reducing the fly pupae available for maturation.[6]

SUMMARY

This article treated some of the modes of actions of ionophores in beef feedlot diets. It should be strongly emphasized that the predominant literature cited pertains to work with monensin sodium and more recently lasalocid sodium. There is ample evidence that the mode of action of these two ionophores is somewhat different and as new ionophores are cleared, it should not be assumed they follow the same mode of actions as described in this article.

REFERENCES

1. Bergen WG, Bates DB: Ionophores: Their effect on production efficiency and mode of action. J Anim Sci 58:1465, 1984
2. Branine ME, Galyean ML: Influence of grain and monensium supplementation on ruminal fermentation, intake, digesta connectics and incidence in severity of frothy bloat in steers grazing winter wheat pasture. J Anim Sci 68:1139, 1990
3. Branine ME, Galyean ML: Influence of grain and monensium supplementation on ruminal fermentation, intake, digesta connectics and incidence in severity of frothy bloat in steers grazing winter wheat pasture. J Anim Sci 68:1139, 1990
4. Chen M, Walin MJ: The effect of monensin and lasalocid sodium on the growth of the methanogenic and rumen saccharolytic bacteria. Appl Environ Microbiol 38:72, 1979
5. Goodrich RD, Garrett JE, Gast DR, et al: Influence of rumensin on the performance of cattle. J Anim Sci 58:1484, 1984
6. Harold F, Knapp FW: Effect of monensium on development of the face fly and horn fly. J Econ Entomol 73:762, 1980
7. Hartley EE, Herod EL, Bechtle RM et al: Effect of monensium or lasalocid, with or without niacin on amicloral, on rumen fermentation and feed efficiency. J Anim Sci 49:1067, 1979

8. Nagaraja TG, Avery TB, Bartley EE, et al: Prevention of lactic acidosis in cattle by lasalocid or rumensin. J Anim Sci 53:206, 1981
9. Newbold CJ, Wallace RJ, McKain N: Effects of the ionophore tetronasin on nitrogen metabolism by ruminal microorganisms in vitro. J Anim Sci 68:1103, 1990
10. Olentine C: Ionophores for beef cattle. Feed Management 33:14, 1982
11. Scwingel RW, Bates DB, Denham SC, et al: Effect of potassium and sodium on in vitro ruminal fermentations in the presence of ionophores. Florida Beef Cattle Research Report, 1989
12. Spears JW, Harvey RW: Lasalocid and dietary sodium and potassium effects on mineral metabolism, ruminal volatile fatty acids and performance on finishing steers. J Anim Sci 65:830, 1987
13. Stock R, Mader T: Feed additives for beef cattle. Great Plains Beef Cattle Handbook Fact Sheet, 1987
14. Wagner D: Ionophore comparisons for feedlot cattle. The Bovine Practitioner 19:151, 154

Address reprint requests to

Larry R. Corah, PhD
Weber Hall
Kansas State University
Manhattan, KS 66506-0201

0749-0720/91 $0.00 + .20

Nutritional and Dietary Interrelationships with Diseases of Feedlot Cattle

Bill Johnson, DVM*

The rumen was designed to convert roughage of variable quality into energy and protein using microbial fermentation, which can be then digested by the host. Economics have forced us to push this intricate process to the edge by feeding large quantities of high quality plant feeds that are processed to exploit this microbial fermentation to its full potential. Consequently, in our manipulation of this natural process, we have created metabolically related problems such as bloat, ruminal lactic acidosis, and sequelae to acidosis including mycotic rumenitis, hepatic abscesses, and caudal vena thrombosis and pulmonary arterial thromboembolism. It's not clear whether feedlot feeding practices are involved in the pneumonic condition, acute bovine pulmonary emphysema.

RUMINAL LACTIC ACIDOSIS

Ruminal lactic acidosis, rumen overload, grain overload, acidosis, and lactic acidosis are synonyms describing a condition in ruminants that results in an overproduction of lactic acid in the rumen due to the overingestion of highly fermentable starches.[2] Clinically, the condition is the result of a combination of separate but interrelated events. Ruminal lactic acidosis is a summation of the effects of the overingestion of rapidly fermentable starches that result in rapid overproduction of lactic acid and increased concentrations of volatile fatty acids (VFA), which are accompanied by ruminal atony, increased ruminal osmolality, and decreased salivation. Depending on severity, the absorbed lactic acid and VFA may cause a metabolic acidosis and the increased ruminal osmolality can cause dehydration.

*Diplomate, American College of Veterinary Pathologists; Pathologist, California Veterinary Diagnostic Laboratory System, University of California, Davis, California

The rumen typically functions at a pH range of 5.5 to 7.5.[2] Usually the fast amylolytic (starch splitting) fermentation will occur at the lower end of the pH range. This type of fermentation is common in the feedlots because concentrates and high quality roughages are used. Cellulolytic fermentation (more common with pasture grasses) occurs at a higher pH. The total VFA produced are low with cellulolytic fermentation and higher with amylolytic fermentation.[21] Normally, a rumen's lactic acid is produced slowly, with metabolism easily keeping pace with production.

The ingestion of highly fermentable grains results in more amylolytic fermentation and also results in a population shift of ruminal bacteria. This new bacterial population, which includes high numbers of Streptococcus bovis and Lactobacillus spp., uses the overabundant carbohydrates to cause a rapid overproduction of lactate.[9] Amylolytic fermentation also results in increased production of VFA, which contribute to reducing the ruminal pH. The lactic acid is the dominant force, being 10 times stronger than VFA.[9] However, VFA, especially butyric acid, play an important role in the development of metabolic acidosis because as the ruminal pH reaches 5, rumen stasis develops, due to what is thought to be butyric-acid stimulus of rumeno-reticular, epithelial receptors.[8] The rate of lactate absorption across healthy ruminal wall at a higher pH is slow.[21] As the ruminal concentrations of lactic acid increase and the ruminal pH decreases to 4, the absorption of lactate increases.[9] Absorbed lactate is metabolized by the liver. The L-lactate isomer is easily metabolized while the D-lactate isomer is difficult to metabolize.[9] In one study, the L-isomer was predominant, but as grain intake increased, the D-lactate became the predominant isomer.[25] The rapid production of lactates quickly overrides the buffering capacity in the rumen.[21] In addition, the VFA (increased because of amylolytic fermentation) become more undissociated at the lower ruminal pH resulting in more rapid rumen absorption of the VFA.[21] The normal bicarbonate buffering capacity of the blood is quickly overwhelmed by the increased amounts of lactate and VFA in the circulation resulting in metabolic acidosis.[2,21]

The by-products of fermentation cause the osmolality of the rumen to reach more than twice the normal value.[9] This increase in osmolality can result in a significant transfer of fluids from the plasma into the rumen, contributing to dehydration of an animal that is already becoming metabolically acidotic. The effects of the acidosis and dehydration, if left untreated, quickly lead to shock and death.

The milder the episode of ruminal acidosis and the better the host's ability to buffer and metabolize these products, the less the animal is affected. Some animals may simply become inappetent and appear listless for a day or two followed by quick recovery. This is in contrast to the animal that staggers then lays with its head turned back into its flank.

There are numerous factors that can trigger or contribute to the development of ruminal lactic acidosis. Typically it takes about 2 weeks for a microbial population to adapt from one food substrate to another.[28] When weaned, pasture-acclimated, young calves are introduced to the feedlot; the animal must be allowed to adapt to the low roughage, high concentrate feedlot ration in a slow incremental pattern. This allows the beneficial ruminal flora to adjust to this change in feed and at the same time remain as the predominant population. One proposed safe method is to start with a 50/50 mixture of milled roughage/grain ration as a starter for 7–10 days. If no problems are noted, then decrease the amount of roughage by 10% every 2–4 days down to the level of 10–15% roughage in the ration.[2]

The amount of concentrate needed to produce lactic acidosis is variable due to many factors, including condition of the animal, previous ration, how the feedstuff is processed (flaked, cracked, rolled), and the coarseness of the roughage in the ration.[9,28] Animals that are in poorer condition and acclimated to a low concentrate, high roughage diet are the most susceptible.[9,28] Feedstuffs that are processed to allow quicker fermentation in the rumen increase the risk of initiating ruminal acidosis.[9] In addition to these factors the ruminant's saliva has an important buffering effect.[2,32] When Utley et al fed steers 80% concentrate and 20% whole peanut hulls, only 3.7% of the steers had liver abscesses, but 56% had abscesses when hulls were ground and 59% had abscesses when hulls were pelleted.[32] It appears that the chewing time is an important factor in the amount of saliva produced.[6,32] Thus, as the percentage of concentrates in the ration increases and roughage decreases or is pelleted, the animal loses part of this natural buffering protection.

Any one of several different events that cause an interruption or change in routine eating habits can trigger a lactic acidosis event. In experimental work with singly housed animals, it is rare that the individual animal will overingest.[9] It appears that group competition and hierarchy play a role in feedlot cattle overingesting.[9] A breakdown in the feedmill or a truck-driver error may result in a particular pen feeding being missed. Subsequent delivery of the normal amount of feed for that pen will result in overconsumption by several in the pen. Any feeding interruptions like this can be particularly devastating if the pen contains animals of varying sizes, which allows for more feed to be ingested by larger, more aggressive individuals. If a bunk of feed gets wet, the animals may not ingest all of that particular feeding. When the bunks are cleaned out and fresh dry feed added, the rush and competition for feed may result in some ruminal acidosis cases.[2] Changes to a cooler temperature may cause some to over-indulge.[9] Putting dry hay in the bunks on top of concentrates may result in larger more aggressive animals filling up on hay while other animals later overload on concentrates.

There are no definitive gross postmortem lesions seen in an animal whose death was caused by ruminal acidosis. Sloughing of the ruminal mucosa is a result of postmortem autolysis and not necessarily a result of acidosis or toxicity. Reddening under the ruminal mucosa is often misleading because it is common in a number of other conditions. Checking the pH of the rumen with a pH meter or pH paper within 2 hours of death is the best way of determining ruminal lactic acidosis postmortem. Typically, the ruminal pH is above 5.5 in feedlot animals on high concentrate. Ruminal pH values in lactic acidosis are often in the range of 3.9–4.5.[9] A pH below 5 is usually considered evidence of a ruminal acidosis.[2] However, interpretation of the ruminal pH in animals that have been dead for any length of time is difficult and less reliable. Limited clinical observations suggest that fermentation continues for awhile after death causing the pH to continue to decrease approximately one half of a pH unit.[15] After a few hours, the fermentation rate will decrease and the ruminal pH will start to increase. In animals that have been dead for 4 to 12 hours, a ruminal pH between 4.9 and 5.2 is difficult to interpret with any certainty.

Histologic sectioning of the ruminal mucosa can provide evidence of acidosis. Acidosis is one of the few conditions that cause a laminar ballooning degeneration and necrosis to the middle layer of the stratum spinosum of the squamous epithelium of the ruminal mucosa.[18] Histopathologic examination of sections of ruminal mucosa can be used to help diagnose acidosis. However, because it may take from 24 to 48 hours to get a diagnosis back from a laboratory, clinical diagnosis usually rests with one's best judgment based on clinical signs, ruminal pH, lack of other findings, and pen history.

Ruminal ionophores (monensin, lasalocid) have offered some protection for ruminal acidosis by controlling ruminal flora.[2] Generally, the ionophore antibiotics are effective against the growth of gram-positive bacteria. Two such gram-positive bacteria are *Streptococcus bovis* and *Lactobacillus spp.*, which are major lactate producers. It is believed that by controlling major lactate producers, the ionophores can help protect against clinical and subclinical acidosis.[2,23] In one study, salinomycin was more effective than monensin or lasalocid.[23]

Addition of sodium bicarbonate to the rations of feedlot animals has been examined but the results are equivocal. While addition of bicarbonate to the beginning ration may help with adaption to the concentrate, it appears to have little effect later.[10] The best preventive may be a good understanding of the causes and physiology of ruminal acidosis coupled with sound management advice and monitoring.

CONSEQUENCES OF RUMINAL LACTIC ACIDOSIS

Animals that survive an episode of lactic acidosis may be subjected to long term effects that can result in poor performance and death. At slaughter there may be significant condemnation of livers due to hepatic abscesses.[30]

Mycotic Rumenitis

Ruminal acidosis results in large scale destruction of the ruminal mucosa which favors the growth of *Mucoraceous spp.* fungi. Degradation of the ruminal mucosa allows these organisms to invade the submucosa of the rumen wall.[18] These fungal organisms have a predilection for arterioles, initiating a severe vasculitis with resulting thrombosis and infarction of the ruminal wall. Lesions may be so severe that there is complete transmural necrosis of the ruminal wall. Grossly, the rumen can have disseminated subserosal hemorrhage, lesions 2–8 cm in diameter, or massive segments of the wall affected. The underlying mucosa is yellowish gray, often with an adherent, necrotic pseudomembrane. The devitalized ruminal mucosa allows entry of bacterial and fungal organisms into the ruminal wall and subsequently, into the portal blood. Use of thiabendazole, orally, after episodes of ruminal acidosis is thought to be partially effective in preventing mycotic rumenitis.

Liver Abscesses

The entry of bacteria across a devitalized ruminal mucosa following lactic acidosis results in establishment of small bacterial colonies in the ruminal wall.[26] Bacteria gain entry into ruminal vessels, sending bacterial emboli to the liver via the hepatic portal venous system. There the bacteria localize in the hepatic parenchyma with subsequent development of hepatic abscesses.[20,26] These liver abscesses are a concern of the slaughter plants. A 1982 study of feedlots in the Texas/Oklahoma panhandle, eastern New Mexico, southeastern Colorado, and southwestern Kansas recorded 39.4% of the livers condemned out of 56,658 cattle coming from 60 different feedlots.[22] The liver can account for approximately 2% by weight of the carcass, which can add up to a significant financial loss.[30] However, it is not the loss of the liver that is of greatest economic concern to the feedlot manager. A Nebraska study, looking at more than 2500 experimental cattle, revealed average daily gain to be depressed by 0.1 lb. in those cattle with hepatic abscesses. Other trials have shown poorer performances with abscessed cattle compared with healthy cattle.[11]

Fusobacterium necrophorum is the most common isolate, quite often in pure cultures. Some abscesses contain mixed populations of *Corynebacterium pyogenes*, *Streptococcus spp.*, *Staphylococcus spp.*, or *Bacteroides spp.* often in conjunction with *F. necrophorum*. Of the three biotypes, A, B and C, of *F. necrophorum*, only biotypes A and B have been implicated in the disease. Type B is more common in ruminal wall abscesses, while biotype A is more common in liver abscesses.[14] A specific leucotoxin is liberated by *F. necrophorum* which enables this organism to colonize the liver parenchyma.[14]

Prevention is aimed at controlling ruminal acidosis as much as possible. A second possibility is the use of antibiotics in the feed to stop the growth of the bacteria. Commonly used antibiotics are bacitracin, methylene disalicylate, chlortetracycline, oxytetracycline, and tylosin. These antibiotics vary in effectiveness.[20]

Cauda Vena Cava Thrombosis/Pulmonary Arterial Thromboembolism

Infrequently, a hepatic abscess ruptures into the post cava, resulting in thrombosis of the vena cava and bacterial emboli showering the lung. These small pulmonary thrombi can develop into small abscesses that erode the walls of the pulmonary arterioles. Since the pulmonary arterial system lies adjacent to the airways, erosion and rupture of the vessel wall can result in hemorrhage into bronchioles.[12] Clinically, these animals may suddenly develop frank epistaxis, may blow bloody froth from the nostrils, or may cough up blood clots. These animals are usually in good flesh. The course of illness, once clinical signs of hemoptysis appear, is usually 100% fatal, and usually within 24 hours.[18,19] At necropsy, numerous small (0.5–2 cm) abscesses can be palpated bilaterally in all lobes of the lung. There are scattered lobules that are bright red due to aspirated blood. Clumps of clotted blood may be seen in the trachea and rumen.[12,16] Jensen found cauda vena cava thrombosis in 1.3%[17] of 1998 yearling feedlot cattle necropsied. He found 40% to occur in the first 45 days of the feeding period and 28% in the next 45 days.[16] Since the condition is 100% fatal, the only alternatives are to try to control the incidence of hepatic abscesses or to salvage via slaughter as soon as clinical signs are noted.[29]

BLOAT

Neutralization of the fermentation products of ruminal starches by salivary bicarbonate results in the production of large quantities of gases (CO_2, CH_2, N_2). These gases are constantly eliminated by the eructation process. If unencumbered, this process is capable of handling any rate of ruminal gas production.[21] However, for eructation to take place, a normal sequence of events must occur.[35] In order for the cardia to open, the cardiac region of the rumen must be clear of fluid and froth. If not, an inhibitory reflex will override the stimulus for the cardia to open.[21]

Bloat is usually recognized as either primary or secondary. Primary bloat is typically called frothy bloat due to the formation of large numbers of tiny, stable bubbles that occur in cattle on legume pastures and in feedlot cattle on high grain rations. Secondary ruminal tympany is due to large amounts of free gas in the rumen and failure of eructation.[3,31]

When an outbreak of bloat occurs in a feedlot it is most often due to frothy bloat.[31] Individual repeat bloaters are more likely to have a problem with secondary bloat due to some type of mechanical or physiological problem (i.e. esophageal blockage or ruminal atony).[21] Saliva has a natural mucin that acts as a surfactant to disrupt the formation of the tiny bubbles seen in frothy bloat.[31] As mentioned in the section on ruminal acidosis, the lack of roughage in a diet or the pelleting of the roughage will result in less saliva and therefore salivary buffers being produced, leaving the animals predisposed to frothy bloat.[32] Other contributory causes of foam in feedlot animals are not fully understood. Some bacteria such as *Streptococcus bovis* produce an insoluble slime that can entrap the gas bubbles of fermentation.[31] Also, the size of the grain particle being fed can affect the amount of froth and its stability. Fine particles (geometric mean particle size, 388 μm) have been associated with more froth than coarser particles (715 μm).[3]

There is no clear prevention for feedlot bloat. Additives such as poloxalene, which break down the foam, are not as effective in feedlot bloat as they are on typical legume pasture bloat.[3] The ionophore, lasalocid, has shown some early promise as a bloat preventive in feedlot tests in Kansas.[31] Attention should be given to the amount of roughage in the ration and the coarseness of the roughage. If possible, less fermentable roughages such as grass hay should be used rather than leafy alfalfa hay. The addition of tallow to the ration has some promise but the results are equivocal.[3]

ACUTE BOVINE PULMONARY EDEMA AND EMPHYSEMA (ATYPICAL INTERSTITIAL PNEUMONIA)

Acute bovine pulmonary edema and emphysema (ABPE) is one of several terms denoting a pneumonia-causing acute respiratory distress with particularly labored expiration. Other names applied are atypical interstitial pneumonia (AIP), acute respiratory distress syndrome (ARDS), fog fever, and acute bovine pulmonary adenomatosis.[4,5,17,19,24,34] Pathologically, these lungs have combinations of the following: pulmonary congestion, edema, interstitial emphysema, alveolar epithelial hyperplasia, and hyaline membrane formation.[4] Grossly, lesions occur in any or all of the lung lobes. The lungs do not collapse when the thoracic cavity is opened. There is variable subpleural and interlobular emphysema (often bullous). The pleura is smooth and shiny with no fibrin present. The lungs are extremely heavy and wet. Lobules are reddened, have a rubbery texture and are separated by pale yellow interlobular edema. Emphysema may occur in the mediastinal tissue and occasionally subcutaneously.[4,5,17,19,33] Early in the disease, before opportunistic bacterial infections cause a secondary bronchopneumonia, the animal's temperature is variable, ranging from 102.5 to 107° F.[33] Part of the animal's elevated temperature may be dependent on the environmental temperature because respiration is the bovine's main source of temperature regulation. Severely affected animals stand with their heads down, necks extended and have open mouth breathing. These animals often die quickly.[19]

There are several agents or mechanisms that can cause this set of changes therein complicating this respiratory condition. Grossly, this pneumonia could be linked with damage from hypersensitivity diseases (farmer's lung, milk allergy), 3-methylindole (from lush grass rich in L-tryptophan), parasitic diseases (Dictyocaulus viviparus), plants (moldy sweet potatoes, purple mint), and exposure to irritant gases and fumes (nitrogen dioxide, zinc oxide).[4,5,19,24,34] In addition, the infectious pneumonia caused by bovine respiratory syncytial virus (BRSV) can be grossly indistinguishable from any of the previously mentioned causes.[1]

Microscopically, there are subtle differences that can be used to distinguish parasitic pneumonias, allergic pneumonias, and some BRSV pneumonias from the others.[1,4,5,26,27,34] Microscopically, the pneumonias caused by 3-methylindole, 4-ipomeanol from moldy sweet potatoes, and perilla ketones from *Perilla frutescens* (purple mint) can appear identical.[4]

Breeze made the argument that ABPE should be used to describe only those animals that develop this pneumonic condition while grazing lush pastures.[4,5] In these instances the animals are usually adult cows and several are affected due to the ingestion of grasses rich in L-tryptophan. The L-tryptophan is converted in the rumen to 3-methylindole, which when metabolized by the mixed-function oxidase system is toxic to the lung. This condition is common in the United States and is most likely the same condition as fog fever in the United Kingdom. For the proposed renaming of these pneumonias see Breeze.[5]

In the feedlots, a pneumonic condition, commonly referred to as AIP or ABPE, is seen in which the changes are the same as those previously described. The feedlot cases are sporadic; but still are a common cause of feedlot deaths. One study found a mortality from AIP/ABPE to be 0.498% in 18,633 calves and 0.107% in 58,990 yearling cattle during a 4-year period. The mean mortality for the groups was 0.62% and 0.35%, respectively.[14] Another study found 106 yearlings (5.3%) of 1988 yearlings necropsied had AIP/ABPE.[17]

The cause of these pneumonias in feedlot cattle is often not determined.[33] It would be unlikely for feedlot cattle to gain exposure to the plant purple mint. Usually when calves get exposed to 4-ipomeanol from moldy sweet potatoes, several animals in the pen develop respiratory distress and die. It has been shown that feeding monensin to cattle prior to the ingestion of L-tryptophan will protect against the formation of the toxic agent, 3-methylindole.[13] Hjerpe indicated that he did not see a difference in morbidity and mortality from AIP/ABPE in the feedlot even with the addition of 30 gm per ton monensin to the ration.[14] This in addition to the sporadic nature of the problem in the feedlot suggests that factors other than diet may be involved. One group found a higher incidence during summer and fall, suggesting that the problem may be triggered by dust.[17] Hjerpe saw no seasonal change in incidence in animals that were on slats with minimal exposure to dust.[14] Recently, improved diagnostic procedures using immunoperoxidase histochemical techniques on formalin-fixed tissues have shown the presence of BRSV in cases that were previously labeled atypical interstitial pneumonia.[7] It may be that BRSV is responsible for more of these sporadic cases than previously diagnosed.

The condition is basically caused by agents that destroy the thin, delicate, type I pneumoncytes that line the alveolar walls or by affecting the capillary endothelial cells in alveolar walls. The damage results in protein-rich fluid flooding the alveolus and is followed by proliferation of thicker type II pneumonocytes to cover the damaged alveolus. Diffusion of oxygen across this larger alveolar epithelial cell is more difficult. The type II cells plus the alveolar edema inhibit oxygenation of the blood, causing the animal to become more and more hypoxic. The oxygen-starved animal gasps for breath, leading to rupture of alveoli and formation of emphysematous bulla.[24]

At present there is no proven prevention for this condition as it occurs in the feedlot. No single treatment regimen has proved entirely successful. Combinations of antibiotics, atropine, antihistamines, diuretics, corticosteroids, and epinephrine have been used.[14,19,33] These animals are often so ill that any harsh handling will result in rapid death. It is important to submit pieces of lung from different lobes, fresh and fixed, to a diagnostic laboratory to make sure the problem is not due to one of the preventable causes such as BRSV or parasites.

SUMMARY

Feedlot economics dictate that highly fermentable rations be fed, leaving the ruminant constantly on the edge of lactic acidosis. Consequently, a number of subtle changes in feed, environment, or management can tip the balance, causing ruminal acidosis. Even though the animal may not die from the immediate effects of a metabolic acidosis, there are sequelae such as mycotic rumenitis, hepatic abscesses, cauda vena cava thrombosis, and pulmonary arterial thromboemolism that may cause subsequent losses. Another condition, typically referred to as atypical interstitial pneumonia/acute bovine pulmonary emphysema is a sporadic cause of death in feedlot animals. This condition is sometimes linked to the feed or hypersensitivities such as dust. At present, it seems the condition is not linked with the above and part of the problem may be undiagnosed bovine respiratory syncytial virus BRSV infection.

REFERENCES

1. Baker JC, Frey ML: Bovine respiratory syncytial virus. Vet Clin North Am: Large Anim Pract 1:259, 1985
2. Blood DC, Radostits OM: Acute carbohydrate engorgement of ruminants (rumen overload). *In* Veterinary Medicine, ed 7. London, Bailliere Tindall, 1989, p 246
3. Blood DC, Radostits OM: Ruminal tympany (bloat). *In* Veterinary Medicine, ed 7. London, Bailliere Tindall, 1989, p 265
4. Breeze RG, Carlson JR: Chemical-induced lung injury in domestic animals. Adv Vet Sci Comp Med 26:201, 1982
5. Breeze RG, Selman IE, Pirie HM: A reappraisal of atypical interstitial pneumonia in cattle. Bovine Pract 13:75, 1978
6. Brent BE: Relationship of acidosis to other feedlot ailments. J Anim Sci 43:930, 1976
7. Collins JK, Jensen R, Smith GH, et al: Association of bovine respiratory syncytial virus with atypical interstitial pneumonia in feedlot cattle. Am J Vet Res 49:1045, 1988
8. Crichlow EC, Chaplin RK: Ruminal lactic acidosis: Relationship of forestomach motility to nondissociated volatile fatty acids levels. Am J Vet Res 46:1908, 1985
9. Dunlop RH: Pathogenesis of ruminant lactic acidosis. Adv Vet Sci Comp Med 16:259, 1972
10. Emerick RJ: *In* Weinverg MS, Sheffner AS (eds): Buffers in Ruminant Physiology and Metabolism. New York, Church & Dwight, 1976
11. Foster L, Woods W: Liver losses in finishing cattle. *In* Beef Cattle Progress Report. Lincoln, NE University of Nebraska, 70:218:1, 1970
12. Gudmundson J, Radostits OM, Doige CE: Pulmonary thromboembolism in cattle due to thrombosis of the posterior vena cava associated with hepatic abscessation. Can Vet J 19:304, 1980

13. Hammond AC, Carlson JR, Breeze RG: Effect of monensin pretreatment on trypto-
    phan-induced acute bovine pulmonary edema and emphysema. Am J Vet Res
    43:753, 1982
14. Hjerpe CA: Clinical management of respiratory disease in feedlot cattle. Vet Clin
    North Am: Large Anim Pract 5:119, 1983
15. Hollis L, Personal communication, 1990
16. Jensen R, Pierson RE, Braddy PM, et al: Embolic pulmonary aneurysms in yearling
    feedlot cattle. JAVMA 169:518, 1976
17. Jensen R, Pierson RE, Braddy PM, et al: Atypical interstitial pneumonia in yearling
    feedlot cattle. JAVMA 169:507, 1976
18. Jubb KVF, Kennedy PC, Palmer N: Pathology of Domestic Animals, ed 3, vol 2. New
    York, Academic Press, 1985
19. Kerr LA, Linnabary FD: A review of interstitial pneumonia in cattle. Vet Hum
    Toxicol 31:247, 1989
20. Langworth BF: *Fusobacterium necrophorum*: Its characteristics and role as an animal
    pathogen. Bacteriol Rev 41:373, 1977
21. Leek BF: Clinical diseases of the rumen: A physiologist's view. Vet Rec 113:10,
    1983
22. Montgomery TH: Research update—liver abscesses among commercially fed cattle.
    West Texas State University report, 1982
23. Nagaraja TG, Avery TB, Galitzer SJ, et al: Effect of ionophore antibiotics on experi-
    mentally induced lactic acidosis in cattle. Am J Vet Res 46:2444, 1985
24. Pirie HM, Dawson CO, Breeze RG, et al: Fog fever and precipitins to micro-orga-
    nisms of mouldy hay. Res Vet Sci 12:586, 1971
25. Ryan RK: Concentrations of glucose and low-molecular-weight acids in the rumen of
    sheep changed gradually from a hay to hay-plus-grain diet. Am J Vet Res 25:653,
    1964
26. Scanlan CM, Hathcock TL: Bovine rumenitis-liver abscess complex: A bacteriologi-
    cal review. Cornell Vet 73:288, 1983
27. Schiefer B, Jayasekara MU, Mills JHL: Comparison of naturally occurring and tryp-
    tophan-induced bovine atypical interstitial pneumonia. Vet Pathol 11:327, 1974
28. Slyter LL: Influence of acidosis on rumen function. J Anim Sci 43:910, 1976
29. Stober M: Pyogenic thrombosis of caudal vena cava in cattle. World Association for
    Buiatrics, 1967, p 395
30. Tindall B: Liver abscesses hidden losses. Animal Nutrition & Health September–
    October:38:22, 1983
31. Tindall B: Bloat characteristics and control. Animal Nutrition & Health May–
    June:38:44, 1983
32. Utley PR, Hellwig RE, Butler JL, et al: Comparison of unground, ground, and
    pelleted peanut hulls as roughage sources in steer finishing diets. J Anim Sci
    37:608, 1973
33. Wikse SE: Feedlot cattle pneumonias. Vet Clin North Am: Large Anim Pract 1:289,
    1985
34. Wilkie BN: Allergic respiratory disease. Adv Vet Sci Comp Med 26:233, 1982
35. Williams E: A study of reticulo-ruminal motility in adult cattle in relation to bloat
    and traumatic reticulitis with an account of the latter condition as seen in a general
    practice. Vet Rec 67:907, 1955

Address reprint requests to

Bill Johnson, DVM
California Veterinary Diagnostic Laboratory System
UC Davis
Thurman Lab
West Health Sciences Drive
Davis, CA 95616

0749–0720/91 $0.00 + .20

Nutritional and Dietary Interrelationships with Diseases of Grazing Beef Cattle

Steven E. Wikse, DVM,* Thomas M. Craig, DVM, PhD,†
and David P. Hutcheson, PhD‡

Acute Bovine Pulmonary Emphysema and Edema (ABPEE) is a disease that affects cattle that have been changed abruptly from a poor plane of nutrition to lush growths of pasture grasses, alfalfa, or *Brassica* species[6,8,25] such as rape and turnips. Pastures that are irrigated and well fertilized or hay fields with lush regrowth following harvest are especially dangerous. ABPEE occurs throughout the United States, with the highest incidence in Western states where it is responsible for losses of thousands of cows annually.[4,15] All breeds are affected. Herefords are most commonly affected, not because they are more susceptible than other breeds, but probably because they are the predominant beef breed in the Western states where common herd-management practices predispose the herd to ABPEE.[6] Outbreaks occur most frequently in the summer and fall with a peak incidence during August, September, and October.[15] A hard frost or repeated freezing usually results in pastures being safe to graze,[4,5] however, an increase in ABPEE outbreaks has been observed when early fall frosts were followed by warm weather and lush regrowth.[9,12]

The pathogenesis of ABPEE has been shown to involve the conversion of the amino acid L-tryptophan (TRP) in ingested herbage to 3-methylindole (3MI) by rumen bacteria.[6] Rumen 3MI rapidly rises

*Diplomate, American College of Veterinary Pathology, Associate Professor, Large Animal Medicine and Surgery, College of Veterinary Medicine, Texas A&M University, College Station, Texas
†Professor, Department of Veterinary Pathobiology, College of Veterinary Medicine, Texas A&M University, College Station, Texas
‡Professor, Texas Agricultural Experiment Station, Texas A&M University, Amarillo, Texas

after the change to lush pasture, peaks at 3 to 4 days, and declines to relatively low levels by 7 days.[6,13] It is absorbed into the circulatory system and reaches the lung where it is metabolically activated by a mixed function oxidase system in bronchiolar Clara cells and alveolar type I pneumocytes to unidentified reactive intermediates that damage the cells, resulting in desquamation and alveolar edema. The microbial population of the rumen, which is dependent on diet, appears to be a more critical risk factor for the development of ABPEE than the concentration of TRP in the forage, because the TRP content of pastures associated with ABPEE outbreaks has not been found to be higher than control pastures.[16] Cattle that are on a low plane of nutrition prior to being placed on lush pasture seem to have a rumen bacteria population that readily converts TRP to 3MI.

ABPEE occurs mainly in adult cows, however, severe outbreaks can occur in yearlings.[25] Clinical signs generally develop 4 to 10 days after cattle are introduced to lush pastures. Morbidity varies from 3% to 100% but is generally less than 50% and an average of 50% of affected animals succumb. Animals affected with ABPEE display clinical signs of acute respiratory distress. Rumen 3MI levels are elevated in nonaffected as well as affected cattle, however, peak 3MI levels are higher and last longer in clinically affected animals.[13]

The two main concerns in the face of an outbreak of ABPEE are (1) how to enhance the survival chances of affected animals; and (2) how to minimize the number of new cases. Spontaneous recovery generally occurs in mild to moderately affected animals, so treatment should only be considered for severe cases. For severe cases, no treatment may be the prudent course of action because no effective therapy has been identified that will reverse the fully developed lesions of ABPEE and the stress of handling often causes severely affected animals to collapse and die.[22] If severely affected cases are treated, they should be slowly moved as short a distance as possible to a temporary treatment pen. Attempts should be made to reduce the massive pulmonary edema by administering a diuretic such as furosemide (0.4 to 1 mg per kg body weight intravenously or intramuscularly every 12 hours) and by restricting drinking water.[6] Further development of edema should be limited by giving the antiprostaglandin flunixin meglumine (2.2 mg per kg intravenously or intramuscularly every 12 hours). Recently, antiprostaglandin therapy administered intravenously at the onset of experimentally induced ABPEE was shown to alleviate clinical signs and lung pathology.[21] Unfortunately, the degree of lung pathology in severe field cases is no doubt much greater than that of the experimental cases that were treated. Animals that are treated should also be given antibiotics effective against bovine lung pathogens such as *Pasturella* spp. to prevent their proliferation in the protein-rich pulmonary edema.

There is no effective way to minimize the total number of affected animals in an ABPEE outbreak. The first reaction is often to remove the cattle from the offending pasture. This measure has sometimes been recommended in the past, however, clinical observations have shown that removal of cattle will not prevent the development of new cases.[5]

This finding is consistent with the timing of the biochemical events that determines whether an animal will become ill or not — rumen production of 3MI, which has usually peaked prior to the appearance of the first case. Whether the cattle are removed from the pasture or not, new cases can be expected to continue for 4 or 5 days after the index case.[5,25] It is probably best to leave the cattle on the pasture and feed 2 to 3 lb per head per day of poor quality hay or straw. Cattle on lush pastures readily consume dry roughage, which dilutes the intake of ABPEE-inciting pasture.

Prevention is the paramount approach for successful management of ABPEE because, there is no effective treatment and no effective means of minimizing new cases in an outbreak. Preventive measures fall into two categories (1) dietary management and (2) medical measures.[5,6] Optimal success in prevention of ABPEE is dependent on implementing some combination of both practices.

Opportunities for dietary management begin prior to introducing cattle to ABPEE-prone fields. Cattle that have been on a low nutritional plane should be placed on a full diet of good quality hay for 2 to 3 weeks prior to entering lush pastures. This will allow the development of a population of rumen microorganisms capable of properly digesting the high amounts of TRP in the pasture. If that is not possible, then cattle could be fed hay in a corral and only allowed to graze the lush pasture for a few hours a day, gradually increasing grazing time until they are left on the pasture at 10 days.[5] The next best, but still effective alternative is to feed a supplement of 2 to 3 lb of hay or straw per head per day beginning when the cattle are introduced to the potentially offensive pasture. Although the quality need not be high, the palatability of the dry roughage must be good enough that the cattle consume adequate amounts. Pasture management measures that reduce the possibility of ABPEE include grazing the pasture before it becomes particularly lush, section-grazing with portable electric fences, and mowing the pasture before grazing.

Medical steps to prevent ABPEE involve the administration of polyether ionophore antibiotics such as monensin (Rumensin 60, Elanco Products) and lasalocid (Bovatec, Hoffman-LaRoche), which inhibit the gram-positive rumen bacteria that convert TRP to 3MI.[6,7,18] Monensin administered at 200 mg per head per day beginning 1 day before introduction to lush pasture and continued for 10 days is very effective in inhibiting 3MI production.[7,19] Ionophore antibiotics can be given in custom-milled pellets as either an energy supplement (94.85% barley, 0.5% molasses, and 0.15% ionophore) or a protein supplement (10% dehydrated alfalfa, 26.6% dent yellow corn, 0.5% molasses, 58.25% soybean meal, and 0.15% ionophore) formulated to provide 200 mg of monensin or lasalocid per head per day when fed once daily, or as a divided dose, in a total of 1 kg supplement (Lasalocid is also effective in reducing rumen 3MI) production, however, it must be administered for 6 days prior to exposure to lush pasture to allow rumen lasalocid concentrations to reach inhibitory levels.[18] In contrast, monensin must only be given for 1 day prior to exposure, because after

4 days it loses its ability to strongly inhibit the production of 3MI.) Medical supplements should be offered in a sufficient number of tubs or troughs to allow free access by all cattle. Consumption of commercially available lick blocks containing molasses, salt, and monensin has been shown to result in inadequate daily intakes of monensin.[14] No beneficial effect of monensin or lasalocid is to be expected after clinical signs of ABPEE appear, because by that time 3MI-induced pneumotoxicity has occurred. Supplements should be mixed properly, labeled, and stored to prevent ingestion by horses or other animals that are more sensitive than cattle to ionophore antibiotic toxicity. Monensin toxicity has been reported in horses and chickens,[3] cattle,[3] and dogs[29] and is often associated with ingestion of either monensin premix or improperly mixed supplements.

LUNGWORM AND GASTROINTESTINAL NEMATODES IN CALVES

Control of parasites may be directed at the host and/or the environment. Treatment of the host removes parasites and, if given in a timely fashion, may affect the environmental contamination. It is essential to understand the environmental factors that affect parasite development and survival in order to develop programs that will control parasites rather than treating affected animals.[11,24] Parasitism could be said to exist at three levels, those of infection, economic parasitism, and clinical parasitism.[10] The latter is a situation in which definite losses can be measured — death, weight loss, labored breathing, anemia, diarrhea, rough hair coat, etc. Only a small portion of parasitic loss is included in this category, most of the losses are economic. Economic parasitism is defined as that level of parasitism that prevents the host from reaching its genetic potential in growth or other measurable criteria. Economic parasitism may be influenced by many other factors, including the quality and abundance of feed, the competition for the feed, the age, sex, and breed of the host, and its acquired resistance to infection. Infection by parasites in numbers below the economic threshold are a reminder that the potential for disease is still there, but with adequate control will not reach economic levels. Infection by parasites is a normal part of the ecosystem. Ensuring that calves are exposed to infection in limited numbers may be ultimately advantageous to cattle because of immune system stimulation especially if the environment changes.

With most internal parasites, the degree of damage to the host is directly related to the number of parasites that have been able to establish an infection within the host. The level of infection is related to the susceptibility of the host and the exposure afforded from the environment. Acquired resistance to parasitic infection is related to the age, sex, and genetics of the individual animal and requires repeated exposure over several months to stimulate a protective immune response.[20] Resistance to nematodes will wane within a short period of time so exposure at a low level may be desirable to maintain resistance to infection.[17] Genetic variation within and among breeds of livestock indicate a tremendous heterogeneity of response to helminth antigens. Some efforts have been made to detect markers that could select those individuals that will mount an early strong immunity to important parasites in a geographic area.[1] Thus far, useful markers have not been identified in livestock. It could be said that the immunologic consequences of host-parasite interactions are characterized either as those that are damaging to the worm or those that expel the worm. Both phenomena may occur in an individual host concurrently. The damage done to the worm (stunting, decreased fecundity, movement to different areas of the intestine, or changes in acetylcholinesterase or other chemical constituents) appears to be species specific although expulsion may affect other species of helminths in the gastrointestinal tract.[1] Because worm expulsion is chemically mediated, not only will the target species be removed, but also bystanders in the local area.[17]

Even though the immune system will probably protect cattle from clinical disease (at least as adults), stocker cattle never live long enough to have gained solid immunity against the most important parasites of cattle in North America. Because young, rapidly growing animals are at risk (have little acquired immunity) and may be grazed under intensive management systems, economic parasitism becomes one of the major constraints in the efficient production of beef.

Where calves are concerned, control programs must then be directed toward the environmental level. The most obvious answer to controlling parasitic worms in the environment is to extirpate the free living stages from pastures. This is the case when small grain pastures are used for stocker grazing. The only parasites in small grain pastures, which have been turned and a seed bed prepared, are progeny of those present in the calves turned onto the pasture. Treatment 24 hours prior to releasing calves onto the pasture will successfully prevent the contamination of these pastures with larvae of parasitic worms.[10]

Rotation of pastures does not alleviate exposure to worms of livestock on the pasture. A pasture must be rested long enough to allow a die off of infective larvae, (60 to 180 days, depending on the time of year and the environmental condition). Infective larvae cannot replenish their energy reserves and as poikilotherms will expend energy in direct relation to ambient temperature. The higher the temperature the more rapid depletion of energy and subsequent death. Pasture management using rotational systems may increase the quantity of nutritious palatable forage and increased production per unit of area may occur, but this is due to increased nutritional intake, not fewer worms.

A pattern of larval transmission has been observed in various geographic regions of North America. An important factor in these observations are that all helminths do not follow the same epidemiologic pattern in all areas of the country. *Ostertagia ostertagi* is present in most of North America but in warm humid zones *Haemonchus placei* may be tremendously important in wet summers, and the lungworm *Dictyocaulus viviparous* can be devastating when susceptible cattle are exposed to the pasture during rapid forage growth.

Because *Ostertagia* is the most likely candidate to be the primary pathogen, programs designed to control this parasite may well suffice to largely control other species as well. *Ostertagia* has adapted to various areas in North America to avoid the most unfavorable times of the year when outside of the host, winters in the north and summers in the south. During these periods few eggs are deposited into the environment and fewer still will develop to the infective stage and escape the dung pat. The method of avoiding these inclement conditions is by that of hypobiosis or arrested development. Larvae picked up from pastures in the last month or so of the grazing season in the north and in the spring in the south, enter into a period of metabolic inactivity deep in the abomasal glands. While in the glands, little if any damage occurs to the host but it provides a refuge from winter cold and summer heat for the arrested larvae. The larvae are genetically programmed to resume development when conditions are again likely to be favorable for their development and survival on pasture. The development of many arrested larvae to the adult stage takes place within a short time span and many lead to clinical signs of type II ostertagiasis.[28]

If one cannot expose treated cattle to clean (or nearly so) pastures then treating during the period of hypobiosis of larvae is the most logical approach to controlling ostertagiasis.[23] Treatment with a suitable anthelmintic after the autumn grazing season in the north or during the hot, often dry summer in the south will concentrate the population of worms within the cattle and not on the pastures.[26] To be sure, some larvae will survive the unfavorable weather in the soil or dung pat, but will not be in great enough numbers to adversely affect cattle grazing those pastures later. However, there will be sufficient numbers to effectively reseed the pastures with infective larvae.

Strategic deworming in the summer in southern and in the winter in the northern United States should be done with all ages of cattle; adult cows, suckling calves (more than 2 months of age), and stockers. This may be combined with other procedures, i.e., treating for ectoparasites, cattle grubs, pregnancy examinations, vaccinations, implanting, etc. On permanent pastures in the southern United States, stocker calves will benefit from a three time program—going into the winter, early spring, and mid summer.[27]

Unfortunately, there are no good ways of examining cattle to determine whether they have an economic level of parasitism, so empirical treatment is used based upon the veterinarian's knowledge of conditions suitable for the propagation and survival of internal parasites in the local practice area. When calves are introduced from other areas they will bring with them the parasites of the region from which they originated. Treatment at the time of arrival should help relieve stress and prevent contamination of local pastures.

BLOAT

Bloat is a severe problem in both pasture and feedlot conditions. Bloat refers to excessive accumulation of gas in the rumen of cattle and is defined as rumen tympany. The gas that is formed in the rumen may be mixed with ingesta or may be free in the rumen. Development of bloat is related to many factors. Some of the factors are cytoplasmic proteins, plant pectins, development of mucinolytic bacteria, and gas production. Prevention in grazing cattle can be accomplished by increasing dry matter consumption or by use of surfactants.

Bloat has been associated with the mucinolytic activity of anaerobic bacteria. Salivary mucin is an antifoaming agent that aids in the prevention of bloat and is significantly reduced when animals are fed succulent forages such as wheat, clovers, or alfalfa. The content of the mucin activity in the rumen is further diminished and may permit stable bloat foaming organisms to form.

Growing plants contain considerable amounts of pectin and pectin methylesterase. Pectin methylesterase's function is to demethylate pectin. The activity is strongest during stages of rapid growth, when bloat tends to be more prevalent. Pectin methylesterase converts pectin to pectic acid and carbon dioxide. The pectic acid will bind with water and form a stable gel, which in turn may trap bubbles of carbon dioxide as a viscid froth. Increases of surface tension and viscosity in rumen fluid are physical factors that are associated with excessive foaming. The rumen content of cows with bloat may show an increase of *Streptococcus bovis*. Antifoaming agents may not change the number of *Streptococcus bovis*, but in many cases, do prevent bloat in cattle. Secondary bloat may be caused by an obstruction in the esophagus or in some part of the stomach that would allow an accumulation of gas leading to bloat.

Much research has been conducted on legume bloat, but the exact mechanisms that cause bloat have not been determined. There are many factors involved in the bloat syndrome that interact to produce bloat. The roles of volatile fatty acids changes, pH, and buffering capacity are not clear. There are conflicting results when pH is determined during bloat; however, pH tends to decrease during bloating from legume pastures. Volatile fatty acids tend to increase during bloating. There is no evidence that buffering capacity of the rumen changes during bloat. The chemical composition of bloat-inducing forages has been explored. Nitrogen soluble and insoluble fractions have been considered to be involved with bloat provocative pastures. Soluble nitrogen seems to be related to bloat since NH_4 is produced rapidly in the rumen and may be entrapped.

Wheat pasture provides an excellent forage for grazing stocker cattle and the numbers of stockers grazing wheat pasture have increased in past years. However, wheat pasture grazing is not without its problems and bloat is a major problem. There are several variables that are related to wheat pasture bloat such as highly fermentable forage, high amounts of soluble-nitrogen, and low dry matter intake. Table 1 illustrates the relationship of total protein, soluble protein, and nonprotein nitrogen (NPN). The NPN could contribute to the bloat, but studies that show a causative relationship to NPN have not been reported.

Table 1. *Nitrogen Composition of Wheat (Dry Matter Basis)*

MONTH	TOTAL PROTEIN %	SOLUBLE PROTEIN %	NONPROTEIN NITROGEN %
December	23.3	11.2	7.0
January	22.3	8.9	6.1
February	21.5	7.6	5.0
March	20.8	6.9	4.5
April	22.7	9.0	5.5
May	15.1	6.3	4.6

The best known prevention of bloat is poloxalene and the compound is cleared for the prevention of bloat. Poloxalene should be fed continuously at the rate of 1 to 2 g per 100 lb of body weight per day. The ionophore antibiotics, particularly monensin, have been shown to be nearly as effective as poloxalene in pasture bloat prevention. Monensin at a dosage of 0.66 mg per kg per day prevented clinical bloat on legume pasture.[2] The authors also found that for severely bloat provocative pastures, monensin combined with one-fourth to one-half the normal dose of poloxalene would give good protection. Regardless of the drug selected, bloat prevention is best when treatment is begun before exposure to the bloat-inducing pasture.

Increasing dry matter intake is another common practice used for cattle grazing bloat provocative pastures. This is accomplished in several ways, such as allowing grazing of bloat-inducing pastures with free access to corn stalks or other crop residue or dry hay. A method that tends to reduce the incidence of bloat in cattle grazing bloat provocative pastures is feeding of 1 to 2 lb of grain per head per day.

Bloat-inducing pastures tend to be highly productive pastures and present management problems that have to be solved to prevent bloat. Cattle that bloat and do not die are less productive than cattle that do not bloat when grazing these pastures.

CONCLUSION

It is fortunate that the management and medical measures effective in preventing ABPEE and bloat are similar because cases of ABPEE and bloat often develop on the same lush pastures if they contain legumes or *Brassica* spp.[25] The daily intake of monensin needed to prevent bloat in an adult cow over is 300 mg per day, which is higher than the usual dosage used to prevent ABPEE. This higher dose of monensin would result in greater inhibition of rumen production of 3MI. Prevention of diseases by medication that alters populations of rumen bacteria has promise for controlling many diseases of grazing cattle. The ionophores have potential for preventing other diseases that have the activity of gram-positive digestive tract bacteria as key factors in their pathogenesis, such as polioencephalomalacia and enterotoxemia, which are both associated with exposure to lush pastures. More work is needed to determine whether these speculative disease control benefits of ionophore supplementation occur in grazing cattle.

REFERENCES

1. Albers GAA, Gary GD: Breeding for worm resistance: a perspective. Int J Parasitol 17P:559–566, 1987
2. Bartley EE, Nagaraja TG, Pressman ES, et al: Effects of lasalocid or monensin on legume or grain (feedlot) bloat. J Anim Sci 56:1400–1406, 1983
3. Beck BE, Harries WN: The diagnosis of monensin toxicosis: A report on outbreaks in horses, cattle, and chickens. Proc 22nd Ann Meet Am Assoc Vet Diag 269–282, 1979
4. Blake JT, Thomas DW: Acute bovine pulmonary emphysema in Utah. J Am Vet Med Assoc 158:2047–2052, 1971
5. Blood DC, Radostits OM, Arundel JH, et al: Veterinary Medicine. Philadelphia, Baillière Tindall, 1989, p 1432
6. Breeze R: Respiratory disease in adult cattle. Vet Clin North Am - Food Animal Practice 1:311–346, 1985
7. Carlson JR, Hammond AC, Breeze RG, et al: Effect of monensin on bovine ruminal 3-methylindole production after abrupt change to lush pasture. Am J Vet Res 144:118–122, 1983
8. Ciszwski DK, Slocombe RF: Acute bovine pulmonary emphysema and edema. Comp Cont Ed 10:766–774, 1988
9. Cote FT: Rape poisoning in cattle. Can J Comp Med 7:38–41, 1944
10. Craig TM: Impact of internal parasites on beef cattle. J Anim Sci 66:1565–1569, 1988
11. Dunn AM: Veterinary Helminthology ed 2. London, William Heinemann Medical Books Ltd, 1978
12. Evans ETR: Kale and rape poisoning in cattle. Vet Rec 63:348–349, 1951
13. Hammond AC, Bradley BJ, Yokoyama MT, et al: 3-methylindole and naturally occurring acute bovine pulmonary edema and emphysema. Am J Vet Res 140:1398–1401, 1979
14. Heinemann WW, Heinemann HR, Russell TS: Implants, barley straw, and an ionophore for steers grazing turnips (research bulletin XBO942). Pullman, WA, Washington State University Agricultural Research Center, 1984
15. Heron BR, Suther DE: A retrospective investigation and random sample survey of acute bovine pulmonary emphysema in Northern California. Bov Pract 14:2–8, 1979
16. Mackenzie A, Ford JE, Scott KJ: Pasture levels of tryptophan in relation to outbreaks of fog fever. Res Vet Sci 19:227–228, 1975
17. Miller HRP: Gastrointestinal mucus, a medium for survival and for elimination of parasitic nematodes and protozoa. Parasitology 94:S77–S100, 1987
18. Nocerini MR, Honeyfield DC, Carlson JR, et al: Reduction of 3-methylindole production and prevention of acute bovine pulmonary edema and emphysema with lasalocid. J Anim Sci 60:232–238, 1985
19. Potchoiba MJ, Nocerini MR, Carlson JR, et al: Effect of energy or protein supplements containing monensin on ruminal 3-methylindole formation in pastured cattle. Am J Vet Res 45:1389–1392, 1984
20. Rothwell TIW: Immune expulsion of parasitic nematodes from the alimentary tract. Int J Parasitol 19:139–169, 1989
21. Selman IE, Allan EM, Gibbs HA, et al: The effect of anti-prostaglandin therapy on an acute respiratory distress syndrome induced in experimental cattle by the oral administration of 3, methylindole. Bov Pract 20:124–126, 1985
22. Smith JA: Acute bovine pulmonary edema and emphysema. In Smith BP (ed): Large Animal Internal Medicine. Philadelphia, CV Mosby Company, 1990, p 596

23. Suarez VH, Ciminari OE, Bedotti DO, et al: Epidemiology, effects and control of nematode infections on zebra crossbreed, Hereford, and Hereford × Brahman calves of Argentina's western pampas. Vet Parasitol 35:79–91, 1990

24. Thomas RJ: The ecological basis of parasite control: Nematodes. Vet Parasitol 11:9–24, 1982

25. Wikse SE, Leathers CW, Parish SM: Diseases of cattle that graze turnips. Comp Cont Ed 9:F112–F121, 1987

26. Williams JC, Corwin RM, Craig TM, et al: Control strategies for nematodiasis in cattle. Vet Clin North Am: Food Animal 2:(2)247–260, 1986

27. Williams JC, Knox JW, Marbury KS, et al: Three treatments with ivermectin in year-long control of gastrointestinal nematode parasites of weaner-yearling beef cattle. Vet Parasitol 33:265–281, 1989

28. Williams JC: Epidemiologic patterns of nematodiasis in cattle. Vet Clin North Am: Food Animal 2:(2)235–246, 1986

29. Wilson JS: Toxic myopathy in a dog associated with the presence of monensin in dry food. Can Vet J 21:30–31, 1980

Address reprint request to

Steven E. Wikse, DVM
Department of Large Animal Medicine and Surgery
Texas A&M University
College Station, TX 77843-4475

0749–0720/91 $0.00 + .20

Trace Element Deficiencies in Cattle

Thomas W. Graham, DVM, MPVM*

This and a companion article focus on the trace element and vitamin deficiencies that are most likely to occur in beef cattle. Properties, metabolism, and function of cobalt, copper, iodine, iron, molybdenum, manganese, selenium, and zinc are discussed. Each discussion of the nutrients includes the typical clinical parameters associated with deficiency, how to diagnose its adequacy/status, and forms of dietary and parenteral therapy available.

A nutrient is considered essential if its removal from the diet consistently interferes with an organism's ability to survive and reproduce. A nutrient becomes limiting or deficient when the dietary level is insufficient to meet performance goals or physiologic criteria. Dietary requirements are set to meet specific performance criteria such as maintenance, weight gain, reproduction, and lactation. Dietary requirements can be extended to include the level at which that nutrient performance is optimized. At this point, cost-benefit analyses are required to determine whether the levels fed are appropriate for a specific management regimen and are profitable.

Many nutrient requirements have not accounted for relatively new information that describes the effect of nutrition on immune function, and many of the requirements have not been evaluated in terms of optimal reproductive performance. Suggested dietary levels of the trace minerals are listed in Table 1. Deficiencies affecting immune function and reproduction are usually considered subclinical, but these deficiencies can lead to an increased susceptibility to infectious, parasitic, and metabolic diseases. While nutrient deficiencies or infectious/metabolic processes can independently impair maintenance, growth, and production, the combined effects can be doubly damaging. Thus, inability to recognize or respond to opportunistic or highly pathogenic organisms increases grossly apparent morbidity, as well as mortality.

---

*Assistant Veterinarian, Department of Nutrition, University of California, Davis; Davis, California

Table 1. *Current US Governmental Recommendations for Dietary Cobalt, Copper, Iodine, Iron, Manganese, Molybdenum, and Zinc for Beef Cattle*

	NATIONAL RESEARCH COUNCIL[311]	AGRICULTURAL RESEARCH COUNCIL[5]
Cobalt	0.07–0.11 mg/kg DM	
Growth	----------	0.08–0.11 mg/kg DM
Pregnancy	----------	Not available
Lactation	----------	Not available
Copper	4–10 mg/kg DM	
Growth	----------	8–15 mg/kg DM
Pregnancy	----------	13–20 mg/kg DM
Lactation	----------	8–14 mg/kg DM
Iodine	0.2–2.0 mg/kg DM	0.5 mg/kg DM, but increased to 2 mg/kg DM when goitrogens are suspected
Iron	50–100 mg/kg DM	
Growth	----------	100 mg/kg DM
Pregnancy	----------	40 mg/kg DM
Lactation	----------	30 mg/kg DM
Manganese	20–50 mg/kg DM	20–25 mg/kg DM
Molybdenum	Dietary requirement not established	Dietary requirement not established
Selenium	0.05–0.3 mg/kg DM	0.05–0.1 mg/kg DM
Zinc	20–40 mg/kg DM	
Growth	---------	26–35 mg/kg DM
Pregnancy	----------	13–21 mg/kg DM
Lactation	----------	18–31 mg/kg DM

Some of these effects have been considered in this and other reviews.[126,132,214,355,406]

Requirements of trace elements and vitamins for optimal reproductive performance have not been well characterized. Reasons for this include the fact that large scale trials are required to examine diseases of relatively low frequency. Thus, dose-response trials that evaluate the influence of trace elements and vitamins on factors such as cystic ovarian disease, services per conception, embryonic loss, abortion, and calving difficulty have not been fully examined because of the cost and labor involved. Instead, we must rely on associative evidence that has been obtained from epidemiologic investigations and case reports to begin to understand how individual nutrients can impair reproduction. Because these reports are often confounded by multiple deficiencies, toxicities, or concurrent disease, it is evident that additional research needs to be conducted on the roles of trace elements and vitamins on developmental processes, other than post-natal growth.[193]

Causes of nutrient deficiencies can be divided into primary and secondary deficiencies. Secondary deficiencies can also be called conditioned deficiencies. Primary deficiencies are those in which an inadequate dietary intake of that nutrient occurs. Secondary or conditioned deficiencies are those that occur because of impaired absorption, distribution or retention. Conditioned deficiencies occur because of pre-existing disease states that affect nutrient metabolism, or because of interaction between nutrients (Table 2). Both primary and secondary deficiencies occur in cattle, but deficiency of a single nutrient is unusual. This is because the conditions leading to soil deficiencies or deficiency of a nutrient in forages often are accompanied by simultaneous reduction of other related nutrients. Thus, when green forage is highly restricted or absent, vitamins A and E can become limiting nutrients in production. Similarly, in areas of high rainfall with acidic, well drained soils, multiple trace-element deficiencies are likely to occur. Even when a single nutrient deficiency occurs, the effect of this deficiency on normal gastrointestinal, hepatic, immune, renal, and other organ function often becomes impaired to the extent that it alters the requirements for other nutrients or impairs uptake, distribution, retention, or function. Because of this, a single nutrient deficiency can induce multiple, conditioned deficiencies. For example, high molybdenum and sulfur can induce secondary copper deficiency. Gastrointestinal transit time and mucosal transport of nutrients can be altered by the diarrhea associated with this molybdenum-sulfur induced hypocuprosis. Alterations in gastrointestinal transit and malabsorption can induce secondary deficiencies of protein and energy, as well as other select vitamins and trace elements. Similarly, a deficiency of vitamin A can inhibit normal epitheliogenesis, leading to squamous metaplasia. These mucosal changes can also induce diarrhea and a secondary malabsorption syndrome that can cause conditioned nutritional deficiencies. Table 3.

Because the rumen microflora produce water-soluble vitamins, deficiencies of this group of vitamins are less likely to occur in cattle than are deficiencies of lipid-soluble vitamins or trace elements. However, signs or symptoms of nutrient deficiencies can occur when antimetabolites and factors that degrade water- or fat-soluble vitamins are present because these factors antagonize the action of native vitamins or reduce the concentration of the vitamin. Thus, polioencephalomala-

Table 2. *Types and Examples of Interactions of Trace Elements and Vitamins**

Antagonistic	When one nutrient directly impairs the uptake, utilization/function or retention of another nutrient
	Excess calcium depresses zinc absorption[153]
	High dietary zinc reduces copper absorption[184]
	High dietary iron reduces zinc absorption[393]
	Supplemental folate depresses zinc absorption[246]
	Excess Vitamin E impairs Vitamin K utilization[254]
Synergistic	One nutrient can substitute for or enhance the function of another nutrient
	Vitamin E reduces the requirement for selenium[215]
	Zinc deficiency increases the Vitamin E requirement[246]
	Zinc deficiency impairs Vitamin A metabolism[246]
	Vitamin E acts as an antioxidant, sparing Vitamin A[254]

*Multiple interactions are probably more common than single nutrient interactions, but are much more difficult to characterize.

Table 3. *Principal Conditions and Signs Associated with Trace Element Deficiencies or Trace Element Responsive Disorders of Cattle*

Cobalt	Inappetance, weight loss, hepatic lipidosis, megaloblastic anemia, granulocytopenia, hypoglycemia, chronic wasting/ill thrift, ocular discharge, photosensitivity, immunosuppression
Copper	Immunosuppression, defective connective tissue metabolism (vascular anomalies, abnormal bone formation), achromotrichia, alteration in keratin sulfhydryl groups, growth failure, pancreatic atrophy, falling disease, enzootic ataxia (neuronal necrosis and wallerian degeneration), anemia
Iodine	Hypothyroidism, goiter, delayed and arrested development, variable alopecia, abortion, resorption, altered estrous cycles, weakness, and increased morbidity and mortality of affected stock
Iron	Microcytic, hypochromic anemia; reduced capacity for exertion; tachycardia; acidemia after exertion
Manganese	Small birth weights; limb and spinal deformities in newborn calves; weakness, incoordination, or paralysis in affected calves; increased services/conception; abortion; altered estrous cycles; seminal tubular degeneration
Molybdenum	Supplementation has increased cellulolytic activity and reduced rumen nitrite levels (decreased microbial nitrate reductase), but more commonly, high molybdenum is associated with induction of a secondary copper deficiency
Selenium	Skeletal and myocardial necrosis, immunosuppression, retained placenta, increased services/conception, abortion, weak and stillborn calves, diarrhea, reduced feed efficiency and weight gains, reduced conversion of T4 to T3
Zinc	Skin encrustations and fissures with bleeding (head and neck, teats/udder, foot/pastern, tail head), pruritis of the tail head, abortion, mummification, prolonged calving/uterine inertia, impaired vitamin A metabolism and immunosuppression, thymic hypoplasia/atrophy, marked decline in milk production and weight gain, and reduction in circulating insulin and growth hormone levels

cia occurs in calves fed excess amprolium (antimetabolite of thiamine) or in young and adult cattle ingesting lush feed or concentrate rations. The cause of this latter disease is idiopathic, but if treated early, many cattle respond well to thiamine administration. Water-soluble vitamins are not considered to be required for normal maintenance, growth or production in ruminants. However, improved performance has been noted in cattle supplemented with niacin and biotin.

In contrast to the negative interactions of nutrients, vitamin-vitamin, mineral-mineral, and vitamin-mineral interactions can be beneficial. Thus, vitamin E and selenium can reciprocally reduce dietary requirements for one another. When either vitamin E or selenium is marginally deficient and oxidant challenge would otherwise lead to nutritional myodegeneration (white muscle disease), the nutrient in moderate excess can reduce peroxidative damage and protect the calf from myodegeneration. Similarly, copper toxicity can be treated with supplemental zinc therapy, thereby reducing hepatic copper and increasing survival probability.

Range cattle are principally dependent on native forage for their nutrients. Parent soil type, rainfall patterns, drainage patterns, calcification, salinization, pH, forage type and availability, microbes present, organic matter, and land use will affect availability of trace elements to the plants and, thus, to the animals.[357,439] In feedlot or supplemented range cattle, quality and storage conditions for hay, haylage, silage or green chop can directly affect fat-soluble vitamins and increase the requirements for some trace elements.[183] Similarly, blocks, liquids, loose salts, and other nutritional supplements that alter normal nutrient ratios can lead to conditioned deficiencies by altering availability of nutrients. Minerals can complex with organic or inorganic components in the diet, altering intestinal uptake, transport or retention of other nutrients. Thus, the absolute amount and ratios of directly interacting trace elements will alter nutrient status and directly alter absolute requirements.

Recommendations of the National Research Council[310] and the Agricultural Research Council[5] can be used as guides for minimal requirements. See Tables 1 and 4. Bear in mind that these dietary guidelines were established for animals that are disease free. The highly interrelated nature of intercurrent disease and deficiencies or excesses of other nutrients can alter nutrient requirements and the tissue concentrations of nutrients, metabolites, or products that reflect status. Additional mineral or vitamin supplementation, above that of the National Research Council[310] and Agricultural Research Council[5] suggested dietary intake may be appropriate, but proper dietary and animal assessment is necessary before diagnosing a nutrient deficiency.

Table 4. Current US Governmental Recommendations for Dietary Vitamins A, D, and E for Beef Cattle

	NATIONAL RESEARCH COUNCIL[311]	AGRICULTURAL RESEARCH COUNCIL[5]
Vitamin A*		
Growth	2200 IU/kg DM	20 μg retinol/kg BW or 120 μg β-carotene/kg BW
Pregnancy	2800 IU/kg DM	30 μg retinol/kg BW/day or 180 μg β-carotene/kg BW/day
Lactation	3900 IU/kg DM	30 μg retinol/kg BW/day or 390 μg β-carotene/kg BW/day
Breeding Bulls	3900 IU/kg DM	Not available
Vitamin D†	250 IU/kg DM	0.1 μg/kg BW/day
Vitamin E‡	15–60 IU/kg	10–15 mg/kg DM if adequate selenium 15–28 mg/kg DM if selenium deficient

*1 IU of vitamin A = 0.3 μg retinol, 0.55 μg vitamin A palmitate, or 2.5 μg β-carotene.
†1 IU of vitamin D = 0.025 μg cholecalciferol.
‡1 IU of vitamin E = 1 mg dL-α-tocopherol acetate.

COBALT

Properties and Metabolism

Cobalt is a group VIIIA element that exists in animal tissues covalently bound in cobalamins (cobamides) and has an atomic weight of 58.9. Deficiency of cobalt, in cattle, induces a vitamin B_{12} deficiency because of an inability of rumen mircobes to synthesize adequate quantities of cobalamins. Thus, signs and symptoms of cobalt deficiency reflect defects in enzyme pathways requiring B_{12}. Active forms present in animal cells are methylcobalamin and adenosylcobalamin[392] and, in cattle, proprionate metabolism and methyl transfer are the principal biochemical functions that involve cobalt/B_{12}. Cattle are more susceptible to cobalt deficiency than are nonruminants, presumably because microbial sequestration reduces efficiency of absorption.[392] Iron and cobalt interact, and iron deficiency enhances cobalt absorption.[215]

In humans, absorption of B_{12} is mediated primarily by a complex of intrinsic factor and B_{12} in the ileum. Intrinsic factor is secreted by the parietal cells of the gastric mucosa, and diseases of either the gastric mucosa or ileum can cause pernicious anemia. Diseases of the bovine gastric mucosa or ileum have not been reported to cause pernicious anemia. Parasitic diseases in cattle, such as infestations with *Haemonchus spp.*, *Ostertagia spp.*, or *Trichostrongylus spp.*, and infectious diseases, such as Mycobacterium paratuberculosis (Johne's disease), could induce B_{12} deficiency if mechanisms of ruminant B_{12} absorption are similar to those in people. Thus, B_{12} deficiency may contribute to the pathogenesis of these diseases. However, in cattle infected with *Ostertagia ostertagia*, B_{12} concentration was not affected, even though liveweight gain was depressed in parasitized as compared with control steers.[255] Worm counts in this trial were low (100–800 adult *Ostertagia ostertagi*/calf). Thus, abomasal mucosal damage may not have been severe enough to alter intrinsic-factor release.

Function

Cobalt-activated reactions are thought to be limited to those pathways that contain B_{12}. In ruminants, gluconeogenesis and hemopoiesis are critically affected by cobalt deficiency, and carbohydrate, lipid, and nucleic acid metabolism are all dependent on adequate B_{12} and folate metabolism.[27] Regeneration of tetrahydrofolic acid is necessary for both purine metabolism and for the synthesis of choline. Regeneration of tetrahydrofolic acid is required for transfer of the formimino group of formiminoglutamic acid to tetrahydrofolic acid as one step in purine biosynthesis. Additionally, methyl transfer from 5′-methyl-tetrahydrofolate is required for the regeneration of tetrahydrofolic acid and methyl-B_{12} in the reaction catalyzing the conversion of homocysteine to methionine. This reaction is catalyzed by 5′-methyltetrahydrofolate-homocysteine methyltransferase and is integrally tied to regeneration of s-adenosyl-methionine for the production of choline. Glucose metabolism in ruminants is integrally tied to proprionate metabolism, which requires the molecular rearrangement of methylmalonyl-CoA to succinyl-CoA before entry into the tricarboxylic acid cycle for gluconeogenesis. This is catalyzed by the B_{12}-containing methylmalonyl-CoA mutase. Impairment of these two critical enzymes will increase methylmalonic acid, formiminoglutamic acid and reduce glucose, purine, and choline synthesis.

Assessment of Status

Deficiencies. Suggested dietary intakes of cobalt for cattle are listed in Table 1. Expected liver concentrations of cobalt in cattle range between 0.2 to 0.3 μg/g dry matter (DM) (3.4–5.1 nmol/g DM), and concentrations under 0.04 to 0.08 μg/g DM (0.68–1.37 nmol/g DM) are considered to be deficient.[426] However, determination of cobalt status is problematic because of the low concentration of cobalt in tissues. Mills[299] has recently reviewed indicators of cobalt status in ruminants and these are briefly summarized. Quantitation of plasma B_{12} concentrations can accurately discriminate between adequate and severely deficient cobalt status, but cattle have a large number of circulating cobalamins with low bioactivity.[157] Expected plasma concentrations of B_{12} in lactating dairy cows have been reported to range from 60 to 80 μg/mL (44.2–59.0 μmol/L),[268] which is much higher than those concentrations reported to be adequate for sheep (1–3 ng/mL; 0.74–2.21 nmoL/L).[426] Judson et al[205] reported that cobalt-supplemented calves and cows had an expected range of serum B_{12} from 0.12 to 0.27 ng/mL (88.53 to 199.2 pmol/l) and 0.1 to 4.0 ng/mL (73.78 to 2,951.2 pmol/l) respectively, which is similar to the sheep data. A decline in circulating B_{12} in cobalt supplemented and nonsupplemented lactating dairy cows has been reported to occur between the fourth and 28th week of lactation,[268] suggesting a physiologic effect of lactation. This may have important implications in the interpretation of plasma B_{12}.

There are many low activity cobalamins, and the validity of using plasma cobalamins as a reflection of cobalt status has been questioned. Carlos et al[77] have compared methods for determining vitamin B_{12} concentrations in cattle and discussed some of the problems with determining plasma B_{12} concentrations in bovine tissues. It has been suggested that metabolic intermediates of pathways requiring B_{12}, such as plasma methylmalonic acid and urinary methylmalonic acid or formiminoglutamic acid, better reflect physiologic adequacy. While criteria for defining cobalt adequacy based on plasma cobalamin and methylmalonic acid concentrations have been established for sheep, these criteria have not been as well defined for cattle.[299] Suttle[408] has recommended the following as a baseline for cattle. Plasma B_{12} is marginally deficient at 380 to 760 pmol/L and deficient when under 380 pmol/L. Liver B_{12} concentrations between 22 to 110 nmol/kg are marginal and deficient when under 20 nmol/kg. Plasma methylmalonic acid concentrations greater than 5 μmol/L are considered diagnostic of cobalt deficiency. As with most trace element deficiencies, response to supplementation (i.e., with cobalt or injections of B_{12}) is rapid and is considered diagnostic. Determination of urinary methylmalonic acid or formiminoglutamic acid concentrations is not considered to be of practical value in cattle at this time. Limitations of these procedures were recently discussed.[298]

Clinical Parameters. There is an initial period in B_{12} depletion when no changes in circulating B_{12}, methylmalonate or formiminoglutamic acid may be detected, but tissue B_{12} concentrations decline. MacPherson et al[255] have suggested that polymorphonuclear function can be impaired during the preclinical period (i.e., before anorexia and weight loss). This can predispose cattle to other infections and may contribute to the pathogenesis of cobalt deficiency, as has been suggested by Suttle.[411] Overt signs of deficiency are anorexia, impaired growth in young, weight loss, listlessness, diarrhea, and cachexia, often in the face of apparently adequate feed. Anemia and granulocytopenia occur late in the course of the disease and do not appear to make a marked contribution to its pathogenesis.[215,392] Typical necropsy findings include a marked wasting, a pale, fatty liver, and a mild normocytic, normochromic anemia.[219]

Two other conditions attributed to cobalt deficiency are ovine white liver disease and Phalaris staggers.[392] Ovine white liver disease is characterized by hepatic lipidosis and emaciation. Alteration in choline synthesis presumably leads to impaired lipid mobilization, but white liver disease may be complicated by other factors. Similarly, the persistent neural effects of *Phalaris spp.*, inducing Phalaris staggers, have been shown to be preventable with oral cobalt supplementation, but not with B_{12}. The mechanism by which oral cobalt supplementation prevents the neural symptoms of Phalaris staggers is not clearly understood. Auricular myocardial necrosis has been reported in cobalt-B_{12} deficient sheep.[303] Reduced activity of 5'-methyltetrahydrofolate-homocysteine methyltransferase presumably increased homocysteine concentrations, and elevated homocysteine has been associated with intimal injury, reduced platelet survival, and arterial thrombosis.

Dietary Sources and Fortification

Treatment of pastures with cobalt sulfate is practical in small, intensively managed systems, but it is impractical on extensive ranges. Reid and Horvath[357] have reviewed the soil conditions that affect cobalt metabolism in plants and animals. Granitic, calcareous, sandy soils and soils high in manganese are associated with cobalt deficiency. Supplementation of pastures with 500 to 600 g cobalt sulfate/acre/year maintains adequate levels, and pastures with greater than 1000 μg manganese/g soil will benefit from cobalt treatment.[4] Intraruminal boluses are the most convenient supplementation for range cattle, but they are not commercially available in the United States. Only small amounts of cobalt are required (1–2 mg/day), and soluble glass boluses,[101] cobalt oxide/iron boluses, trace element cements,[344] and cobalt glucoheptonate all appear effective in supplying adequate amounts of cobalt. An injection of vitamin B_{12} is critical for rapid correction of cobalt deficiency, and typical doses are in the range of 500 to 3000 μg/head, which may be repeated weekly.

If accidental oversupplementation is suspected, both calves and adult cattle may manifest signs of toxicity. In calves given intravenous cobalt the signs are salivation, lacrimation, dyspnea, incoordination, defecation, and urination.[401] Oral toxicity in adult cattle was marked by anorexia, reduced water consumption, incoordination, increased packed cell volume, and elevated hemoglobin and red cell counts.[401]

COPPER

Properties and Metabolism

Copper is a group IB element with an atomic weight of 63.5. Copper deficiency is a common disease of ruminants, both as a primary and a conditioned disorder. It impairs ruminant productivity extensively throughout the world. Molybdenum/sulfur-induced copper deficiency is well described, but excess iron, zinc, and calcium can also contribute to the development of hypocuprosis. Because of these interactions, dietary recommendations of the National Research Council[310] and the Agricultural Research Council[5] can only be considered guidelines, and hypocuprosis often occurs, even when estimated minimum requirements are provided. A variety of enzymes contain copper, and these enzymes are involved in energy, peroxide, connective tissue, amino acid, vitamin, and lipid metabolism.[95,215] Thus, signs and symptoms of copper deficiency are varied, and hypocuprosis can affect virtually all stages of growth and production.

Copper metabolism in ruminants has recently been reviewed, including specific discussions of molybdenum's role in hypocuprosis.[140,411] Usually, availability of dietary copper is less than 10%[408] and other dietary factors will further reduce copper absorption/retention. Copper thiomolybdates ($CuMoOS_3$ and $CuMoS_4$) are particularly responsible for antagonizing copper absorption in ruminants and, for this reason, dietary sulfur intake is also important in determining the degree of interaction. Stable complexes of copper thiomolybdates are insoluble and impair copper absorption from the gastrointestinal tract,[411] but absorbed oxythiomolybdates may be responsible for some of the systemic manifestations of secondary hypocuprosis, including infertility and growth failure.[57,189] Studies by Humphries et al[189] and Bremner et al[57] strongly support the idea that iron directly interferes with copper metabolism, but that the signs of copper deficiency are primarily manifested when calves are also fed excess molybdenum. Zinc can also induce copper deficiency, but it appears that the diet must be fed at a level that is only marginally adequate in copper.[148] Additionally, high dietary protein is associated with reduced copper availability and retention,[198] but this may also be related to the sulfur content. After gastrointestinal mucosal uptake, copper is carried to the liver, bound to albumin and histidine. Once in the hepatocyte, copper is transferred to metallothionein and metalloenzymes, retained in lysosomes, or excreted via bile.[140,215] Extrahepatic copper uptake is presumably mediated by the copper carrier protein, ceruloplasmin, and, to a lesser degree, albumin and histidine.[111] Once inside the cell, copper can again be stored on metallothionein, be available for copper activated reactions, or be incorporated covalently into proteins.

Function

Copper functions primarily in a catalytic capacity in enzymes, but alterations of protein and lipid metabolism that have not been characterized biochemically have been noted. Cytochrome oxidase is the copper dependent terminal enzyme in the electron transport chain, which is required for ATP production. Reductions in activity of this enzyme have been suggested to be one factor underlying the pathogenesis of enzootic ataxia in sheep.[121] While it has been argued that reduction in the activity of cytochrome oxidase could result in the neuronal necrosis, wallerian degeneration, and demyelination of enzootic ataxia, it is possible that reduced cytochrome oxidase is a consequence of degenerating and necrotic cells. Thus, metabolic lesions proximal to the loss of cytochrome oxidase may actually lead to degeneration and necrosis of neurons and oligodendroglia, which results in defects in mitochondrial enzyme function. Mechanisms of neonatal ataxia are still controversial,[278] but once neurologic symptoms appear they are presumably refractory to treatment.[215] Although neonatal ataxia has been reported in cattle,[371] it is an infrequent manifestation of hypocuprosis.

Bovine copper deficiency has been associated with immunosuppression. Reduced activity of cytochrome oxidase[52] and copper-zinc superoxide dismutase[22,203] has been suggested to reduce killing capacity of phagocytized organisms. Superoxide dismutase catalyzes the dismutation of superoxide to hydrogen peroxide, which is then metabolized to water and oxygen. Thus, with a reduction in activity, increased peroxidation of cellular constituents can potentially reduce cell viability or function. Reduced lymphocytic mitogen responsiveness in vitro is another suggested mechanism for enhanced susceptibility to infection associated with copper deficiency.[202,355,406] Immunoglobulin concentrations have been variably affected by copper deficiency,[355] but one report suggests that copper ions are required for optimal antigen-antibody interactions.[333] In the field, reduced lymphocyte responsiveness, antigen-antibody interaction, and phagocyte killing increase susceptibility to infection.[202,406] Mild copper deficiency has been associated with significantly greater mortality in mice challenged with *Pasteurella hemolytica*.[204] Thus, copper deficiency is associated with reduced responsiveness to antigens and increased susceptibility to bacterial infections.

Copper-deficiency induced anemia in cattle is inconsistent and only manifests after a prolonged course. The mechanism of impaired erythropoiesis is still poorly characterized. Many cases of copper deficiency are associated with chronic inflammation. Increased reticuloendothelial iron storage secondary to chronic inflammation[116-119] is one mechanism that can help explain a defect in erythrocyte production. Observed increases in tissue iron in the face of a microcytic hypochromic anemia suggest that intracellular iron mobilization is impaired during hypocuprosis. Similarly, copper-deficient reticulocytes are associated with reduced iron uptake and heme synthesis.[445] The observation that copper-deficient erythroblasts accumulate iron[139] helps substantiate the hypothesis that one mechanism involved in the anemia of copper deficiency is impaired intracellular iron mobilization. Williams et al[444] have suggested that heme synthesis is impaired within the mitochondria, before incorporation of iron into heme, and before export to the cytosol. Another mechanism that has been suggested to contribute to the anemia of copper deficiency in cattle was reported by Suttle et al.[405] In their experimental model of copper deficiency in lambs, they observed a Heinz body mediated anemia. The proposed mechanism for initiating the observed anemia was attributed to a reduction in copper-zinc superoxide dismutase activity. Reduced copper-zinc superoxide dismutase activity presumably resulted in an increased oxidation of hemoglobin and subsequent formation of Heinz bodies. Jain and Williams[199] have reported that copper-deficient rats have increased red blood cell fragility, viscosity, malonyldialdehyde adduct, and altered membrane lipid composition, which they have attributed to membrane peroxidation. They suggested that these changes result in reduced deformability of the erythrocytes, which increases splenic removal because of impaired erythrocyte sinusoidal transit. Hebbel and Miller[167] have demonstrated that treatment of human erythrocytes with malondialdehyde will promote macrophage erythrophagocytosis, but other mono- and dialdehydes failed to do so. Thus, malondialdehyde appears to have a specific biologic relevance to premature red cell destruction. These studies support the hypothesis that inflammatory conditions or a reduced capacity to metabolize oxidized products will promote the anemia of copper deficiency.

Abnormal sulfhydryl cross-linkage in keratin is characteristic of copper deficiency and results in weak and coarse hair fibers.[95] Similarly, abnormal collagen and elastin metabolism alters the integrity of connective tissue and is associated with reduced lysyl oxidase activity. Achromotrichia, or alteration in hair color, is associated with a reduced activity of tyrosinase and this impairs melanin synthesis. Another enzyme associated with copper metabolism is dopamine β hydroxylase, which catalyzes the oxidation of dopamine to norepinephrine. Reduction in norepinephrine levels is one mechanism by which hypocuprosis can alter cardiac and central nervous system function, but some of the observed reductions in activity may be structural loss of tissue, rather than alteration in enzyme kinetics. Additionally, dopamine and norepinephrine have been noted to be lower in whole-brain homogenates, but norepinephrine has been noted to be higher in the hypothalamus of copper deficient rats.[278] Other biochemical aspects of copper metabolism have recently been reviewed.[95,140,215]

Comparative effects of molybdenum, iron, and molybdenum/iron supplementation on copper status in cattle have been examined by Phillippo et al.[331] In this series of feeding trials, delayed puberty, altered estrous cycle length (occasionally leading to anestrous), cystic ovarian disease, impaired ovulation, and reduced conception rates were associated with molybdenum treatment, rather than copper deficiency per se. Iron treatment appeared to reduce the copper status to an equivalent level (3.9–5.2 μg copper/g liver DM; 61.37–81.83 nmol copper/g liver DM) as that of the molybdenum treatment (3.6–4.6 μg/g DM; 61.37–72.39 nmol copper/g liver DM), but did not cause the marked impairment of fertility associated with high molybdenum. The authors concluded that disturbances of luteinizing-hormone (LH) release were the cause of infertility and they documented lower pulsatile release during the cycle, as well as lower peak LH concentrations at ovulation. There is support for the concept that copper alters release of gonadotropin-releasing hormone from median eminence explants and that this process is dependent on chloride ions for activity.[28] Phillippo et al[331] have reported that repeated injections of copper (40 mg copper sulfate) did not correct molybdenum induced infertility in an experimental setting. Commercial beef cows, with a mean herd plasma copper concentration less than 0.3 μg/mL (4.7 μmol/L), were injected with 100-mg copper as copper calcium edetate and serially examined over a 3 year period.[332] No significant improvement in reproductive performance was noted in copper-supplemented cows as compared to control cows. In both of these experiments, the amount of systemic copper may have been insufficient to overcome chronically high dietary molybdenum, and trials examining the efficacy of oral copper supplementation for the treatment of excess molybdenum are needed. Thus, the roles of copper and molybdenum in bovine fertility need further clarification so that appropriate therapy can be designed. If it is molybdenum, per se, that directly causes molybdenosis, and it is not mediated via a secondary copper deficiency, then supplementation with tungsten may be a reasonable alternative for a direct antagonism of molybdenum. The safety and efficacy of tungsten treatment of antagonizing molybdenum has not been fully investigated, but it appears to be useful for prevention of nitrate poisoning (see molybdenum following).

Pancreatic acinar cell degeneration and apoptosis, resulting in acinar atrophy and fatty replacement, was noted in copper-deficient cattle.[120] It was anticipated that one mechanism of diarrhea associated with copper deficiency could be attributed to exocrine pancreatic insufficiency, but none of the cattle in this study developed diarrhea. If exocrine pancreatic function is altered during the course of hypocuprosis, then maldigestion could contribute to some of the alterations in feed conversion and weight gain discussed subsequently.

Assessment of Status

Deficiencies. Dietary recommendations of copper for cattle are listed in Table 1. Expected liver concentrations of copper for cattle range between 30 and 120 μg/g liver on a wet weight basis (0.47–1.88 μmol/g). Copper concentrations between 10 and 25 μg/g liver (0.15–0.39 μmol/g) are considered marginally adequate and deficient when less than 10 μg/g (0.15 μmol/g).[346]

Liver biopsy in cattle is a safe technique, but many producers are reluctant to allow this procedure to be performed on their animals. Additionally, field conditions in many beef operations make the technique less practical. For these reasons, blood constituents are more desirable, but still require interpretation. Claypool et al[83] have examined the correlation between 540 paired liver and plasma copper concentrations in beef and dairy cows and heifers. They concluded that plasma copper concentrations below 0.6 μg/mL plasma (9.4 μmol/L) indicate deficiency, but concentrations above this are not necessarily sufficient. Suttle[408] and Mills[299] have reviewed an approach to interpreting copper status in cattle, particularly deficiency. Both reviewers emphasized the limited use of plasma copper or ceruloplasmin, because both will increase with inflammatory disease. Suttle and McMurray[407] have suggested that erythrocyte copper-zinc superoxide dismutase activity can be useful for interpreting copper status, because it is copper activated and is correlated with duration of copper deficiency. Suttle[408] recommended that adult cattle that have an erythrocyte copper-zinc superoxide dismutase activity less than 2 U/g hemoglobin and plasma copper less than 0.2 μg/mL (3.1 μmol/L) are frankly deficient. Additionally, when erythrocyte copper-zinc superoxide dismutase activity is greater than 5 U/g hemoglobin and the plasma copper concentration is greater than 0.6 μg/mL (9.4 μmol/L), cattle can be considered adequate. The sensitivity and specificity of these tests for diagnosing copper deficiency are not established. Therefore, the number of false positive and negative tests is currently unknown.

Gooneratne and Christensen[142] recently reported maternal-fetal copper concentrations in cattle throughout gestation. Fetal liver copper concentrations were approximately 4 to 22 times higher than corresponding maternal levels, and fetal copper increased through gestation, while maternal levels declined. The authors stated that greater than 50% of these cows were copper deficient,[142] which limits the usefulness of these data. In previous work, Pryor[345] reported no variation in fetal liver copper concentration with fetal size, but did report a decrease in maternal liver copper through gestation. Importantly, both studies reported a positive correlation of fetal with maternal liver copper concentration, which strongly suggests that maternal copper status directly influences fetal copper status.

Clinical Parameters. Clinical signs and symptoms of copper deficiency may take as long as 170 days to appear[296] and are most severe when molybdenum is in excess.[57,189] Typical signs associated with copper deficiency have been described by Mills et al.[296] A summary of these conditions follows. A decline in both whole blood and liver copper concentrations preceded the manifestations of clinical deficiency by 100 days or more. Similarly, ceruloplasmin activity declined with whole blood copper. Liver iron concentration was higher in copper deficient cattle. In this experiment they noted alterations in gait manifested by various deformities, over extension of the flexor tendon, and epiphyseal exostosis of the metacarpophalangeal and carpal-metacarpal joints. Mechanistically, these changes would be compatible with alteration in activity of lysyl oxidase, a copper-dependent enzyme.

Reduced activity of tyrosinase, another copper-dependent enzyme, was responsible for the observed changes in coat color. In affected cattle, normally black hair was grey-brown, and eyes were encircled by grey hair. Increased feed intake per body weight gain and reduced weight gain were important in terms of production loss. An observed diarrhea may have contributed to both the increased feed to gain ratio and weight loss. Small intestinal villus atrophy was suggested as the cause of diarrhea, but the mechanism of villus atrophy was not documented. As discussed previously, Fell et al[120] suggested that exocrine pancreatic insufficiency may contribute to the pathogenesis of diarrhea associated with hypocuprosis. Myocardial hypertrophy and degeneration were noted at necropsy, and one animal died of a rupture of the vena cava. Alteration in elastin content of cardiovascular tissue may weaken vascular integrity and contribute to falling disease. Falling disease is a sudden death syndrome that occurs in copper-deficient cattle that has been attributed to alteration in cardiac function. In addition to defective connective tissue synthesis, reduced cardiac function can occur because of altered catecholamine levels[343] or increased elastin degradation by serum proteases.[365]

Reproductive dysfunction, manifested as alteration in estrous-cycle length, anestrous, increased services per conception, suspected early embryonic loss, and cystic ovarian disease, has been associated with copper deficiency, but may be caused by excess molybdenum per se.[331] Two additional syndromes associated with low copper concentrations in plasma and liver are polioencephalomalacia and abomasal ulcers. Gooneratne et al[140] have reviewed the evidence for these associations and possible mechanisms that could lead to the conditions. Briefly, polioencephalomalacia has been suggested to be induced by a three-way interaction of high dietary sulfur reducing thiamine concentrations, exacerbated by copper deficiency.[140,144,318] Affected animals in this case report[144] had plasma copper concentrations of less than 0.5 μg/mL (7.86 μmol/L), but the mechanisms of how copper could induce thiamine deficiency were not discussed. An association of abomasal ulcers and low hepatic copper concentrations has been reported in the Wyoming-Nebraska region. In this report, affected calves had much lower liver copper concentrations (45–48 μg/g DM; 0.71–0.76 μmol/g DM), than did unaffected calves (243–245 μg/g; 3.82–3.86 μmol/g DM) and the authors suggested that hypocuprosis was a factor in the cause of abomasal ulcers in calves.[241] Thus, evaluation of copper status is warranted when either polioencephalomalacia or abomasal ulcers are noted. This may help clarify the roles of copper in both disorders.

Dietary Sources and Fortification

As emphasized by Gooneratne et al,[140] prediction equations derived for estimating copper requirements have limited applicability and, in most cases, will require correction factors. As with other trace elements, monitoring the response to therapy with clinical evaluations, as well as follow-up samples, is recommended. This precautionary measure will aid in verifying a diagnosis, ensure efficacy of treatment, and prevent toxicity. Therefore, concrete recommended dosages are not currently appropriate, and follow-up examinations are critical. It is important to recall that seasonal and regional variation in copper, molybdenum, and sulfur will alter requirements. Thus, while the need for dietary copper will greatly exceed the recommended 10 μg copper/g when molybdenum concentrations are in the range of 10–15 μg/g, 10 μg/g will be sufficient if the molybdenum concentrations fall less than 1 μg/g.

Copper supplementation can be done parenterally or orally. Copper glycinate[47] is commercially available in the United States for subcutaneous use. Soluble glass boluses,[13] acid-base cements,[344] and copper oxide wires[73,409,410] are forms that can be administered periodically. Of these three oral products, only the copper oxide wires are commercially available in the United States. Addition of copper salts (i.e., copper sulfate or copper lysinate) to water supplies,[190] in blocks, liquid supplements, or complete rations have all been effective in correcting hypocuprosis. Additionally, application of 5 to 10 kg copper sulfate/ha has been shown to maintain adequate copper status on noncalcareous soils.[13,426] Typically, copper sulfate licks contain 0.5% to 1.9% copper sulfate for the prevention of copper deficiency.[426] Parenteral copper edetate has been associated with acute copper toxicosis and death in cattle.[46,66] Copper glycinate has been associated with abcessation and irritation at the injection site.[46] One recent report examining the comparative efficacy of copper oxide wires and copper glycinate injections concluded that 50 g of copper oxide was more efficacious in maintaining plasma copper concentrations than was a standard 120-mg dose of copper glycinate.[98] Typically, between 20 and 30 g of copper oxide wires are used for therapy. When rations are fed, daily additions of mineral supplements are included, and this allows for greater control of nutrient balance. Copper oxide is poorly available (<1%), copper sulfate is more soluble than the oxide form and more readily available (<10%), and the newer mineral chelates, such as copper lysinate, are designed to enhance absorption.

Copper toxicosis in adult cattle is rare, but has been reported in one cow ingesting a 200 μg/g diet.[43] Signs of copper toxicosis are most likely to occur in cattle that have received parenteral copper supplements rather than oral preparations, but young stock are susceptible to oral overdose of copper sulfate.[401] In calves, copper fed in excess of 115 μg/g has been associated with increased thirst, hemolysis, icterus, hepatic necrosis, hemoglobinuria, and death.[401]

IODINE

Properties and Metabolism

Iodine is a group VIIB halide that is critical for the synthesis of the thyroid hormones 3,5,3',5'-tetraiodothyronine (thyroxine; T4) and 3,5,3'-triiodothyronine (T3). Signs of iodine deficiency can be accompanied by grossly evident thyroid enlargement or goiter and, when extreme, by hypothyroidism. Ingestion of feed ingredients with low iodine concentration causes primary iodine deficiency, and secondary iodine deficiency can occur because of interfering substances called goitrogens.

Hemken,[170] Bustad, Fuller,[70] and Miller et al[289] have reviewed the metabolism of iodine in cattle. Iodine is efficiently extracted from the digesta and is primarily absorbed as iodide, but it can also be complexed to organic compounds such as amino acids or thyroxine. Approximately 70% to 80% of dietary iodine is absorbed by the rumen and another 10% from the abomasum.[29] In addition to absorption, the abomasum secretes large quantities of iodide, and the ability of the abomasum to concentrate iodide is much greater than for chloride.[29,279,280] Most of this secreted abomasal iodide is reabsorbed as it passes through the small intestine, but absorption takes place along the entire gastrointestinal tract.[29] Once absorbed, iodine can exist free in the blood as inorganic iodide, or it can be bound to proteins.[244,284] Iodine is efficiently and preferentially concentrated in the thyroid gland for the synthesis of T4 and T3. The only known physiologic function of iodine is as a component of the thyroid hormones, and iodine is primarily located in the thyroid gland. Other tissues also retain iodine, but at very low concentrations.[288]

An important aspect of iodine metabolism in domestic animals and humans is related to altered neural function induced by hypothyroidism during fetal life. Sheep have been used extensively as a model of cretinism, specifically to examine the mechanism of impaired fetal neural development. Placental thyroid-hormone transfer appears to be minimal, at least in women and ewes.[368] On the other hand, iodide is transported readily to the bovine fetus,[25,284] and thyroid function develops early in fetogenesis.[145,449] Fetal T4 is higher than maternal T4, and fetal T3 is lower than maternal T3 in many species, including cattle.[400]

Iodine is excreted primarily by the kidneys, with fecal and milk excretion minor routes of iodine loss. The proportions of dietary iodine lost are about 40% in urine, 30% in feces, and 10% in milk. Milk iodine is directly affected by dietary iodine and stage of lactation,[128,35] and transfer coefficients of iodine to milk are directly correlated to milk production.[90] Thus, milk can be a significant source of iodine loss in lactating cattle, particularly in high producing cows.[287,289] While simple iodine deficiency occurs in cattle,[114] hypothyroidism or exacerbation of the effects of low dietary iodine intake occurs when goitrogens are fed.

Goitrogens are compounds that interfere with the synthesis, processing, or release of the thyroid hormones and cause goiter.[70,130,174,232] Normally, a decrease in circulating T4 and T3 causes the basophilic thyrotrophs in the adenohypohysis to secrete thyroid stimulating hormone (TSH). After chronic stimulation by TSH, a hyperplastic and hypertrophic response by the follicular thyroid cells leads to thyroid enlargement and goiter. There are many naturally occurring and synthetic compounds that are goitrogenic or have antithyroid effects.

Three major groups of goitrogenic substances include thiocyanate and isothiocyanate, goitrins (L-5-vinyl-2-thio-oxazolidone) and aliphatic disulfides.[130,174] Cyanogenic glucosides are found in many feeds, such as beet pulp, cassava, corn, sweet potatoes, lima beans, soybeans, and millet. Once ingested, these cyanogenic glucosides can be metabolized to the goitrogenic compounds, thiocyanate and isothiocyanate. Progoitrins and goitrins are found in plants of the family cruciferae (rape, kale, cabbage, broccoli, cauliflower, turnips, mustard), and aliphatic disulfides are found in garlic and onions. The mechanism by which thiocyanate causes goiter is related to its ability to alter iodide transport across the thyroid follicular cell membrane, inhibiting thyroidal iodide retention and incorporation into tyrosine/thyronine.[108] Goitrin and, possibly, the aliphatic disulfides inhibit thyroperoxidase, which in turn prevents the formation of mono and diiodotyrosine.[108] Inhibition of peripheral T4 5'-monodeiodination will also cause goiter by blocking the normal T4 to T3 conversion. Additionally, glucocorticoids, estrogens, other antagonists of iodide transport, excessive iodine and lithium, and hypomagnesmia can affect thyroid hormone synthesis, release, or peripheral metabolism, and these factors have been reviewed.[130,232,308]

Typically, one type of goitrogen will predominate in a feed or ration, but there can be more than one goitrogen present. This is important because the goitrogenic effects of thiocyanates can be overcome by supplemental iodine, while iodine supplementation has no effect on the goitrogenic action of goitrin and aliphatic disulfides. When goitrin is identified as the primary cause of hypothyroidism, an alternate feed source must be used in order for the thyroid to regain normal function. Alternatively, exogenous T4 or T3 can also correct the defects induced by many goitrogenic agents. Corn silage, soybean, and other feeds containing cyanogenic glucosides are commonly fed to cattle.[168,169] Thiocyanate is a common cause of goiter that also affects cattle.[283,285] When potentially goitrogenic feeds are grazed or are used in a ration, cattle should be monitored for signs of hypothyroidism, and identification of the source of thyroid impairment will be required before appropriate therapy can be started.

Function

Iodine is integrally related to thyroid hormone production, and recent reviews have examined the regulation and synthesis of the thyroid hormones.[174,258,341,369] Thyroglobulin is a protein dimer that contains tyrosine residues for the synthesis of the two thyronine hormones, T4 and T3. A hypothalamic–pituitary feedback loop controls the concentrations of circulating T4 and T3. Thyroglobulin synthesis, posttranslational modification, and release of T4 and T3 are controlled by the pituitary hormone thyrotropin (TSH). Release of TSH is primarily regulated by thyrotropin releasing hormone (TRH), somatostatin, and T4 and T3. Normal thyroid function is dependent on an adequate iodine supply, and iodine is efficiently removed from blood by the follicular cells of the thyroid.[53,76] After TSH binds to its thyroid follicu-

lar cell receptor, TSH activates adenylate cyclase, resulting in cAMP
release. Release of cAMP is the intracellular signal that activates the
cell. Follicular cell stimulation results in an increase in T4/T3 synthesis
and release.[136,326] The mechanism of iodide transport is active and
requires an ATPase driven sodium-potassium transporter.[220,221] Once in
the follicular cells of the thyroid, iodide is transported to the follicular
lumen where thyroperoxidase catalyzed oxidation occurs.[6,258,341,414]
The mechanism of iodide oxidation is similar to that described for
myeloperoxidase. This is discussed in the section on iron. In part, the
activity of thyroperoxidase is controlled by TSH.[341] In the follicular
lumen, highly reactive iodine will bind to tyrosine groups on the thyroglobulin molecule to form monoiodinated (MIT) and diiodinated tyrosine (DIT). Further oxidation couples the MIT and DIT to form T3 and
T4, the active thyroid hormones.[258] After iodination, and in response to
TSH, the follicular cells begin pinocytosis of lumenal thyroglobulin.
Lysosomal fusion with the endocytic vacuole, and subsequent proteolysis, result in release of amino acids, T4 and T3. After diffusion of T4 and
T3 into the capillaries surrounding the follicle, the thyroid hormones
are carried into the systemic circulation.[242,369]

Both T4 and T3 are lipophilic hormones that circulate in blood
bound to thyroxine binding protein (TBG, 70%), thyroxine binding
prealbumin (5%–20%), albumin (10%–25%), and other proteins.
Transthyretin is a protein complex (2.5:1) of the vitamin A binding
protein, retinol binding protein, and thyroxine binding prealbumin.[352]
A kinetic model of thyroid hormone metabolism has been reviewed,
and this model is based on the hypothesis that only protein free T4 and
T3 are available for cellular uptake.[276] In cattle and many other mammals,[313] the concentration of free T4 and T3 is several times less (0.03%
and 0.3% respectively) than proteinbound T4 and T3.

The actions of thyroid hormone are regulated by an intracellular
receptor that has a 10-fold greater affinity for T3 than T4,[96,421] and the
concentration of T3 is regulated by T4 5'-monodeiodinase. Monodeio-
dination of T4 to T3 and reverse T3 (rT3; 3, 3', 5'-triiodothyronine) can
occur in the liver, which can then secrete T3 back into the plasma, or
T4 is deiodinated within the target cells in the periphery.[336,352] Activity
of the thyroid hormones is T3 > T4, and rT3 is presumably nonfunctional. Chromatin associated nuclear T3 receptors bind T3, and these
DNA binding proteins are related to the erb A oncogene family of
proteins. The erb A proteins contain 7 to 11 zinc atoms per molecule
and bind steroid hormones, retinoids, and T3 to affect cell division,
growth, maturation, and maintenance.[97,137] Zinc can affect binding of
T3 to its receptor, and this is briefly discussed in the section on zinc
function. It is by this interaction of T3 with its nuclear receptor that
thyroid responsive nuclear elements are activated and that T3 affects
cell function.

Thyroid hormones affect virtually every organ at some stage of
development, growth, or maturation. The effects of thyroid hormone
are organ specific, but generally, increased lipolysis, glycolysis, cardiac
function, cardiac output, oxygen consumption, and metabolic rate are

observed when circulating concentrations of T4 and T3 are high. Additionally, epithelial maturation, reproductive function, bone development, and embryo/fetogenesis are critically affected by thyroid status. Iodine deficiency is also one of the few well described human teratogens. Iodine deficiency and goitrogens can induce a hypothyroid state that is characterized by reduced basal metabolic rate, muscle weakness, reduced growth, decreased cardiac output and reduced myocardial contractility, alterations in skin and hair formation, and reduced apocrine secretions.

It is important to recall that lactation and environmental temperature affect circulating thyroid hormone concentrations, and this can influence interpretation of laboratory results. Nonlactating cattle have relatively stable concentrations of T4 and T3,[3] and lactating cows have less circulating T4 and T3 than nonlactating cows. Additionally, milk production is proportional to T4 release.[394] In response to environmental changes outside the thermal neutral zone, lactating cows have more widely fluctuating rT3/T4 and T3/rT3 ratios than nonlactating cows.[3] It can be anticipated that the rT3/T4 ratio will decline, and the T3/rT3 ratio will rise in response to heat or cold.[3] As lactation progresses, T4 and T3 levels will increase,[7,313] and the ratios of T3/T4, rT3/T4, and T3/rT3 will consistently decline through lactation.[7] Normal T4 concentrations are 62 to 75 nmol/L; normal T3 levels are 1.3 to 2 nmol/L; normal rT3 levels are 0.25 to 0.60 nmol/L; the expected ratio of T3/T4 is 0.03; the ratio of rT3/T4 is 0.004 – 0.13; and the ratio of T3/rT3 is 2 to 8.[3]

Other uses of iodine in cattle are as a preventative for infectious pododermatitis (foot rot),[34,249] as an antiseptic for external wounds, as a treatment for *Actinobacillus lignieresi* (woody tongue), as a uterine infusion for treatment of endometritis, and to induce uterine release of $PGF_{2\alpha}$ for the purpose of altering estrous cycle length. These uses are not related to dietary essentiality, but can contribute to the total iodine stores in the animal.

Assessment of Status

Deficiencies. Suggested dietary concentrations of iodine are listed in Table 1. The recommended dietary concentrations (0.2 – 2 mg/kg) correspond to a daily iodine intake of about 2.7 to 27 mg/animal/day, assuming a dietary intake of 13.6 kg dry matter/day. The range of dietary iodine intake considered safe is relatively narrow. Dietary iodine intake less than 7 mg/animal/day has been associated with iodine deficient goiter,[8] and iodine toxicity has been noted in cattle fed in excess of 68 mg/animal/day.[320] Goitrogens, such as thiocyanate, will increase the requirement for iodine. Supplementation of iodine in these cases would require dose-response evaluations, including monitoring for signs of iodine toxicosis (see clinical parameters). For lactating dairy cattle, the combination of feed additives and sanitizing products can increase the iodine content of milk to levels that are unacceptable for its use as a product intended for human consumption.

Milk is a significant source of iodine for the human population, and thyrotoxicosis from excess iodine can occur.[127] Thus, the public health aspects of iodine supplementation for cattle must be kept in mind when altering dietary levels.

Dietary iodine intake is correlated to both serum (r = 0.81) and milk (r = 0.66) iodine concentration.[35,248] Thus, evaluation of serum and milk are useful tools for determining the iodine status of cattle. Total serum iodine in the range of 10 to 40 μg/dL (787.99–3151.98 nmol/L) appears to be adequate and less than 5 μg/dL (393.98 nmol/L) appears to be deficient.[10,38,346] It can be anticipated that, when the dietary intake is less than 7 mg/animal/day, milk iodine will fall below 20 μg/L (157 nmol/L), and cattle will be at risk for developing goiter.[8] Milk iodine was associated with goiter when less than 10 μg/L (78.8 nmol/L), but goiter was not commonly observed when milk iodine was greater than 20 μg/L (157 nmol/L).[39] Others have recommended that milk iodine in the range of 30 to 300 μg/L (236.4–2363.98 nmols/l) appears to be adequate and deficient when less than 25 μg/L (197 nmol/L).[346] The dairy industry has imposed a maximum allowable iodine content of 500 μg/L (3939.97 nmol/L), and Berg et al[35] have evaluated the effect of dietary ethylene-diamine-dihydoriodide (0–45 mg/animal/day) on milk iodine concentration. Dietary iodine in excess of 25 to 30 mg/animal/day can cause the milk iodine concentration to exceed 500 μg/L (3939.97 nmol/L).

Thyroid weight can be used as an index of congenital goiter, and the log-log relationship between fetal crown to rump length and thyroid weight is linear.[312] Comparing thyroid weights of goitrous calves[10] with thyroid weights from fetal calves collected at slaughter[312] suggests that a two-fold increase in thyroid weight is diagnostic of goiter. At term, thyroids should weigh 6 to 6.5 g.[312,449] Histology of the thyroid gland can be another useful tool for diagnosing hypoiodinism.[10] Hyperplastic and colloid goiter are commonly associated with low dietary iodine or goitrous feeds, but iodine excess can also induce thyroid hyperplasia.[75] Thus, both feed and tissue chemical analyses, along with anatomic pathology, are required to substantiate the diagnosis of goiter and to correctly diagnose the cause. A confounding factor in the diagnosis of endemic goiter is a hereditary congenital goiter of Afrikander cattle, but these calves typically lack colloid in the follicular lumen.[324] The genetic defect is a nonsense mutation in which a cytosine is replaced by thymine. This mutation creates a stop codon, and only a partial thyroglobulin molecule is translated.[361]

Clinical Parameters. Good experimental descriptions of acute, subacute and chronic effects of iodine deficiency for both sexes of cattle at each successive stage of development are not readily available. Most of the experimental models in ruminants have been developed in sheep. However, there are case reports that compared the effects of iodine administration in cattle with unsupplemented controls. A hallmark sign of bovine iodine deficiency is reduced fertility, including cessation of estrous, irregular interestral intervals, higher first service conception rates, abortion, retained placenta, and birth of stillborn or weak, goitrous, and sometimes hairless calves.[10,114,207,302,436,437] Cattle may be less susceptible to iodine deficiency than are horses, pigs, sheep, or goats,[114,207,436] and this may explain the relative paucity of information regarding iodine deficiency for cattle.

There is a seasonal pattern of iodine deficiency, and a seasonal change in iodine content of the thyroid was noted in beef cattle at slaughter. Summer and fall thyroid iodine concentrations were higher than values derived from thyroids obtained in the winter and spring.[114] Newborn goitrous calves born during cold weather are more likely to die than are nongoitrous calves, but in good weather most affected calves survive.[207,436] Affected calves can have hemorrhage and edema around the thyroid, and many calves have a clearly visible jugular pulse.[207] Some goitrous calves will show symptoms of respiratory difficulty and grow poorly compared to calves without goiter, but a majority of affected calves appear normal at 8 to 10 months.[436] Myxedema is another manifestation of hypothyroidism that can accompany iodine deficiency in sheep, goats, and pigs. Myxedema is an edematous condition of the connective tissues that is not commonly reported as a sign of hypothyroidism for cattle, but does occur in goitrous, hairless calves.[436] These myxedematous calves are either born dead or die soon after birth.[207,436]

An autosomal recessive trait in Afrikander calves is associated with goiter, respiratory difficulty, pica, and a predisposition to osteoporosis.[379] The initial descriptions of this inherited goiter indicated that thyroid enlargement would develop after birth and that calves grew poorly.[265] Thus, while the causes of the iodine-deficient and inherited forms of goiter in cattle differ, manifestations of the two disease states appear similar.

Thyroidectomy has been associated with absence of libido in bulls, and bulls with poor breeding performance have been noted to have increased sexual function after thyroprotein supplementation.[260] In people, hypothyroidism can be accompanied by an increase in prolactin secretion and mild hypogonadism. Whether reduction in libido and alteration in prolactin is commonly manifested in iodine-deficient bulls needs to be assessed, but if iodine deficiency is diagnosed in calves, it can be assumed that iodine supplementation of all breeding stock is warranted.

Cretinism is common in lambs born of severely iodine-deficient ewes. This has been used as a model of iodine deficiency or goitrogen-induced cretinism in humans.[175,259,272,273,337,338] Impairment of neuroblast migration and myelination results in anatomic and functional impairment of the cerebellum and cerebrum. Additionally, lower birth weight, brain mass, cell number per mg DNA, and protein/DNA ratios were observed in iodine deficient compared to control lambs. Cretinism is not commonly recorded as a manifestation of iodine deficiency in calves.

Dietary Sources and Fortification

Because iodine is readily absorbed, most sources of iodine are adequate for supplementation. Thus, sodium and potassium iodide, calcium iodate, pentacalcium orthoperiodate, and EDDI are useful for increasing iodine stores in cattle. Pentacalcium orthoperiodate may be preferred when mineral blocks are used because of volatilization of iodine with subsequent loss to the atmosphere or leaching from the blocks when the other forms of iodine are used.[14] Injectable forms of iodide (400 mg) are efficacious for alleviation of iodine deficiency in sheep.[18,259,338] Volatilized iodine appears to alleviate signs of iodine deficiency in cattle,[302] and topical forms of iodine, including the organic soaps and disinfectants, can be absorbed.[127] When total dietary iodine intakes exceed 50 mg/animal/day, routine examination of cattle for signs of iodine toxicity should be made. Signs and symptoms of iodine toxicity include pneumonia, increased mortality, reduced milk production, hyperthermia, nasal and lacrimal discharge, salivation, coughing, and dry, scaly, unthrifty coats.[320] In contrast to humans, cattle do not appear to be highly susceptible to iodine-induced thyrotoxicosis.[238] When each animal was fed 1250 mg of iodine, decreased T4 and T3 secretion was observed. This reduction in thyroid hormones has been observed with excess lithium and iodine.[104,130,396]

IRON

Properties and Metabolism

Iron is a Group VIIIA element required for normal heme synthesis. Iron deficiency is one of the most common nutritional disorders in human populations. Iron is ubiquitous in the environment, and because cattle normally ingest large quantities of iron as forage and soil, iron deficiency in adult cattle is rare.[426] When iron deficiency occurs, it can usually be attributed to blood loss. Thus, infections with organisms such as *Haemonchus spp.*, *Bunostomum spp.*, and *Eimerias spp.*, or infestations of biting flies, ticks, and sucking lice can cause significant reductions in iron stores. Similarly, abomasal ulcers and coagulation disorders will result in blood loss and can lead to iron deficiency. In contrast to the relatively rare occurrence of iron deficiency in adult cattle, an induced iron deficiency occurs from feeding milk for commercial veal production.

The metabolism of iron has been reviewed.[122,188,305,389] Similarly, aspects of iron kinetics in cattle have been examined.[160,208-210] Iron homeostasis appears to be controlled by altering intestinal uptake of iron[269,443] with only slight alterations in excretion. Ingested iron exists primarily as oxidized Fe^{3+} (ferric) and is poorly absorbed. Complexes with organic and inorganic compounds can inhibit iron uptake. Exceptions to this are hemoglobin and transferrin.[122] After reduction of inorganic Fe^{3+} to Fe^{2+} (ferrous), iron is taken up by mucosal enterocytes of the duodenum and bound to proteins. Mucosal ferritin and transferrin bind iron, and transferrin contributes to the regulation of iron release into the portal blood. Additionally, when iron stores are adequate to high, enterocytes can accumulate iron-ferritin, and this is lost in the course of normal cell turnover. Factors increasing the reduction of ferric to ferrous iron or enhancing its solubility will favor mucosal uptake. Thus, the acid pH of the abomasum, vitamin C and other organic acids, "meat factor," and various amino acids will enhance mucosal transport of iron. The "meat factor" has not been identified, but iron uptake has been reported to be enhanced above that predicted by the iron concentration when meat is ingested. High intakes of zinc, copper, cobalt, cadmium, manganese, and phosphorous can depress iron absorption. Once iron has been transported across the basolateral membrane to the portal blood it is available for distribution to the major iron containing tissues — bone marrow, liver, and muscle.

Iron uptake from the intestine and within cells can be regulated by the number of externalized transferrin receptors on cell membranes. Cellular storage forms of iron are ferritin and hemosiderin. When bound, iron is prevented from undergoing oxidation reduction cycling with other cellular constituents. The binding of iron prevents free iron catalyzed oxidative destruction of structural and functional components within the cell.[49] In addition to the storage proteins, oxygen carrying and catalytic iron proteins include hemoglobin, myoglobin, cytochrome oxidase, cytochrome P-450 enzymes, peroxidase, and catalase. In plasma, iron is bound to transferrin, and this complex can then bind to membrane transferrin receptors for endocytosis and release within cells. After endocytosis, the iron is released within the endocytic vacuole, then retroendocytosis of transferrin releases transferrin back to the blood for further iron binding and transport. Low concentrations of plasma ferritin also circulate and can reflect tissue iron stores. Iron transport from maternal plasma to the fetus appears to be efficient.[142,186] However, reports of iron deficiency anemia in neonatal calves suggests that utero-placental iron transport can be inadequate for some fetal tissues. Iron deficiency in neonatal calves appears to be relatively common, but will quickly respond if the animals are raised with access to soil or forage, or are given iron supplements.[270,348,350,416]

Iron excretion is limited in all species, but small amounts are lost in feces and urine. The majority of iron is continually recycled by phagocytosis and catabolism in macrophages.[200] Thus, as senescent erythrocytes are removed in the spleen, hemoglobin is degraded in macrophages to free heme, globin, and iron. The heme portion is degraded to biliverdin and then to bilirubin for excretion. The globin is degraded to amino acids, and iron is stored as ferritin or transported to the bone marrow for erythropoiesis. When extravascular hemolysis occurs, free hemoglobin is bound to haptoglobin and removed by the macrophages in the liver, spleen, and marrow, or it is converted to methemoglobin and then to hematin. Hematin then binds to hemopexin or albumin and is removed primarily by the liver. Iron is again released for reutilization, and heme is metabolized for excretion in the bile.

Function

All cells require iron for synthesis of components of the electron transport chain enzymes, including cytochrome oxidase, which generate the high energy phosphate bonds of ATP, GTP, etc. Other heme-containing enzymes requiring iron are the cytochrome P-450 isozymes, involved in degradation or metabolism of endogenous and exogenous compounds, and myeloperoxidase and catalase. Myeloperoxidase reduces hydrogen peroxide and chloride to hypochlorous acid and water, and catalase reduces hydrogen peroxide to water and oxygen. There are a number of non-heme–containing, iron catalyzed or iron-containing enzymes, such as succinate dehydrogenase and nicotinamide adenine dinucleotide dehydrogenase, which are key enzymes in the citric acid cycle and for energy transfer.[91] However, oxygen-carrying hemoglobin is the largest pool of iron, and myoglobin is also critical for normal aerobic muscle function. Thus, an obvious critical role for iron is in oxygen related energy metabolism.

Iron is equally important to many infectious organisms, such as bacteria and protozoa. Bacteria release siderophores for iron chelation, sequestration, and subsequent use for growth. It has been proposed that secretion of lactoferrin in milk and reduced plasma iron, noted during the acute-phase response, decrease the available iron for bacteria during infection.[243] Others have argued that the affinity of siderophores for iron is low compared with transferrin, but iron will be removed slowly from transferrin. In contrast, intracellular iron is readily mobilized by siderophores for bacterial use.[61] Milk lactoferrin will inhibit microbial growth,[61] but its essential role may be to enhance intestinal iron uptake. Specific lactoferrin receptors have been identified on intestinal brush border membrane preparations from Rhesus monkeys,[92,93] and these may facilitate delivery of iron while lactoferrin sequesters iron from bacteria.

An important aspect of iron deficiency is related to immunodeficiency.[37,91,126,385] Marked impairment of phagocytic myeloperoxidase activity has been proposed as one mechanism of iron deficiency induced reduction in phagocytic killing.[37] Myeloperoxidase is critical for oxygen dependent killing in phagocytes. This system uses oxygen and NADPH, generated by the hexose monophosphate pathway, to produce superoxide. The reaction is catalyzed by NADPH oxidase. Superoxide dismutase or Fentonlike reactions can generate hydrogen peroxide. Hydrogen peroxide and halides (Cl, B, I) combine quickly when catalyzed by myeloperoxidase and generate halide acids.[26] Hypochlorous and other acids, produced during the respiratory burst in phagocytic vacuoles of neutrophils and monocytes, are potent oxidizing agents. These oxidants severely damage bacterial cell walls and cause lysis or expose cell wall constituents for further degradation by enzymes. The host is also vulnerable to these oxidant species, and tissues are partially protected by copper-zinc and manganese superoxide dismutase, catalase, glutathione peroxidase, and vitamins E and C.

Specific antibody response has been noted to be depressed, but immunoglobulin concentrations and response to antigen challenge generally appear to be normal during iron deficiency. Susceptibility to parasitic and infectious agents is higher in cases of iron deficiency, and one mechanism for this increase in morbidity can be attributed to depression in cell mediated immunity.[37,91,385] Reduced sensitivity of T cells to in vitro stimulation tests, depressed killer cell activity, and decreased cutaneous hypersensitivity reactions have been proposed as some of the mechanisms involved in iron deficiency induced immuno-suppression. Greater morbidity and mortality are the result of depressed immunity, as has been noted in cases of iron deficiency in humans, rodents,[37,385] and cattle.[68,304,375] Increased morbidity and mortality have been observed even when there was no effect on packed cell volume.

Assessment of Status

Deficiencies. Plasma and liver can be used as indices to determine iron status. Quantifying plasma iron concentration, total iron binding capacity, and plasma ferritin concentration will allow for estimation of stored intracellular iron. Bone marrow iron, erythrocyte protoporphyrin, tissue non-heme iron, and ferrokinetic studies are other useful methods for estimating iron status, and these techniques were reviewed by Smith.[389] Additionally, liver iron concentrations can be useful for estimating stored iron. When deficiency is prolonged, hemoglobin concentration, packed cell volume (PCV), mean corpuscular hemoglobin (MCH), mean corpuscular hemoglobin concentration (MCHC), and mean corpuscular volume (MCV) can be used to help determine the iron status of the animal. These indices can also help differentiate the cause of anemia because chronic disease and other intercurrent nutrient deficiencies differentially affect these parameters.

Liver iron concentrations between 45 and 300 $\mu g/g$ (0.806–5.37 $\mu mol/g$) wet weight are considered adequate, and liver concentrations less than 30 $\mu g/g$ (0.537 $\mu mol/g$) wet weight are deficient.[346] Liver biopsy is a useful tool, and distribution of iron in the liver is fairly uniform.[1] Plasma is more desirable, because collection is easier and less invasive. Plasma iron falls immediately after birth and then increases to a range of 130 to 350 $\mu g/dL$ (23.28–62.67 $\mu mol/L$) as cattle mature.[301,346,438] Total iron binding capacity, a measure of plasma transferrin concentration, is approximately 300–700 $\mu g/dL$ in adult cows.[129,426] When expressed as percent saturation, calves on typical diets increase the saturation of transferrin from 16.8% at birth to 34.6 to 52%, but milk-fed calves have only 11% or less saturation.[438] Total iron binding capacity increases after birth from 300 to 500 $\mu g/dL$ and then declines.[301] Total iron binding capacities for adult cattle range between 250 to 350 $\mu g/dL$.[129] Expected concentration of ferritin in cows is 35–40 ng/mL,[129] but Puls[346] has suggested a range between 30 and 50 ng/mL. When TIBC is used in conjunction with plasma ferritin concentration they can reflect iron status in adult cattle and calves.[129,301]

Physiologic factors affecting plasma iron, TIBC, and ferritin concentrations are inflammation and pregnancy. Plasma iron and total iron binding capacity decline during the periparturient period and then return to previous values.[129] Pregnancy causes a marked increase in plasma ferritin at the time of delivery, which persists for 4 to 8 weeks after parturition.[129] Plasma iron concentrations initially increase and rapidly decrease in the acute phase of inflammation.[147,243] Chronic inflammation can block iron mobilization. The anemia of chronic disease and the effects of chronic disease on iron metabolism have been discussed by Feldman and colleagues.[116-119] Thus, interpretation of measures of iron status must be based on a complete evaluation of the disease and physiologic state of the animal.

Anemia occurs late in the course of iron deficiency, but is a useful sign for diagnosis of inadequate iron status. In calves, hemoglobin (10.2 g/dL at birth) and erythrocyte numbers ($7.72 \times 10^6/\mu L$ at birth) typically increase during the first 15 to 16 weeks after birth, particularly when supplemental iron is administered.[133,176,200,348-350] Mean corpuscular volume usually decreases (46.2 fl at birth) within the same time frame.[200] Normal blood values for adult cows are as follows: mean erythrocyte number is $6.36 \times 10^6/\mu L$; hemoglobin concentration is 10.9 g/dL; PCV is 33.6%; MCV is 52.8 fl; MCH is 17 pg; and MCHC is 32.5 g/dL. Alterations in these parameters can indicate iron deficiency anemia, but the reader is referred to Jain[200] for complete discussions of the differential diagnoses of anemia.

Clinical Parameters. The initial signs of iron deficiency are related to reductions in phagocytic function and depressed cell mediated immunity during the depletion or latent phase.[252] Once tissue stores are depleted, anemia becomes more evident. Reduction in optimal growth has been noted in calves that were iron deficient,[45,55] and response to iron supplementation has been beneficial in some studies,[78,360] but not others.[133,348,349] Increased hemoglobin, erythrocyte numbers, PCV, MCV, MCH, and serum/plasma iron concentrations are commonly noted after beef calves are injected with iron, even though weight gain is not always responsive to supplementation.[133,176,348,349] In general, it must be assumed that calves ingesting typical diets will ingest sufficient quantities of iron to correct or prevent iron deficiency, unless excessive blood loss occurs. However, calf weight in the first and subsequent weeks of life was positively correlated to serum iron during the first week of life.[348] This can imply that maternal iron status will influence subsequent performance of calves.

In addition to microcytic and hypochromic anemia, other clinical pathologic changes that can be attributed to iron deficiency in calves are reduced venous oxygen and lower arterial pH after exercise.[351] Anemic calves have increased cardiac and respiratory rates after exercise,[351] which imply a degree of exercise intolerance.

Dietary Sources and Fortification

Dietary requirements for iron are listed in Table 1. Most feed sources supply adequate amounts of iron, and ingestion of soil will contribute to the dietary intake. Iron is usually supplemented as ferrous sulfate, ferrous carbonate, or as a ferrous-methionine-sulfate complex, but it is doubtful that adult cattle on range or dirt require additional iron, unless parasitism has caused blood loss. Soluble forms of iron in the reduced state (ferrous) are recommended as opposed to oxidized iron (ferric) in the form of insoluble salts.[15,55,56,271] Injection of calves with iron dextran at a rate of 10 to 24 mg/kg body weight should be effective in preventing iron deficiency.[78,348] Usually, doses are 10 mg iron/kg body weight.

Cattle are refractory to severe toxic effects of dietary iron, but it is important to recall the negative interaction of iron with copper. When negative effects of dietary iron are noted they commonly are manifested as reduced rates of gain, feed consumption, and diarrhea.[401] Acute signs of iron toxicity include anorexia, oliguria, diarrhea, hypothermia, shock, and metabolic acidosis that can lead to death.[401]

MANGANESE

Properties and Metabolism

Manganese is a group VIIA metal with an atomic weight of 54.94. Manganese deficiency has caused skeletal abnormalities and abortion in beef calves in the Pacific Northwest.[105] Other reproductive disorders have been observed, including irregular estrus, reduced conception rates, and seminal tubular degeneration. Immune defects in mice have been described, but the effects of manganese deficiency on immune function in cattle have not been investigated. Lipid and carbohydrate metabolism are disturbed with manganese deficiency in laboratory animals, and this was recently reviewed.[192,215]

Adult cattle usually absorb and retain only a small fraction (1–5%) of dietary manganese.[293,356,373] This also appears to be true for young, but not newborn, calves.[295] Absorption has been noted to be as high as 15%[146] to 17%,[161] but retention was 2.2%.[146] Calcium and phosphorous can affect manganese absorption,[235] but the magnitude of this interaction is small.[9] Dietary antagonism of manganese by iron, copper, and zinc has been noted.[40,42,195–197] Additionally, the age of an animal and the dietary concentration of manganese influences the absorption and retention of manganese. Manganese absorption and retention was much higher in calves fed unsupplemented whole milk than when additional manganese (15 μg/g) was added to the whole milk.[79] The higher absorption and retention of manganese implies that ligands or other factors in secreted milk enhance the availability of manganese,[80] or that homeostatic mechanisms alter absorption or retention in calves. Newborn calves will absorb and retain much more manganese than adult cattle[79,187] and this has been observed in other species as well.[212,245]

Manganese absorption and retention appear to be increased by low manganese status of the calf,[79,294] in contrast to observations in other species, suggesting that manganese absorption is not increased with deficiency.[218] Manganese solubility is reduced in the rumen and increased in the abomasum.[198] This was interpreted to be an effect of pH on the dissociation of manganese complexes. Manganese flux appears to occur throughout the intestine.[418,419] Grace[146] has noted a significant amount of manganese absorption in the large intestine of sheep, but a net secretion from the abomasum and small intestine.[146]

After absorption from the gastrointestinal tract, manganese is transported by blood through the portal vein to the liver. This can be as a free ion (Mn^{2+}) or bound to $\alpha2^-$ macroglobulin.[372,376] Transferrin will also transport manganese, but as Mn^{3+}.[135] The liver efficiently removes and retains a majority of absorbed manganese.[135] Once in the liver manganese can be oxidized to Mn^{3+} and bound to transferrin, where it can enter the general circulation.[135] Mechanisms of manganese uptake into cells are poorly understood,[54] but pancreatic, renal, adrenal, pituitary, and skeletal tissues retain a significant amount of manganese.[79] In one study, manganese concentrations have been reported to be lower in maternal liver compared with fetal liver,[161] but the reverse was true in another investigation.[140]

Fecal excretion is the major route for manganese loss in cattle, and urinary excretion is only a minor route.[187,294,434] Carter et al[79] noted that as dietary manganese was increased, biliary secretion also increased. Biliary excretion is rapid and presumably controls manganese retention.[79,294] Distribution and control of manganese metabolism is still poorly understood,[115] but some aspects of the cellular distribution were recently reviewed.[215]

Function

Manganese function in mammals has been summarized.[192,215] Well characterized metabolic roles for manganese are described for skeletal development and involve the glycosyltransferases.[236] This family of enzymes catalyzes the transfer of sugar moieties, bound to uridine diphosphate, to an acceptor molecule to form the proteoglycan matrix of cartilage. Thus, bone deformities occur with abnormal proteoglycan synthesis, and this is consistently observed in manganese-deficient young animals.

Alterations in glucose metabolism have been noted, and it is possible that enzymes in the gluconeogenic pathway, pyruvate carboxylase and phosphoenolpyruvate carboxykinase, or insulin metabolism can be responsive to manganese in some situations.[215,217,363] The function of manganese in pyruvate carboxylase is not currently defined, but its activity is manganese dependent.[381] In contrast, catalytic activity of phosphoenolpyruvate carboxykinase appears to be obligatory.[314] The effect of manganese on insulin metabolism appears to be at the level of the insulin receptor protein kinase.[377] Insulin release could also be affected by manganese.[217]

Other manganese enzymes include manganese superoxide dismutase,[36,215] arginase,[48] and glutamine synthetase.[435] Manganese superoxide dismutase has a role similar to copper-zinc superoxide dismutase within mitochondria and catalyzes the reduction of superoxide to hydrogen peroxide. Arginase is involved in ureagenesis, and glutamine synthetase is involved in ammonia metabolism. In contrast to the suggestion that glutamine synthetase is manganese activated in vivo, Maurizi et al[266] gave evidence that magnesium is more likely to induce glutamine synthetase in bovine and ovine brains.

Manganese deficiency induced infertility has been described for cattle.[105,364] A mechanism that can explain some of the defects in fertility is related to cholesterol metabolism. Cholesterol is required for ruminant luteal steroidogenesis and is derived from plasma lipoproteins.[447] Alterations in lipoprotein metabolism have been noted in manganese deficiency,[211] and manganese-activated farnesyl pyrophosphate synthetase is one step that can control cholesterol synthesis.[32] Manganese has been noted to reduce plasma lipid concentrations and alter hepatic lipid composition in pregnant sheep.[180] Anestrous and irregular estrous cycles in females[105,178,181,446] and abnormal sperm have been attributed to manganese deficiency. Ruminant sperm adenylate cyclase activity[62,172,399] appears to be a manganese dependent enzyme. Gossypol-induced infertility can be related to inhibition of adenyl cyclase, and manganese can reverse the inhibitory effects of gossypol on adenyl cyclase.[442] Thus, the mechanisms of manganese deficiency induced infertility can be multiple.

In mice injected with manganese chloride, enhanced immunoresponsiveness and immune dysfunction have been noted with addition of manganese,[397] but whether this has any practical importance for cattle has not been established. Alterations in macrophage function, T-cell responsiveness to lectins, mixed lymphocyte responsiveness, and antibody production have been noted. Further investigations of the effects of manganese on the immune system in cattle are warranted.

Assessment of Status

Deficiencies. Recommended dietary manganese levels are presented in Table 1. Because there are not any consistent biochemical changes that occur with manganese deficiency, alteration in activity of enzymes such as manganese superoxide dismutase, pyruvate kinase, and insulin concentrations are not useful. Whole blood manganese may be useful for diagnosing manganese deficiency,[85,213] and this has been recognized as a useful measure of manganese status in early studies of manganese deficiency in cattle.[33,166] In wethers and lambs, strong correlations between soft tissue or serum concentrations of manganese and dietary manganese have been noted.[41,451] Thus, liver and whole blood manganese are the most practical measures of status, but dietary concentrations and a response to manganese supplementation will help confirm a diagnosis of deficiency.

Liver manganese levels less than 1 μg/g (18.2 nmol/g) wet weight are deficient. Hepatic manganese concentrations between 1.5 and 3 μg/g (27.30–54.61 nmol/g) are considered marginal, and concentrations between 2.5 and 6 μg/g (45.51–109.21 nmol/g) can be considered adequate. Similarly, whole blood manganese concentrations less than 0.02 μg/mL (364.1 nmol/L) or serum less than 0.005 μg/mL (91.01 nmol/l) are considered deficient. Whole blood manganese in the range of 0.07–0.09 μg/mL (1.27–1.64 μmol/L) and serum in the range of 0.006–0.07 μg/mL (0.11–1.27 μmol/L) are considered adequate.[346]

Clinical Parameters. Calves fed 1 μg manganese/g diet for 1 year had signs of severe manganese deficiency.[166] Clinical signs were excessive salivation, lacrimation and nasal discharge, diarrhea, buckling of the carpal-metacarpal joint with enlargement and weakening of the pasterns, and spreading of the hooves. The most severe signs were seizures, obtundation, and death. Rojas et al[364] did not see any gross manifestation of manganese deficiency in pregnant cows, but they did note increased services per conception. Calves born to manganese-deficient cows had gross limb deformities, which included shortened limbs with enlarged swollen joints and angular deformities. This was manifested by stiffness and apparent weakness. Bentley and Phillips[33] noted an increase in bile duct proliferation, abscesses, fatty degeneration, and hyalinized vessels in livers of manganese-deficient heifers. Kidneys were normal on gross and histopathologic examination in deficient heifers. Also noted were lower concentrations of manganese in ovarian tissue and a slight but consistent increase in services per conception in manganese-deficient compared with supplemented heifers. Manganese supplementation has been noted to increase first service conception rates and reduce services per conception when compared with unsupplemented controls.[446] Additionally, manganese can reduce the rates of abortion in some situations, but the actual effects of manganese on luteal function are not characterized.[182] Thus, the primary lesions that are consistently described for cattle are limited to limb deformities and weakness in calves and reproductive dysfunction in mature females.

Future manganese research should be directed toward further examination of the effects of manganese on follicular and luteal function, as well as examining the role of manganese in diseases such as hepatic lipidosis and ketosis. Examining the degree to which manganese affects lipid and carbohydrate metabolism in the bovine could be an exciting area of research that has direct practical implications for production of meat and milk.

Dietary Sources and Fortification

Manganese supplementation is effective for reversing the reproductive signs of manganese deficiency and can prevent the skeletal changes in calves. Some of the available forms for manganese supplementation are manganese oxide (MnO, MnO_2), manganese sulfate ($MnSO_4$), manganese carbonate ($MnCO_3$),[451] and manganese methionine. Manganese sulfate is the most biologically available inorganic form for supplementation, and it is also the most soluble.[451] This is convenient because it can be readily used in liquids and blocks, or mixed in loose salts. Soil pH can directly alter the retention of manganese in plants, and acid conditions will increase manganese availability.[426] Thus, if manganese deficiency is suspected, soil amendment practices, such as applications of $CaCO_3$, can contribute by increasing calcium and pH. Supplementation of $MnSO_4$ with greater than 250 μg manganese/g diet is unwarranted because toxicity in sheep has been noted above this level.[197] Thus, when evaluating the effect of manganese supplementation on adult cattle, a dose of 0.5 g per day should be adequate for an observable response.

Manganese can be toxic to cattle, and the effects are generally related to reduction in rates of gain or negative interactions with iron and calcium.[401] Additional signs, noted in cattle fed high levels of manganese, are reduced hemoglobin concentrations and alteration of the normal microflora, with subsequent reduction of volatile fatty acid production.[401]

MOLYBDENUM

The important factors regarding molybdenum metabolism in ruminant health were discussed with copper in this review. Molybdenum deficiency has been diagnosed or experimentally produced in monogastric animals, but this is unlikely to occur as a practical problem in ruminants.[215] Molybdenosis is problematic in cattle, but there are a few comments about molybdenum deficiency that are worthwhile mentioning. Nitrate reductase is a microbial molybdoenzyme that reduces nitrate to nitrite. In a series of papers examining nitrate toxicity in cattle it was noted that tungsten markedly inhibited ruminal nitrite production and prevented nitrate poisoning.[134,227,228] Nitrite production is presumably reduced by a direct antagonism of microbial molybdenum metabolism by tungsten, which results in depression of nitrate reductase activity. This is further supported by the observations of Johnson et al (as reported by Gooneratne et al[140]) who noted that ruminal nitrite and ammonia production are higher when molybdenum is high.

An additional use of molybdenum is in the form of thiomolybdates to treat copper toxicosis.[143,298] Systemic thiomolybdates and dietary sulfur and molybdenum will form copper complexes and increase net loss of copper. The interactions and metabolism of copper, molybdenum, and sulfur have been recently discussed.[140,141]

SELENIUM

Properties and Metabolism

Selenium is a group VIB element with an atomic weight of 78.96. Selenium deficiency and selenium-responsive disorders have been reported frequently throughout the world. The principal lesions are attributed to reduced glutathione peroxidase activity and immune deficiency. Selenium is absorbed primarily in the duodenum.[239,454] In ruminants, selenium absorption is approximately 40% of the dietary selenium, presumably because selenium is reduced in the rumen from selenite and selenate to insoluble forms of selenium.[71] Organic forms of selenium are apparently better absorbed than are inorganic forms, but the rumen can convert calcium and sodium selenite to biologically available forms of selenium.[173] Elemental selenium and selenium sulfide are not well absorbed.[384,420]

A number of elements have been reported to influence selenium metabolism. Among these elements are arsenic, mercury, cadmium, and copper.[185] In sheep and cattle, interactions of selenium with copper, molybdenum, and sulfur have been suggested, but it appears that the overall influence of these elements on selenium metabolism is small.[224,441] Additionally, oxalate can decrease selenate transport in sheep.[450] Seasonal factors will also alter the availability of selenium in sheep.[440]

Amino acids, particularly the sulfur amino acids, will alter selenium metabolism. Dietary methionine will directly influence the proportion of selenomethionine incorporation into proteins.[72] Waschulewski and Sunde[433] have suggested that dietary selenomethionine may decrease availability of selenium for incorporation into glutathione peroxidase, particularly when methionine is limiting. Additionally, increased dietary methionine will increase conversion of selenomethionine to selenocysteine for incorporation into selenium specific proteins.[72] In addition to dietary protein and sulfur amino acids, other factors influencing retention of selenium are phosphorous and the selenium content of the diet.[152] Thus, multiple factors affect absorption and retention of selenium, with high dietary protein tending to increase absorption, while increasing urinary loss. Higher fecal selenium losses occur in ruminants compared to nonruminants,[454] and this probably relates to reduction of selenium in the rumen, as previously described. Additionally, selenium can form complexes or interact with other components of the digesta, which could render it less available for absorption.

Water-soluble compounds containing selenium are redistributed throughout the body from sites of absorption in the intestine. A selenocystein–containing protein found in rat plasma has been identified as a selenium transport protein.[307] Selenoprotein P, as it has been called, has been shown to vary directly with dietary selenium up to 0.1 mg selenium/kg diet.[455] Burk[69] has suggested that selenoprotein P could serve in an antioxidant capacity, in addition to its putative selenium carrier protein capacity. In sheep, selenium is apparently sulfhydrylbound, and the plasma proteins identified in sheep may differ from those identified in rats.[94] Calves were fed labeled selenite, and blood fractions were analyzed for location of selenium. In blood, selenium is transported loosely bound to erythrocyte and plasma proteins.[412] The ^{75}Se labeled plasma fraction in cattle was tentatively identified[201] as one related to selenoprotein P.[307] Mechanisms for transfer of selenium from plasma constituents to cells and intracellular metabolism of selenium are still poorly characterized. Selenocystein can be synthesized from selenomethionein via the cystathionine pathway.[110] The incorporation of selenocystein into glutathione peroxidase has been suggested to occur via a specific transfer RNA.[164] Recent evidence suggests that *de novo* production of selenocysteine occurs by incorporating selenium into a serine carbon skeleton, and this may be via a specified tRNA.[112,402]

Placental transfer of selenium is positively correlated to maternal selenium status.[427] While placental selenium transfer is dependent on maternal selenium status, fetal liver concentrations are uniformly higher than maternal liver selenium throughout gestation.[427] In contrast, maternal α-tocopherol was generally higher than fetal α-tocopherol, and fetal α-tocopherol declined through gestation.[428] An adequate maternal dietary supply of selenium during pregnancy is critical to the newborn calf.

In addition to fecal losses described earlier, a reciprocal relationship between selenium retention and urinary excretion has been documented in pigs.[154] Urinary excretion has been identified as a major route for selenium excretion, and a renal threshold appears to control excess concentrations of plasma selenium.[412,413] Kinetic models for selenium excretion in cattle and sheep have been developed and describe the relative pool sizes within ruminant animals.[229,412,413] Selenium can be lost from the respiratory route, and this can have a garliclike smell. Injectable forms of selenium can cause increased respiratory loss,[319] but this is thought to be minimal.

Function

Selenium deficiency is associated with degeneration and necrosis of several tissues, including myocardial necrosis and myonecrosis of the muscles of the extremities. In addition to these classic lesions of white muscle disease, immune dyscrasia, alteration of reproduction in males and females, and impaired growth have been associated with selenium deficiency.

The reduction of organic peroxides and hydrogen peroxide to the alcohol form of the organic molecule and water is catalyzed by glutathione peroxidase. This is the only well characterized function for selenium, although many other selenoproteins are being identified.[112,403] When selenium deficiency occurs, reduction in GSH-Px activity can lead to excessive increases in cellular peroxidation because of impaired free radical scavenging. Increased peroxidation of cellular constituents can be the biochemical lesion that leads to the multiple defects observed in natural cases of selenium deficiency discussed later. Deficiencies of other antioxidants (vitamin E and A) can increase expression of selenium deficiency,[177,215] particularly with concurrent inflammation.[138]

Increased erythrocyte fragility can be one consequence of increased membrane lipid peroxidation. Morris et al[306] have noted that anemia can be associated with selenium deficiency. Depression in erythrocyte glutathione peroxidase, with subsequent Heinz body formation,[405] can be one mechanism that can induce anemia similar to that described for copper deficiency.

Many of the conditions associated with selenium deficiency may be related to alterations in normal immunoresponsiveness or control of inflammation. Diarrhea and ill thrift seen in newborns, mastitis, metritis, and other infectious processes are most likely exacerbated by a reduced ability to respond to and kill pathogens.

Normal immunoresponsiveness is dependent on selenium adequacy in cattle[50,52,102,353,354] and sheep.[233,234] Selenium deficiency has been associated with increased mortality and an increase in the severity of pulmonary damage in cattle with bovine ephemeral fever.[317] Conversely, Phillippo and others[329,330] have reported that pneumonia in housed calves was not associated with selenium status or supplementation. They appropriately recommended that controlled trials be used to evaluate in vivo immunoresponsiveness to selenium supplementation in cattle.[329]

Neutrophils obtained from selenium-deficient steers had an impaired ability to kill ingested *Candida albicans* and lacked detectable glutathione peroxidase activity.[50] Similarly, defective intracellular killing of *Staphylococcus aureus* was noted in selenium deficient cattle.[155] Recently, lymphocyte responsiveness to lectins was determined in selenium deficient compared with selenium adequate mice.[226] A decreased mixed lymphocyte reaction and response to stimulation by phytohemaglutinin in selenium deficient mice indicated that a defect in response to stimulation is a consequence of selenium deficiency. This was attributed to reduced responsiveness to interleukin-1 and 2 (IL-1 and IL-2) and not decreased production. Concentrations of IL-1 and IL-2 did not differ between selenium deficient and adequate mice. In addition, selenium deficiency decreased cell mediated cytotoxicity and release of lymphotoxin compared to controls, and selenium supplementation increased both cell mediated cytotoxicity and lymphotoxin release.[370] Selenium deficiency has been associated with lower antibody concentrations in cattle, and antibody production is dependent on adequate selenium status.[102,353,354] The observation that immunosuppression can occur before overt manifestations of other signs of selenium deficiency[50] suggests that routine evaluation of selenium status is necessary to prevent production losses attributed to selenium deficiency.

In addition to observed immune defects caused by selenium deficiency, thyroid function can also be impaired. Conversion of T4 to T3 appears to be impaired in selenium deficient cattle.[23] This has been suggested to be one mechanism contributing to observed growth reductions of selenium deficient calves.

Selenium supplementation has been shown to increase fertility and improve reproductive disorders. Reduced rates of abortion and fewer weak and stillborn young have been recorded for selenium supplemented compared with unsupplemented beef cattle in California.[253] Lower selenium concentrations have been suggested to occur in a group of aborted fetuses (<0.25 μg/g; 3.166 nmol/g). However, the proportion of nonaborted control fetuses that have the same low selenium concentrations as selenium deficient aborted fetuses was not stated.[415] Supplementation of barium selenate significantly increased the first and second service conception rates of selenium deficient heifers.[255]

Selenium deficiency has been attributed to weak calves that were depressed, were reluctant to stand or move, failed to nurse, and had diarrhea and crusting or reddening of the muzzle.[398,415] However, in herds with a history of weak calves, response to selenium supplementation has not always proved beneficial.[358]

An increase in the prevalence of retained placentas has been associated with selenium deficiency.[163,206,423,424] Expected rates of retained placenta are about 10%,[163] and Trinder et al[423] have noted incidence rates of up to 50% in selenium deficient herds. Reductions in the prevalence of retained placenta have been noted in selenium and vitamin E supplemented cows 1 month before calving. Supplementation with selenium alone was only slightly less effective than supplementation with both selenium and vitamin E.[423,424]

Reduced sperm production and testicular degeneration have been induced by dietary selenium deficiency in rats, but the mechanism for this has not been established. Evenson and Sunde[112] describe a testicular selenoprotein that may underlie the defect in spermatogenesis or maturation and may be associated with testicular atrophy. This selenoprotein has been identified in bulls[323] and increases six-fold at maturity in rats.[31]

Improvement in rates of abortion or infertility, reduced numbers of weak and stillborn calves, increased immunoresponsiveness, and improvement of other conditions that have been associated with selenium deficiency have not always been noted after supplementation. This is most likely related to the multifactorial nature of these conditions. Mechanisms by which selenium deficiency can induce infertility, abortion, weak and stillborn young, and retained placenta have not been explained.[215,383]

Assessment of Status

Deficiencies. Recommended dietary concentrations for selenium in cattle have been increasing. The most recent recommendations from the National Research Council[311] suggest that 0.2 μg selenium/g diet is adequate. While the National Research Council[311] and Agricultural Research Council[5] (see Table 1) have suggested that diets with as low as 0.05 μg/g can be adequate, others[346] have suggested that rations containing less than 0.1 μg/g are deficient.

Ullrey[425] has recently reviewed the biochemical and physiologic indicators of selenium status. Dietary selenium is strongly correlated to plasma and muscle selenium concentrations. Plasma selenium will reflect current dietary intake, and erythrocyte glutathione peroxidase activity is strongly correlated to long standing selenium deficiency.[239,425] In general, cattle are selenium deficient when whole blood selenium falls in the range of 0.01 to 0.04 μg/mL (0.13–0.51 μmol/mL) whole blood. Selenium intake is in the marginal range when the range of whole blood selenium is between 0.05 and 0.06 μg/mL (0.63–0.76 μmol/mL). Adequate selenium intake is indicated when whole blood selenium is in the range of 0.07 to 0.10 μg/mL (0.87–1.27 μmol/mL).[250] Similarly, glutathione peroxidase activity less than 15 U/mg hemoglobin/minute in cattle is considered selenium deficient. A marginally adequate selenium consumption is indicated when glutathione peroxidase activity is in the range of 15 to 25 U/mg hemoglobin/

minute. Adequate selenium consumption is indicated when glutathione peroxidase activity is in the range of 25 to 500 U/mg hemoglobin/minute.[250]

Liver levels of selenium in cattle have been reported by Puls.[346] Hepatic concentrations less than 0.17 μg selenium/g (2.15 nmol/g) wet weight are considered deficient. Selenium concentrations in the range of 0.12 to 0.25 μg/g liver (1.52–3.17 nmol/g) indicate marginal dietary intake, and adequate dietary selenium intake is indicated when liver selenium concentrations are in the range of 0.25 to 0.5 μg/g (3.17–6.33 nmol/g). Ullrey[425] suggested that adequate hepatic concentrations of selenium range from 0.2 to 0.8 μg/g (2.53–10.13 nmol/g) wet weight.

Clinical Parameters. A generalized picture of a selenium-deficient herd would include a range of disorders in cows and their calves. Thus, fewer calves born than expected could reflect abortion and subfertility within the herd. An increased incidence of retained placenta, stillborn or weak calves that die soon after birth, and calves that fail to thrive are typical of herds affected by selenium deficiency. In dairy cows, mastitis has been reported to be responsive to selenium[109,391] and vitamin E supplementation, for reasons discussed earlier and reviewed by Smith and Conrad.[390] It can be expected that animals with the greatest growth and production demands will manifest selenium deficiency first. Thus, calves or yearlings with evidence of white muscle disease are commonly observed in problem herds.

Nutritional myodegeneration (white muscle disease) is a degenerative disease of the myocyte in skeletal muscle and the heart, typically affecting young calves. The calves appear stiff and weak, diarrhea is often present, and mortality can be high.[222,378] In experimental nutritional myodegeneration, teeth grinding, constant shifting of weight bearing between limbs, difficulty rising, arched backs, and persistent sternal recumbency were commonly noted signs.[222] Other signs that were observed as the disease progressed were lassitude, anorexia, increased respiration rate, dyspnea, dark urine, muscle tremors, cardiac conduction disturbances, and death.[222,223] Elevations in plasma creatine kinase activity up to 100-fold have been observed. Additionally, increased plasma aldolase and lactic dehydrogenase activity[12] and decreased alkaline phosphatase activity,[23] along with myoglobinuria, can be observed in selenium-deficient cattle.[12]

Typically, post mortem examination shows evidence of white streaks and foci of calcification in the skeletal and cardiac muscles. When severely affected, the muscle takes on the appearance of chicken flesh with edema and occasional hemorrhage.[12] Typically, muscles of locomotion are most severely affected.[12] Nutritional myodegeneration has been observed in yearling cattle. In these cases, myonecrosis has been associated with lush pastures that have been assumed to be high in polyunsaturated fats.[12,16,222,223,359] Arthur[24] has suggested that other factors, in addition to increased polyunsaturated fats, contribute to selenium-deficiency induced myodegeneration of older calves. He has suggested this because housed calves, fed high polyunsaturated diets, did not develop the white muscle disease until they were turned out to pasture. Exercise was discussed as one possibility.

Dietary Sources and Fortification

Parenteral supplementation in the form of injectable selenium products will adequately treat clinical deficiency in a herd, but more frequent injections can be required if dietary intake of selenium is low or interactions of other nutrients result in severe deficiency. After injection with these products, cattle must be held from slaughter for 30 days. Adequate maternal selenium status is required to ensure that the newborn has adequate selenium stores. Intramuscular or subcutaneous injection of the cow 1 month before calving, or of the calf at birth, can increase selenium status. This can be critical when nutritional myodegeneration is problematic. Typically, 3 mg selenium/kg body weight, repeated every 3 to 4 months will correct clinical signs of deficiency.

Usual forms of oral selenium supplements are sodium selenite, selenate, and potassium, or barium selenate. Oral supplementation of whole rations or as blocks, liquids, or loose salts will overcome deficiency, and 2 to 3 mg selenium/animal/day will usually be adequate. Occasionally, supplementation with dosages as high as 7 to 8 mg/day has been necessary to avoid signs of deficiency.[251] If prescription levels of selenium supplementation are used, the veterinarian must assume responsibility for monitoring supplement consumption and for establishing tissue measures of selenium status. This is necessary because the veterinarian assumes all liability for extralabel use of the product. Because of the risk of selenium toxicity, current federal regulations limit supplements to 3 mg/animal/day. Thus, the maximum nonprescription limit is 0.3 μg selenium/g diet and 30 μg selenium/g supplement.[250]

Recently, a new sustained release selenium product (approximately 3 mg/day) has been approved for use in cattle. The duration of action for these osmotic pumps is about 4 months and blood selenium concentrations remained elevated for at least 8 months,[74] and this is somewhat shorter than the older iron-elemental selenium composite boluses, which lasted about a year. These products have proved to be effective in the prevention of selenium-responsive diseases in cattle.

Selenosis occurs in cattle that graze in regions with a high concentration of selenium in their soil or that ingest selenium-concentrating plants. Because supplementation of selenium compounds has become commonplace, it is likely that more cases of iatrogenic selenosis will occur. The classic signs associated with chronic selenium toxicity are impaired vision or blindness; lameness with moderate to severe disturbances in the hoof wall; hair loss; and emaciation. Acute selenium toxicity can occur with ingestion of large quantities of selenium or after parenteral injection. Respiratory distress, ataxia, abnormal stance, diarrhea, prostration, and death have been observed in selenium-poisoned cattle.[401]

ZINC

Properties and Metabolism

Zinc is a group IIB element with an atomic weight of 65.38. Zinc deficiency or zinc responsive conditions in ruminants have been reported in many areas of the world, and interest in zinc metabolism has been high because zinc is involved in carbohydrate, lipid, protein, and nucleic acid metabolism. The severe consequences of zinc deficiency in terms of reproduction and growth have suggested that zinc may be a common limiting nutrient in animal agriculture, even though clinical disease is not apparent.[426] Thus, recent investigations have begun to examine production parameters using levels of zinc supplementation above those suggested by the National Research Council.[311] Zinc deficiency can occur as a primary disorder or as a conditioned deficiency secondary to competition with copper, calcium, or iron. Routine forage analysis of pasture or hay from Arizona, California, Colorado, Idaho, Nevada, and Utah has documented that greater than 90% of the samples had zinc concentrations less than 20 μg/g dry matter (DM) (Benton A, personal communication, 1990), but this is in contrast to information summarized by Miller[291] suggesting that zinc concentrations are usually higher than 30 μg/g. It is apparent that deficiency of zinc in the western United States could be very widespread, but the clinical implications of this have not been fully investigated.

Zinc is absorbed mainly in the small intestine.[125,159] In the enterocyte, zinc is bound to the putative copper and zinc storage protein, metallothionein, transferred to plasma constituents, and transported through the portal system to the liver.[86] Zinc will induce metallothionein synthesis to a greater extent than copper, but the effect of increased dietary zinc and copper is additive.[44] Albumin is the major zinc binding ligand in plasma, but transferrin, α-2macroglobulin, and other low molecular weight ligands such as histidine and cysteine can also bind zinc.[162] Mechanisms of membrane transport of zinc are not well characterized, but once in the cell, zinc is available to bind to membranes and other structural components, or zinc can be incorporated into metallothionein or other proteins. Unlike copper, zinc absorption in cattle can vary from 10% to 80% of the dietary zinc and appears to be dependent on zinc status of the animal.[291] Fecal loss appears to be the major excretory pathway for zinc, and urinary excretion is usually a minor route.[291]

Function

The principal biochemical functions of zinc in animals were recently reviewed[158,215] and are only briefly summarized here. In addition to the role of zinc as a catalytic or stabilizing component of metalloenzymes, such as copper-zinc superoxide dismutase, carbonic anhydrase, alcohol dehydrogenase, carboxypeptidase, alkaline phosphatase, and RNA polymerase, zinc is also required as a structural component for stability of the cell. Membrane stability,[82,316] microtubule polymerization,[321] DNA, and RNA structure or function[81,84] appear to be zinc dependent. Additionally, signal transduction may be critically altered by zinc because of zinc's regulatory interaction with calmodulin,[300] protein kinase C,[88,309] inositol phosphate formation,[387] Na-K ATPase activity,[382] protein phosphatase activity,[325] thyroid hormone binding,[404] and estradiol receptor binding.[275] Zinc deficiency alters prostaglandin metabolism, and this can be a direct effect of zinc on the arachidonic acid cascade. In a series of experiments, O'Dell's group[63,240,315] has reported that zinc deficiency is associated with higher $PGF_{2\alpha}$ and PGE_2 concentrations and a higher $PGF_{2\alpha}/PGE_2$ ratio in vivo, and Meydani and Dupont,[277] using an in vitro model in rats, have reported that $PGF_{2\alpha}$ was elevated. Similarly, PGI_2 has also been reported to be lower in zinc deficient than control animals.[63] Given the multiple effects of prostaglandins, particularly on luteal function and myometrial contractility, it is apparent that zinc deficiency has the potential to directly alter ruminant reproductive function.

The involvement of zinc in virtually every phase of cell growth suggests that each organ system can be severely affected by zinc deficiency. Marked defects in production are observed in zinc deficient cattle. Improved carcass quality has been noted in steers fed zinc methionine, but this may be an effect of methionine rather than an effect of zinc.[151] Increased growth has been noted in cattle on practical diets supplemented with zinc,[30,267,327,342] and field cases of zinc deficiency in cattle[2,237,395] and sheep[334] have been documented. Additionally, a tendency to increase feed consumption in stressed calves has been noted, and zinc supplementation increased rates of gain and response to therapy in sick feedlot cattle.[194] Thus, clinical zinc deficiency and zinc-responsive conditions have been reported in cattle under practical feeding regimens. A genetic defect in zinc metabolism has been reported to occur in Friesian[17,274] and Shorthorn[429] cattle. The defect appears to be one of impaired intestinal uptake[123,124] and is discussed in more detail subsequently.

Zinc deficiency has been associated with endocrine dysfunction, particularly insulin metabolism, growth hormone function, and reproduction. Experimental zinc deficiency has been associated with persistently low circulating insulin concentrations, which can be reversed by zinc supplementation.[225] In rats, zinc deficiency can be characterized by abnormal glucose tolerance and lowered serum insulin when compared with pair-fed controls.[367] Thus, one mechanism of zinc deficiency that could affect growth is an alteration in insulin metabolism. As mentioned above, thyroid hormone binding[404] is affected by zinc concentration, and experimentally induced zinc deficiency can reduce circulating TSH and T4.[430] As discussed in the section on iodine, normal thyroid function is critical for optimal growth, reproduction, and production in cattle. Thus, the ramifications of zinc deficiency on thyroid hormone function in cattle need to be investigated.

Growth hormone directly alters growth, and zinc affects growth hormone metabolism. An inverse relationship between zinc status and growth hormone concentration and a direct relationship between urinary zinc and plasma growth hormone have been reported.[171] Acromegalic individuals had depressed zinc concentrations while individuals with growth hormone deficiency had elevated plasma zinc concentrations. Supplemental bovine growth hormone reduced plasma zinc in the growth hormone deficient individuals. In another study that examined hypophysectomized male rats, the effect of zinc and growth hormone activity on growth were independent, but appeared to be additive.[339] Additionally, zinc deficiency is associated with lower growth hormone concentrations, and plasma growth hormone concentrations increased with zinc supplementation. Growth hormone will not correct the effects of depressed growth in nonhypophysectomized zinc-deficient rats unless zinc is supplemented simultaneously.[339] Recently, this same reciprocal relationship of growth hormone with zinc has been observed when lambs were injected with exogenous somatotropin. Hepatic zinc concentrations in somatotropin treated compared with saline injected control lambs were reduced to almost 50% of control values.[47] With the advent of recombinant bovine growth hormone for commercial use, it is evident that further evaluation of dietary zinc requirements are needed.

Zinc deficiency severely affects reproduction in both males and females. Hidiroglou and Knipfel[179] and Apgar[20] have reviewed the effect of zinc deficiency on male reproduction. Reproductive dysfunction in zinc deficient males includes degeneration of the seminiferous tubules and abnormal Leydig cell number and morphology, which are associated with reduced circulating testosterone and abnormal sperm development. Reduction in size or function of male accessory sex glands has been noted, but this is most likely a consequence of the reduced testosterone production. Root et al[366] examined the pituitary hormones in zinc-deficient male rats and noted that follicle stimulating hormone and luteinizing hormone were higher. The testicular defects associated with zinc deficiency are not at the level of the pituitary, but zinc deficiency directly affects testicular development. In cattle, fertility is responsive to zinc supplementation. Following experimentally induced zinc deficiency, testicular growth was persistently impaired after five weeks of resupplementation,[282] which indicates that adequate zinc supplementation during early growth of bull calves may be critical. In another study, after short periods of zinc deficiency, response to zinc supplementation was complete and without permanent effects on fertility or testicular function.[335]

Abnormal outcome of pregnancy occurs as a consequence of zinc deficiency and includes abortion, fetal mummification, lower birth weight, teratogenic defects, altered myometrial contractility with prolonged labor, increased hemorrhage at delivery, and reduced viability of offspring.[20,216,247] The effects of zinc deficiency, from preconception through parturition, have not been recorded for cattle, but significant increases in the number and weight of lambs born to grazing sheep supplemented with zinc have been reported.[107,262] In experimentally induced zinc deficiency, weight of lambs born to deficient ewes was less than control lambs,[19,263] and resorption, abortion, fetal mummification, fetal malformations and weak lambs were reported,[19] as they have been for laboratory animal species.[216] Dystocia, reportedly associated with lower serum zinc concentrations in cattle, responded to zinc supplementation before calving began.[103] Mechanisms by which zinc can affect uterine contractility have been investigated in the rat. Lower uterine $PGF_{2\alpha}$[113] and total prostaglandin concentration[89] have been documented in zinc deficient rats, as well as reduced uterine contractility and blood flow.[89] Further investigations of the mechanism of decreased uterine contractility have noted increased uterine estrogen receptor retention.[67] Reductions in numbers of myometrial gap junctions have been reported for zinc deficient rats, which presumably reduces synchronous contractility.[106] Investigations of zinc's role in bovine reproduction are needed, specifically the role of zinc in pregnancy outcome from preconception through parturition.

It has been reported that zinc deficiency impairs hepatic mobilization of vitamin A,[388] and this has been observed in ruminants.[21,340,374] Zinc deficiency in sheep can induce night blindness, and this has been attributed to impaired vitamin A metabolism.[21] Impairment of vitamin A mobilization has been related to alterations in hepatic retinol binding protein metabolism.[388] Vision loss noted in calves with experimentally induced zinc deficiency[281] may be caused by reduced retinol binding protein mobilization.

Effects of zinc on the immune system have recently been reviewed.[214] Changes associated with zinc deficiency are principally restricted to the cellular components, but also affect humoral immunity. In experimental animals, lymphopenia and lymphoid depletion are characteristic of zinc deficiency. Responsiveness to lectins is depressed during zinc deficiency. Production of or responsiveness to interleukins can be one mechanism by which cellular immunity is depressed. Additionally, macrophage and neutrophil function can be altered by zinc deficiency, as well as antibody formation.

Similar to laboratory animal models of zinc deficiency, thymic aplasia has been reported[65] in cattle with a hereditary defect in zinc metabolism, lethal trait A46. This defect is expressed as a marked lymphoid depletion and depression in cellular immunity.[64,123,328] The immunologic defects can be corrected by supplementing affected calves with high oral doses of zinc.[123] Many of the immunologic disturbances described for A46 calves are similar to the defects noted in laboratory animals after inducing zinc deficiency.[214] A majority of the A46 calves that are left untreated will die as a consequence of infection with common pathogens, even after treatment with antibiotics and supportive care.[64] Depression in hypersensitivity responses[64,123] and specific response to antigens are lower in affected compared with unaffected calves.[64,328] Similarly, the proportion of circulating CD4 positive T lymphocytes (helper) and B lymphocytes is lower in calves affected by congenital zinc deficiency.[328] Effects on the immune system in zinc deficient cattle without genetic defects need to be assessed.

Zinc can be used therapeutically for other clinical conditions in cattle. Young bulls affected with foot-rot (infectious pododermatitis) had consumed a diet that contained up to 56 μg zinc/g[99] and foot lesions responded to addition of 4.5 to 7 mg zinc/kg body weight per day. Recovery was complete and did not require antibiotic therapy in 11 of 12 animals. One animal did not respond to either zinc or tetracycline therapy. As emphasized by Demertzis and Mills[99] and reviewed subsequently, detection of subclinical zinc deficiency is difficult. On pastures with a high incidence of foot rot, a response trial may be worthwhile to assess the efficacy of zinc supplementation. Zinc has been used therapeutically for the treatment of copper toxicosis in sheep, and this has been identified as a safe mode of therapy with few side effects.[58] Treatment of cadmium toxicity by supplementing affected calves with zinc has been reported.[347] Additionally, zinc has proved to be efficacious in prevention of lupinosis/facial eczema, a hepatotoxic disease of ruminants, in New Zealand and Australia. The condition is caused by *Phomopsis spp.*, and sheep and cattle in affected regions respond to zinc supplementation.[11,386,422]

Assessment of Status

Deficiencies. Minimum dietary requirements for beef cattle are listed in Table 1. As already mentioned, zinc responsive conditions have occurred on rations with as high as 56 μg zinc/g diet, and requirements for zinc can be higher than those predicted by experimental studies.[310] Expected liver zinc concentrations range from 25 to 100 μg/g (0.38–1.5 μmol/g) wet weight. However, marginal status has been suggested to range from 25 to 40 μg/g (0.38–0.61 μmol/g), and deficiency can occur from below 20 to as high as 40 μg/g liver (0.31–0.61 μmol/g).[346] Thus, liver zinc is not considered a good indicator of zinc adequacy, but can reflect status when low. Plasma zinc is lowered by many inflammatory conditions, presumably because glucocorticoids, epinephrine, glucagon, IL-1, and tumor necrosis factor will induce metallothionein and sequester zinc in tissues.[87,100] Inflammation in cattle is associated with these same reductions in plasma zinc,[146,194,243] and inflammation stimulates urinary excretion of zinc.[194] Mills[299] has summarized the important factors that complicate diagnosis of zinc deficiency in cattle. Zinc-responsive conditions occur before accurate detection of zinc deficiency can be made, based on liver or plasma zinc concentrations or other biochemical parameters. Identification of the limiting pools of zinc have not been well characterized, and the effect of diet and disease on the zinc flux in these pools is incompletely identified. The expected range of plasma zinc is 0.8 to 1.4 μg/mL (12.2–21.4 μmol/L). Marginal levels of zinc range between 0.4 and 0.8 μg/mL (6.1–12.2 μmol/L) plasma, and cows can be considered deficient if plasma zinc is consistently below 0.4 μg/mL (6.1 μmol/L). An accurate biochemical index of zinc status has not been established, because enzymes such as carbonic anhydrase and alkaline phosphatase are influenced by intercurrent disease. Thus, diagnosis of zinc deficiency is difficult.

In the laboratory of Justine Garvey,[131,417,448] a radioimmunoassay and enzyme-linked-immunosorbent assay have been developed for quantifying metallothionein in physiologic fluids. Bovine metallothionein cross reacts with the metallothionein antibody,[448] and this may be a useful tool for estimating zinc status in cattle. Induction of metallothionein appears to be primarily zinc dependent, but cadmium will also induce metallothionein synthesis.[59,87] Because other factors induce metallothionein, interpretation will be required. However, plasma, red blood cell, leukocyte, and hepatic metallothionein concentrations may provide useful information on zinc status in the future.

Clinical Parameters. Typical signs of zinc deficiency in young[281,282,297,322] and mature cattle[380] have been described. Plasma zinc concentration declines rapidly after removal of dietary zinc and is quickly restored with supplementation.[297] Initial symptoms of zinc deficiency are listlessness and excessive salivation. Diarrhea and anorexia occur early in the course of zinc deficiency in calves,[328] which is manifested by reduced rates of gain or cessation of growth. Zinc-deficient calves develop mucosal redness and inflammation of the nose and gums, a stiff gait with swelling of the distal extremities (hocks and above the hooves), alopecia (especially around the muzzle, ears, and eyes), cutaneous erythema and crusting with fissures and hemorrhage, horny overgrowth of the lips and dental pads, and loss of vision.[281,282,322] Hooves of affected animals are deformed, and the hair appears abnormal.[297] The animals appear to have ring-worm lesions and a rough starry coat, and skin lesions can be pruritic or painful. Histologically, the characteristic skin lesion is a retention of nuclei in the outer layers of the epidermis (parakeratosis). On necropsy, thymic atrophy is characteristic of zinc deficiency, and lymphoid depletion of the spleen, lymph nodes, Peyer's patches, and other gut associated lymphoid tissue are evident.[64]

Adult cattle have signs and symptoms of zinc deficiency that are very similar to those of immature cattle. Schwarz and Kirchgessner[380] have summarized their findings of experimentally induced zinc deficiency in Friesian cattle. In addition to the lesions described for the calves, teat and udder lesions were present in affected cows, and occasional lesions were noted on the tail. This has been reported in natural cases of zinc deficiency.[156]

Dietary Sources and Fortification

As already discussed, absolute requirements for zinc in cattle cannot be made because of interactions with other elements in the diet, environmental factors, and animal factors that alter the requirement for zinc. In terms of mineral interactions, calcium supplementation has been associated with reductions in serum zinc in yearling steers.[327] This can be of practical importance when $CaCO_3$ is used as a ruminal buffer and particularly when high levels of calcium are fed (e.g., dairy cattle). While death from zinc toxicosis occurs in preruminant calves fed 700 μg zinc/g diet for 30 days,[148,149] mature cows can tolerate diets of 1000 μg zinc/g for 40 weeks without apparent effect.[292] Sources for zinc supplementation in cattle include injectable forms, a zinc-iron bolus, and addition of zinc to water, salt-mineral blocks, and rations. Addition of zinc sulfate to drinking water was associated with an increased growth rate in beef cattle, but variability in water consumption will influence total intake.[453] Intraruminal zinc pellets have been used in sheep for short term zinc response trials,[264] but this may not be efficacious in cattle because the absolute requirement for zinc in cattle is much greater. Injections of 200-mg zinc oxide suspended in olive oil have been used for the prevention[230,231] or treatment of zinc deficiency in sheep.[257] In most situations, practical zinc supplementation will require its addition to blocks, liquids, concentrates, or in a complete ration. Zinc sulfate, zinc oxide, and mineral chelates, such as zinc methionine, will be efficacious in prevention or treatment of zinc deficiency in cattle. Assuming that feed consumption is 15 kg DM/day, supplementation with 30 μg zinc/g diet will increase the daily zinc intake to 450 mg zinc/day. If zinc deficiency or a zinc responsive condition is suspected in adult cattle, a daily intake of 0.5 g zinc per day should alleviate signs of deficiency. This is a useful approach in assessing whether zinc is related to specific disorders, but adequate numbers of control animals are needed to prove causality.

If accidental oversupplementation occurs, cattle can develop signs of zinc toxicosis. Adult cattle are much less susceptible than are calves, and the signs of zinc toxicosis are as follow: diarrhea, anorexia, pica, polyuria, polydipsia, pneumonia, cardiac arrythmia, and seizures.[149] Gross and clinical pathologic changes are as follow: severe diffuse bronchopneumonia, noninflammatory pancreatitis, nephrosis, hepatosis, adrenal cortical fibrosis, infarcts, and petechiation involving many organs, with accompanying reductions in activated partial thromboplastin time and prothrombin time, and leukocytosis with a regenerative left shift.[148,150]

SUMMARY

Deficiency of cobalt, copper, iron, iodine, manganese, selenium, or zinc can cause a reduction in production. Reduced production occurs most commonly when a deficiency corresponds to the phases of growth, reproduction, or lactation. Because of environmental, nutrient, disease, genetic, and drug interactions, deficiencies of single or multiple elements can occur even when the levels recommended by the National Research Council for these nutrients are being fed. Additionally, random supplementation of trace elements above National Research Council recommendations is not justified because of the negative interaction among nutrients and potential toxicosis. Evaluation of trace element status can be difficult because many disease states will alter blood analytes used to evaluate nutrient adequacy. Proper dietary and animal evaluation, as well as response to supplementation, are necessary before diagnosing a trace element deficiency.

REFERENCES

1. Abdelrahim AI, Wensing T, Schotman AJH: Distribution of iron and copper in the liver and spleen of veal calves in relation to the concentration of iron in the diet. Res Vet Sci 40:109, 1986
2. Abu Damir H, Barrie MES, El Hassan SM, et al: Clinical zinc and copper deficiencies in cattle of Western Sudan. Trop Anim Health Prod 20:52, 1988
3. Aceves C, Romero C, Sahagun L, et al: Thyroid hormone profile in dairy cattle acclimated to cold or hot environmental temperatures. Acta Endocrinol (Copenh) 114:201, 1987
4. Adams SN, Honeysett JL, Tiller KG, et al: Factors controlling the increase of cobalt in plants following the addition of a cobalt fertilizer. Aust J Soil Res 7:29, 1969
5. Agricultural Research Council Working Party: The Nutrient Requirements of Ruminant Livestock. Farnham Royal, Slough, Commonwealth Agricultural Bureaux, 1980
6. Ahn C-S, Rosenberg IN: Prompt stimulation of the organic binding of iodine in the thyroid by adenosine 3′,5′-phosphate in vivo. Proc National Acad Sci USA 60:830, 1968
7. Akasha MA, Anderson RR, Ellersieck M, et al: Concentration of thyroid hormones and prolactin in dairy cattle serum and milk at three stages of lactation. J Dairy Sci 70:271, 1987
8. Alderman G, Stranks MH: The iodine content of bulk herd milk in summer in relation to estimated dietary iodine intake of cows. J Sci Fd Agric 18:151, 1967
9. Alfaro E, Neathery MW, Miller WJ, et al: Influence of a wide range of calcium intakes on tissue distribution of macroelements and microelements in dairy calves. J Dairy Sci 71:1295, 1988
10. Allcroft R, Scarnell J, Hignett SL: A preliminary report on hypothyroidism in cattle and its possible relationship with reproductive disorders. Vet Rec 66:367, 1954
11. Allen JG, Masters HG: Prevention of ovine lupinosis by the oral administration of zinc sulphate and the effect of such therapy on liver and pancreas zinc and liver copper. Aust Vet J 56:168, 1980
12. Allen WM, Bradley R, Berrett S, et al: Degenerative myopathy with myoglobinuria in yearling cattle. Br Vet J 131:292, 1975
13. Allen WM: Therapy for deficiency and excess of copper. In Howell JMcC, Gawthorne JM (eds): Copper in Animals and Man, Vol II. Boca Raton, CRC Press, 1987, p 123
14. Ammerman CB, Miller SM: Biological availability of minor mineral ions: A review. J Anim Sci 35:681, 1972
15. Ammerman CB, Wing JM, Dunavant BG, et al: Utilization of inorganic iron by ruminants as influenced by form of iron and iron status of the animal. J Anim Sci 26:404, 1967
16. Anderson PH, Bradley R, Berrett S, et al: The sequence of myodegeneration in nutritional myopathy of the older calf. Br Vet J 133:160, 1977
17. Andresen E, Flagstad T, Basse A, et al: Evidence of a lethal trait, A 46, in black pied Danish cattle of Friesian descent. Nord Vet-Med 22:473, 1970
18. Andrews ED, Sinclair PD: Goitre and neonatal mortality in lambs. New Zealand Society of Animal Production Proceedings 22:123, 1962
19. Apgar J, Fitzgerald JA: Effect on the ewe and lamb of low zinc intake throughout pregnancy. J Anim Sci 60:1530, 1985
20. Apgar J: Zinc and reproduction. Ann Rev Nutr 5:43, 1985
21. Arora SP, Hatfield EE, Hinds FC, et al: Influence of dietary zinc on the activity of blood vitamin A, alcohol dehydrogenase and carbonic anhydrase in lambs. Indian J Anim Sci 43:140, 1973
22. Arthur JR, Boyne R: Superoxide dismutase and glutathione peroxidase activities in neutrophils from selenium deficient and copper deficient cattle. Life Sci 36:1569, 1985
23. Arthur JR, Morrice PC, Beckett GJ: Thyroid hormone concentrations in selenium deficient and selenium sufficient cattle. Res Vet Sci 45:122, 1988

24. Arthur JR: Effects of selenium and vitamin E status on plasma creatine kinase activity in calves. J Nutr 118:747, 1988

25. Aschbacher PW, Cragle RG, Swanson EW, et al: Metabolism of oral iodide and 3,5-diiodosalicylic acid in the pregnant cow. J Dairy Sci 49:1042, 1966

26. Babior BM, Curnutte JT, Okamura N: The respiratory burst oxidase of the human neutrophil. In Halliwell B (ed): Oxygen Radicals and Tissue Injury. Bethesda, Federation of the American Societies for Experimental Biology, 1988, p 43

27. Babior BM, Krouwer JS: The mechanism of adenosylcobalamin-dependent reactions. CRC Crit Rev Biochem 6:35, 1979

28. Barnea A, Colombani-Vidal M, Cho G, et al: Evidence for synergism between copper and prostaglandin E-2 in stimulating the release of gonadotropin-releasing hormone from median eminence explants: $Na+/Cl-$ requirements. Mol Cell Endocrinol 56:11, 1988

29. Barua J, Cragle RG, Miller JK: Sites of gastrointestinal-blood passage of iodide and thyroxine in young cattle. J Dairy Sci 47:539, 1964

30. Beeson WM, Perry TW, Zurcher TD: Effect of supplemental zinc on growth and on hair and blood serum levels of beef cattle. J Anim Sci 45:160, 1977

31. Behne D, Duk M, Elger W: Selenium content and glutathione peroxidase activity in the testis of the maturing rat. J Nutr 116:1442, 1986

32. Benedict CR, Kett J, Porter JW: Properties of farnesyl pyrophosphate synthetase of pig liver. Arch Biochem Biophys 110:611, 1965

33. Bentley OG, Phillips PH: The effect of low manganese rations upon dairy cattle. J Dairy Sci 34:396, 1951

34. Berg JN, Maas JP, Paterson JA, et al: Efficacy of ethylenediamine dihydroiodide as an agent to prevent experimentally induced bovine foot rot. Am J Vet Res 45:1073, 1984

35. Berg JN, Padgitt D, McCarthy B: Iodine concentrations in milk of dairy cattle fed various amounts of iodine as ethylenediamine dihydroiodide. J Dairy Sci 71:3283, 1988

36. Beyer WF, Fridovich I: Manganese catalase and manganese superoxide dismutase: spectroscopic similarity with functional diversity. In Schramm VL, Wedler FC (eds): Manganese in Metabolism and Enzyme Function. Orlando, Academic Press, 1986, p 193

37. Bhaskaram P: Immunology of iron-deficient subjects. In Chandra RK (ed): Nutrition and Immunology. New York, Alan R Liss, 1988, p 149

38. Bide RW: Clinical chemistry of grain-fed cattle. III. Plasma thyroid profiles with notes on interference by EDDI and hypothyroid values in Herefords. Can J Anim Sci 56:457, 1976

39. Binnerts WT, Brouwer E: Analysis of milk in deficiency diseases and intoxications of cattle. Nature 174:973, 1954

40. Black JR, Ammerman CB, Henry PR, et al: Influence of dietary manganese on tissue trace mineral accumulation and depletion in sheep. Can J Anim Sci 65:653, 1985

41. Black JR, Ammerman CB, Henry PR: Effect of quantity and route of administration of manganese monoxide on feed intake and serum manganese in ruminants. J Dairy Sci 68:433, 1985

42. Black JR, Ammerman CB, Henry PR: Effects of high dietary manganese as manganese oxide or manganese carbonate in sheep. J Anim Sci 60:861, 1985

43. Blakley BR, Berezowski JA, Schiefer HB, et al: Chronic copper toxicity in a dairy cow. Can Vet J 23:190, 1982

44. Blalock TL, Dunn MA, Cousins RJ: Metallothionein gene expression in rats: Tissue-specific regulation by dietary copper and zinc. J Nutr 118:222, 1988

45. Blaxter KL, Sharman GAM, MacDonald AM: Iron-deficiency anemia in calves. Br J Nutr 11:234, 1957

46. Bohman VR, Poole SC, Kvasnicka WG, et al: The toxicology and composition of bovine tissues after parenteral administration of high levels of copper salts. Vet Hum Toxicol 29:307, 1987

47. Boila RJ, Devlin TJ, Drysdale RA, et al: Supplementary copper for grazing beef cattle—injectable copper glycinate, and copper sulfate in free-choice mineral supplements. Can J Anim Sci 64:675, 1984

48. Bond JS, Unger DF, Garganta CL: Properties and regulation of mouse liver arginase. *In* Schramm VL, Wedler FC (eds): Manganese in Metabolism and Enzyme Function. Orlando, Academic Press, 1986, p 239

49. Borg DC, Schaich KM: Iron and iron-derived radicals. *In* Halliwell B (ed): Oxygen Radicals and Tissue Injury. Bethesda, Federation of the American Societies for Experimental Biology, 1988, p 20

50. Boyne R, Arthur JR: Alterations of neutrophil function in selenium-deficient cattle. J Comp Pathol 89:151, 1979

51. Boyne R, Arthur JR: Effects of molybdenum or iron induced copper deficiency on the viability and function of neutrophils from cattle. Res Vet Sci 41:417, 1986

52. Boyne R, Arthur JR: Effects of selenium and copper deficiency on neutrophil function in cattle. J Comp Pathol 91:271, 1981

53. Brabant G, Ocran K, Ranft U, et al: Physiological regulation of thyrotropin. Biochimie 71:293, 1989

54. Brandt M, Schramm VL: Mammalian manganese metabolism and manganese uptake and distribution in rat hepatocytes. *In* Schramm VL, Wedler FC (eds): Manganese in Metabolism and Enzyme Function. Orlando, Academic Press, 1986, p 3

55. Bremner I, Dalgarno AC: Iron metabolism in the veal calf. The availability of different iron compounds. Br J Nutr 29:229, 1973

56. Bremner I, Dalgarno AC: Iron metabolism in the veal calf. 2. Iron requirements and the effect of copper supplementation. Br J Nutr 30:61, 1973

57. Bremner I, Humphries WR, Phillippo M, et al: Iron-induced copper deficiency in calves: dose-response relationships and interactions with molybdenum and sulphur. Anim Prod 45:403, 1987

58. Bremner I, Young BW, Mills CF: Protective effect of zinc supplementation against copper toxicosis in sheep. Br J Nutr 36:551, 1976

59. Bremner I: Interactions between metallothionein and trace elements. Prog Food Nutr Sci 11:1, 1987

60. Britton JW, Goss H: Chronic molybdenum poisoning in cattle. J Am Vet Med Assoc 108:176, 1946

61. Brock JH, Mainou-Fowler T: Iron and immunity. Proc Nutr Soc 45:305, 1986

62. Brown MA, Casillas ER: Manganese and manganese-ATP interactions with bovine sperm adenylate cyclase. Arch Biochem Biophys 244:719, 1986

63. Browning JD, Reeves PG, O'Dell BL: Effect of zinc deficiency and food restriction on the plasma levels of prostaglandin metabolites in male rats. J Nutr 113:755, 1983

64. Brummerstedt E, Andresen E, Basse A, et al: Lethal trait A 46 in cattle. Immunological investigations. Nord Vet-Med 26:279, 1974

65. Brummerstedt E, Flagstad T, Basse A, et al: The effect of zinc on calves with hereditary thymus hypoplasia (lethal trait A 46). Acta Path Microbiol Scand [A] 79:686, 1971

66. Bulgin MS, Maas J, Anderson BC, et al: Death associated with parenteral administration of copper disodium edetate in calves. J Am Vet Med Assoc 188:406, 1986

67. Bunce GE, Vessal M: Effect of zinc and/or pyridoxine deficiency upon oestrogen retention and oestrogen receptor distribution in the rat uterus. J Steroid Biochem 26:303, 1987

68. Bunger V, Schmoldt P, Ponge J: Orale und parenterale Eisenmangelbekaempfung in Beziehung zum Ablauf von Erkrankungen bei Traenkkaelbern aus verschiedenen Herkunsftsbetrieben. Mh Vet-Med 41:302, 1986

69. Burk RF: Recent developments in trace element metabolism and function: Newer roles of selenium in nutrition. J Nutr 119:1051, 1989

70. Bustad LK, Fuller JM: Thyroid function in domestic animals. Laboratory Animal Care 20:561, 1970

71. Butler GW, Peterson PJ: Aspects of the faecal excretion of selenium by sheep. NZ J Agric Res 4:484, 1962

72. Butler JA, Beilstein MA, Whanger PD: Influence of dietary methionine on the metabolism of selenomethionine in rats. J Nutr 119:1001, 1989

73. Cameron HJ, Boila RJ, McNichol LW, et al: Cupric oxide needles for grazing cattle

consuming low-copper, high-molybdenum forage and high-sulfate water. J Anim
Sci 67:252, 1989

74. Campbell DT, Maas J, Weber DW, et al: Safety and efficacy of two sustained-release intrareticular selenium supplements and the associated placental and colostral transfer of selenium in beef cattle. Am J Vet Res 51:813, 1990

75. Capen CC: The endocrine glands. In Jubb KVF, Kennedy PC, Palmer N (eds):
Pathology of Domestic Animals, ed 3, vol 3. Orlando, Academic Press, 1985,
p 272

76. Carayon P, Amr S: Mechanisms of thyroid regulation. In DeGroot LJ (ed): Endocrinology. Philadelphia, WB Saunders Co, 1989, p 530

77. Carlos GM, Telfer SB, Johnson CL, et al: Microbiological assay of blood serum for
the vitamin B_{12} status of dairy cows. J Dairy Res 54:463, 1987

78. Carlson RH, Swenson MJ, Ward GM, et al: Effects of intramuscular injections of
iron-dextran in newborn lambs and calves. J Am Vet Med Assoc 139:457, 1961

79. Carter JC Jr, Miller WJ, Neathery MW, et al: Manganese metabolism with oral and
intravenous 54-Mn in young calves as influenced by supplemental manganese.
J Anim Sci 38:1284, 1974

80. Chan WY, Bates JM, Raghib MH, et al: Bioavailability of manganese in milk studied
in in vitro and in vivo systems. In Schramm VL, Wedler FC (eds): Manganese in
Metabolism and Enzyme Function. Orlando, Academic Press, 1986, p 17

81. Chesters JK: Developments in studies of zinc essentiality. In Hemphill DD (ed):
Trace Substances in Environmental Health — XXI. Proceedings of the University
of Missouri's 21st Annual Conference on Trace Substances in Environmental
Health, 1987, p 473

82. Chvapil M: Effect of zinc on cells and biomembranes. Med Clin North Am 60:799,
1976

83. Claypool DW, Adams FW, Pendell HW, et al: Relationship between the level of
copper in the blood plasma and liver of cattle. J Anim Sci 41:911, 1975

84. Clegg MS, Keen CL, Hurley LS: Biochemical pathologies of zinc deficiency. In
Mills CF (ed): Zinc in Human Biology. London, Springer-Verlag, 1989, p 129

85. Clegg MS, Lonnerdal B, Hurley LS, et al: Analysis of whole blood manganese by
flameless atomic absorption spectrophotometry and its use as an indicator of
manganese status in animals. Anal Biochem 157:12, 1986

86. Cousins RJ: Absorption, transport, and hepatic metabolism of copper and zinc:
Special reference to metallothionein and ceruloplasmin. Physiol Rev 65:238,
1985

87. Cousins RJ: Molecular biology and micronutrient-disease relationships — zinc as a
prototype. In Halstead CA, Rucker RB (eds): Nutrition and the Origins of Disease. San Diego, Academic Press, 1989, p 1

88. Csermely P, Szamel M, Resch K, et al: Zinc can increase the activity of protein
kinase C and contributes to its binding to plasma membranes in T lymphocytes.
J Biol Chem 263:6487, 1988

89. Cunnane SC, Majid E, Senior J, et al: Uteroplacental dysfunction and prostaglandin
metabolism in zinc deficient pregnant rats. Life Sci 32:2471, 1983

90. Daburon F, Fayart G, Tricaud Y: Caesium and iodine metabolism in lactating cows
under chronic administration. Sci Total Environ 85:253, 1989

91. Dallman PR: Biochemical basis for the manifestations of iron deficiency. Ann Rev
Nutr 6:13, 1986

92. Davidson LA, Lonnerdal B: Fe-saturation and proteolysis of human lactoferrin:
Effect on brush-border receptor-mediated uptake of Fe and Mn. Am J Physiol
257:G930, 1989

93. Davidson LA, Lonnerdal B: Specific binding of lactoferrin to brush-border membrane: Ontogeny and effect of glycan chain. Am J Physiol 254:G580, 1988

94. Davidson WB, McMurray CH: 75-Selenium-labeled sheep plasma: The time course
of changes in 75-selenium distribution. J Inorg Biochem 34:1, 1988

95. Davis GK, Mertz W: Copper. In Mertz W (ed): Trace Elements in Human Health
and Disease, vol 1, ed 5, San Diego, Academic Press, 1987, p 301

96. DeGroot LJ, Torresani J: Triiodothyronine binding to isolated liver cell nuclei.
Endocrinology 96:357, 1975

97. DeGroot LJ: Thyroid hormone nuclear receptors and their role in the metabolic action of the hormone. Biochimie 71:269, 1989
98. Deland MPB, Lewis D, Cunningham PR, et al: Use of orally administered oxidised copper wire particles for copper therapy in cattle. Aust Vet J 63:1, 1986
99. Demertzis PN, Mills CF: Oral zinc therapy in the control of infectious pododermatitis in young bulls. Vet Rec 93:219, 1973
100. Dinarello CA: Interleukin-1 and its biologically related cytokines. Adv Immunol 44:153, 1989
101. Driver PM, Eames C, Telfer SB: The effects of differing compositions of soluble phosphate glass boluses on the copper, cobalt and selenium status of Swaledale ewes. In Hurley LS, Keen CL, Lonnerdal B, et al (eds): Trace Elements in Man and Animals 6. New York, Plenum Press, 1988, p 637
102. Droke EA, Loerch SC: Effects of parenteral selenium and vitamin E on performance, health and humoral immune response of steers new to the feedlot environment. J Anim Sci 67:1350, 1989
103. Dufty JH, Bingley JB, Cove LY: The plasma zinc concentration of nonpregnant, pregnant and parturient Hereford cattle. Austral Vet J 53:519, 1977
104. Dunn JT: Iodine deficiency and excess as environmental goitrogens. In Gaitan E (ed): Environmental Goitrogenesis. Boca Raton, FL, CRC Press, 1989, p 139
105. Dyer IA, Rojas MA: Manganese requirements and functions in cattle. J Am Vet Med Assoc 147:1393, 1965
106. Dylewski DP, Lytton FDC, Bunce GE: Dietary zinc and parturition in the rat II. Myometrial gap junctions. Biol Trace Elem Res 9:165, 1986
107. Egan AR: Reproductive responses to supplemental zinc and manganese in grazing Dorset Horn ewes. Aust J Exp Agric Anim Husb 12:131, 1972
108. Ermans A, Bourdoux P: Antithyroid sulfurated compounds. In Gaitan E (ed): Environmental Goitrogenesis. Boca Raton, FL, CRC Press, 1989, p 15
109. Erskine RJ, Eberhart RJ, Hutchinson LJ, et al: Blood selenium concentrations and glutathione peroxidase activities in dairy herds with high and low somatic cell counts. J Am Vet Med Assoc 190:1417, 1987
110. Esaki N, Nakamura T, Tanaka H, et al: Enzymatic synthesis of selenocysteine in rat liver. Biochemistry 20:4492, 1981
111. Ettinger MJ: Copper metabolism and diseases of copper metabolism. In Lontie R (ed): Copper Proteins and Copper Enzymes, vol III. Boca Raton, FL CRC Press, 1984, p 175
112. Evenson JK, Sunde RA: Selenium incorporation into selenoproteins in the Se-adequate and Se-deficient rat. Proc Soc Exp Biol Med 187:169, 1988
113. Everett G, Apgar J: Effect of zinc deficiency on prostaglandin levels in pregnant rats. Nutr Res Suppl I:335, 1985
114. Evvard JM: Iodine deficiency symptoms and their significance in animal nutrition and pathology. Endocrinology 12:539, 1928
115. Failla ML: Hormonal regulation of manganese metabolism. In Schramm VL, Wedler FC (eds): Manganese in Metabolism and Enzyme Function. Orlando, Academic Press, 1986, p 93
116. Feldman BF, Kaneko JJ, Farver TB: Anemia of inflammatory disease in the dog: Ferrokinetics of adjuvant-induced anemia. Am J Vet Res 42:583, 1981
117. Feldman BF, Kaneko JJ, Farver TB: Anemia of inflammatory disease in the dog: Availability of storage iron in inflammatory disease. Am J Vet Res 42:586, 1981
118. Feldman BF, Kaneko JJ, Farver TB: Anemia of inflammatory disease in the dog: Clinical characterization. Am J Vet Res 42:1109, 1981
119. Feldman BF, Keen CL, Kaneko JJ, et al: Anemia of inflammatory disease in the dog: Measurement of hepatic superoxide dismutase, hepatic nonheme iron, copper, zinc and ceruloplasmin and serum iron, copper and zinc. Am J Vet Res 42:1114, 1981
120. Fell BF, Farmer LJ, Farquharson C, et al: Observations on the pancreas of cattle deficient in copper. J Comp Pathol 95:573, 1985
121. Fell BF, Mills CF, Boyne R: Cytochrome oxidase deficiency in the motor neurones of copper-deficient lambs: A histochemical study. Res Vet Sci 6:170, 1965

122. Finch CA: Regulation of iron exchange. *In* Halsted CH, Rucker RB (eds): Nutrition and the Origins of Disease. San Diego, Academic Press, 1989, p 57

123. Flagstad T, Andersen S, Nielsen K: The course of experimental fasciola hepatica infection in calves with a deficient cellular immunity. Res Vet Sci 13:468, 1972

124. Flagstad T: Intestinal absorption of ^{65}Zinc in A46 (adema disease) after treatment with oxychinolines. Nord Vet-Med 29:96, 1977

125. Flagstad T: Lethal trait A 46 in cattle intestinal zinc absorption. Nord Vet-Med 28:160, 1976

126. Fletcher MP, Gershwin ME, Keen CL, et al: Trace element deficiencies and immune responsiveness in humans and animal models. *In* Chandra RK (ed): Nutrition and Immunology. New York, Alan R Liss, 1988, p 215

127. Fradkin JE, Wolff J: Iodide-induced thyrotoxicosis. Medicine 62:1, 1983

128. Franke AA, Bruhn JC, Osland RB: Factors affecting iodine concentration of milk of individual cows. J Dairy Sci 66:997, 1983

129. Furugouri K, Miyata Y, Shijimaya K: Ferritin in blood serum of dairy cows. J Dairy Sci 65:1529, 1982

130. Gaitan E, Cooksey RB: General concepts of environmental goitrogenesis. *In* Gaitan E (ed): Environmental Goitrogenesis. Boca Raton, FL, CRC Press, 1989, p 3

131. Garvey JS: Metallothionein: Structure/antigenicity and detection/quantitation in normal physiological fluids. Environ Health Perspect 54:117, 1984

132. Gershwin ME, Beach RS, Hurley LS: Nutrition and Immunity. Orlando, Academic Press, 1985

133. Getty SM, Beck CC, Brown LD, et al: Effect of iron on hematology and growth of calves. J Anim Sci 27:712, 1968

134. Geurink HJ, Malestein A, Kemp A, et al: Nitrate poisoning in cattle. 7. Prevention. Neth J Agric Sci 30:105, 1982

135. Gibbons RA, Dixon SN, Hallis K, et al: Manganese metabolism in cows and goats. Biochim Biophys Acta 444:1, 1976

136. Gilman AG, Rall TW: Studies on the relation of cyclic 3',5'-AMP (CA) to TSH action in beef thyroid slices. Fed Proc 25:617, 1966

137. Goldberg Y, Glineur C, Bosselut R, et al: Thyroid hormone action and the erbA oncogene family. Biochimie 71:279, 1989

138. Golden MHN, Ramdath D: Free radicals in the pathogenesis of kwashiorkor. Proc Nutr Soc 46:53, 1987

139. Goodman JR, Dallman PR: Role of copper in iron localization in developing erythrocytes. Blood 34:747, 1969

140. Gooneratne SR, Buckley WT, Christensen DA: Review of copper deficiency and metabolism in ruminants. Can J Anim Sci 69:819, 1989

141. Gooneratne SR, Chaplin RK, Trent AM, et al: Effect of tetrathiomolybdate administration on the excretion of copper, zinc, iron and molybdenum in sheep bile. Br Vet J 145:62, 1989

142. Gooneratne SR, Christensen DA: A survey of maternal and fetal tissue zinc, iron, manganese and selenium concentrations in bovine. Can J Anim Sci 69:151, 1989

143. Gooneratne SR, Howell JMcC, Gawthorne JM: An investigation of the effects of intravenous administration of thiomolybdate on copper metabolism in chronic Cu-poisoned sheep. Br J Nutr 46:469, 1981

144. Gooneratne SR, Olkowski AA, Klemmer RG, et al: High sulfur related thiamine deficiency in cattle: A field study. Can Vet J 30:139, 1989

145. Gorbman A, Lissitzky S, Michel O, et al: Metabolism of radioiodine by the near-term bovine fetus. Endocrinology 51:546, 1952

146. Grace ND: Studies on the flow of zinc, cobalt, copper and manganese along the digestive tract of sheep given fresh perennial ryegrass, or white or red clover. Br J Nutr 34:73, 1975

147. Graham TW, Giri SN, Cullor J, et al: Mechanisms of endotoxin-induced abortion in cows: PGF2α and hypozincemia. FASEB J 3:A1137, 1989

148. Graham TW, Holmberg CA, Keen CL, et al: A pathologic and toxicologic evaluation of veal calves fed large amounts of zinc. Vet Pathol 25:484, 1988

149. Graham TW, Thurmond MC, Clegg MS, et al: An epidemiologic study of mortality in veal calves subsequent to an episode of zinc toxicosis on a California veal calf

operation using zinc sulfate-supplemented milk replacer. J Am Vet Med Assoc 190:1296, 1987

150. Graham TW, Feldman BF, Farber TB, et al: Zinc toxicosis in Holstein veal calves and its relationship to an associated thrombotic state. Comp Haematol International, in press

151. Greene LW, Lunt DK, Byers FM, et al: Performance and carcass quality of steers supplemented with zinc oxide or zinc methionine. J Anim Sci 66:1818, 1988

152. Greger JL, Marcus RE: Effect of dietary protein, phosphorus, and sulfur amino acids on selenium metabolism of adult males. Ann Nutr Metab 25:97, 1981

153. Greger JL: Effect of variations in dietary protein, phosphorous, electrolytes, and vitamin D on calcium and zinc metabolism. In Bodwell CE, Erdman JW (eds): Nutrient Interactions. New York, Marcel Dekker, 1988 p 205

154. Groce AW, Miller ER, Hichcock JP, et al: Selenium balance in the pig as affected by selenium source and vitamin E. J Anim Sci 37:942, 1973

155. Gyang O, Stevens JB, Olson WG, et al: Effects of selenium-vitamin E injection on bovine polymorphonucleated leukocytes phagocytosis and killing of Staphylococcus aureus. Am J Vet Res 45:175, 1984

156. Haaranen S: The effect of zinc on itching tail root eczema in cattle. Nord Vet-Med 14:265, 1962

157. Halpin CG, Harris DJ, Caple IW, et al: Contribution of cobalamin analogues to plasma vitamin B_{12} concentrations in cattle. Res Vet Sci 37:249, 1984

158. Hambidge KM, Casey CE, Krebs NF: Zinc. In Mertz W (ed): Trace Elements in Human Health and Disease, vol 2, ed 5. San Diego, Academic Press, 1986, p 1

159. Hampton DL, Miller WJ, Neathery MW, et al: Absorption of zinc from small and large intestine of calves. J Dairy Sci 59:1963, 1976

160. Hansard SL, Foote LE, Dimopoullos GT: The physiological behavior of iron in the calf. J Dairy Sci 42:1970, 1959

161. Hansard SL: Physiological behaviour of manganese in gravid cattle, sheep and swine. In Isotope Studies on the Physiology of Domestic Animals. Vienna, International Atomic Energy Agency, 1972, p 351

162. Harris WR, Keen CL: Calculations of the distribution of zinc in a computer model of human serum. J Nutr 119:1677, 1989

163. Harrison JH, Hancock DD, Conrad HR: Vitamin E and selenium for reproduction of the dairy cow. J Dairy Sci 67:123, 1984

164. Hawkes WC, Tappel AL: In vitro synthesis of glutathione peroxidase from selenite translational incorporation of selenocysteine. Biochim Biophys Acta 739:225, 1983

165. Hawkes WC, Wilhelmsen EC, Tappel AL: Abundance and tissue distribution of selenocystein-containing proteins in the rat. J Inorg Biochem 23:77, 1985

166. Hawkins GE Jr, Wise GH, Matrone G, et al: Manganese in the nutrition of young dairy cattle fed different levels of calcium and phosphorus. J Dairy Sci 38:536, 1955

167. Hebbel RP, Miller WJ: Unique promotion of erythrophagocytosis by malondialdehyde. Am J Hematol 39:222, 1988

168. Hemken RW, Vandersall HJ, Brown AC: Occurrence of goiter in calves from cows fed corn silage. J Anim Sci 24:886, 1965

169. Hemken RW, Vandersall JH, Sass BA, et al: Goitrogenic effects of a corn silage-soybean meal supplemented ration. J Dairy Sci 54:85, 1971

170. Hemken RW: Iodine. J Dairy Sci 53:1138, 1970

171. Henkin RI: Growth hormone-dependent changes in zinc and copper metabolism in man. In Hoekstra WG, Suttle JW, Ganther HE, et al (eds): Trace Element Metabolism in Animals-2. Baltimore, University Park Press, 1974, p 652

172. Henry D, Ferino F, Tomova S, et al: Inhibition of the catalytic subunit of ram sperm adenylate cyclase by adenosine. Biochem Biophys Res Commun 137:970, 1986

173. Henry PR, Echevarria MG, Ammerman CB, et al: Estimation of the relative biological availability of inorganic selenium sources for ruminants using tissue uptake of selenium. J Anim Sci 66:2306, 1988

174. Hetzel BS, Mabley GF: Iodine. In Mertz W (ed): Trace Elements in Human Health and Disease, vol 2, ed 5. San Diego, Academic Press, 1986, p 139

175. Hetzel BS, Mano MT: A review of experimental studies of iodine deficiency during fetal development. J Nutr 119:145, 1989

176. Hibbs JW, Conrad HR, Vandersall JH, et al: Occurrence of iron deficiency anemia in dairy calves at birth and its alleviation by iron dextran injection. J Dairy Sci 46:1118, 1963

177. Hidiroglou M, Hartin KE: Vitamins A, E and selenium blood levels in the fat cow syndrome. Can Vet J 23:255, 1982

178. Hidiroglou M, Ho SK, Ivan M, et al: Manganese status of pasturing ewes, of pregnant ewes and doe rabbits on low manganese diets and of dairy cows with cystic ovaries. Can J Comp Med 42:100, 1978

179. Hidiroglou M, Knipfel JE: Zinc in mammalian sperm: A review. J Dairy Sci 67:1147, 1984

180. Hidiroglou M, Williams CJ, Kramer JKG: Fate of labeled choline administered intraruminally to pregnant ewes given manganese-deficient or -supplemented rations. Am J Vet Res 40:1273, 1979

181. Hidiroglou M: ^{54}Mn uptake by the ovaries and reproductive tract of cycling and anestrous ewes. Can J Physiol Pharmacol 53:969, 1975

182. Hidiroglou M: Manganese in ruminant nutrition. Can J Anim Sci 59:217, 1979

183. Hidiroglou M: Trace elements in the fetal and neonate ruminant: A review. Can Vet J 21:328, 1980

184. Hill CH, Matrone G: Chemical parameters in the study of in vivo and in vitro interactions of transition elements. Fed Proc 29:1474, 1970

185. Hill CH: Interrelationships of selenium with other trace elements. Fed Proc 34:2096, 1975

186. Hoskins FH, Hansard SL: Placental transfer and fetal tissue iron utilization in sheep. J Nutr 83:10, 1964

187. Howes AD, Dyer IA: Diet and supplemental mineral effects on manganese metabolism in newborn calves. J Anim Sci 32:141, 1971

188. Huebers HA, Finch CA: The physiology of transferrin and transferrin receptors. Physiol Rev 67:520, 1987

189. Humphries WR, Phillippo M, Young BW, et al: The influence of dietary iron and molybdenum on copper metabolism in calves. Br J Nutr 48:77, 1983

190. Humphries WR: Control of hypocupraemia in cattle by addition of copper to water supplies. Vet Rec 106:359, 1980

191. Hunt DM, Johnson DR: An inherited deficiency in noradrenaline biosynthesis in the brindled mouse. J Neurochem 19:2811, 1972

192. Hurley LS, Keen CL: Manganese. In Mertz W (ed): Trace Elements in Human Health and Disease, vol 1, ed 5. San Diego, Academic Press, 1987, p 185

193. Hurley WL, Doane RM: Recent developments in the roles of vitamins and minerals in reproduction. J Dairy Sci 72:784, 1989

194. Hutcheson DP: Nutritional factors affect immune response in cattle. Feedstuffs 61(15):16, 1989

195. Ivan M, Grieve CM: Effects of zinc, copper and manganese supplementation of high-concentrate ration on digestibility, growth, and tissue content of Holstein calves. J Dairy Sci 58:410, 1975

196. Ivan M, Grieve CM: Effects of zinc, copper, and manganese supplementation of high-concentrate ration on gastrointestinal absorption of copper and manganese in Holstein calves. J Dairy Sci 59:1764, 1976

197. Ivan M, Hidiroglou M: Effect of dietary manganese on growth and manganese metabolism in sheep. J Dairy Sci 63:385, 1980

198. Ivan M, Veira DM: Effect of dietary protein on the solubilities of manganese, copper, zinc and iron in the rumen and abomasum of sheep. Can J Anim Sci 61:955, 1981

199. Jain KJ, Williams DM: Copper deficiency anemia: Altered red blood cell lipids and viscosity in rats. Am J Clin Nutr 48:637, 1988

200. Jain NC: Schalm's Veterinary Hematology, ed 4. Philadelphia, Lea and Febiger, 1986, p 1221

201. Jenkins KJ, Hidiroglou M: Binding of selenium-75 to blood and liver cytosolic proteins in the preruminant calf. J Dairy Sci 71:442, 1988

202. Jones DG, Suttle NF: Copper and disease resistance. *In* Hemphill DD (ed): Trace Substances in Environmental Health—XXI. Proceedings of the University of Missouri's 21st Annual Conference on Trace Substances in Environmental Health, 1987, p 514

203. Jones DG, Suttle NF: Some effects of copper deficiency on leucocyte function in sheep and cattle. Res Vet Sci 31:151, 1981

204. Jones DG, Suttle NF: The effect of copper deficiency on the resistance of mice to infection with *Pastuerella haemolytica*. J Comp Pathol 93:143, 1983

205. Judson GJ, McFarlane JD, Riley MJ, et al: Vitamin B_{12} and copper supplementation in beef calves. Aust Vet J 58:249, 1982

206. Julien WE, Conrad HR, Jones JE, et al: Selenium and vitamin E and incidence of retained placenta in parturient dairy cows. J Dairy Sci 59:1954, 1976

207. Kalkus JW: A study of goitre and associated conditions in domestic animals. Bull Wash Ag Exp Sta 156:4, 1920

208. Kaneko JJ, Mattheeuws DRG: Iron metabolism in normal and porphyric calves. Am J Vet Res 27:923, 1966

209. Kaneko JJ, Mills R: Hematological and blood chemical observations in neonatal normal and porphyric calves in early life. Cornell Vet 60:52, 1970

210. Kaneko JJ: Erythrokinetics and iron metabolism in bovine porphyria erythropoietica. Ann N Y Acad Sci 104:689, 1963

211. Kawano J, Ney DM, Keen CL, et al: Altered high density lipoprotein composition in manganese-deficient Sprague-Dawley and Wistar rats. J Nutr 117:902, 1987

212. Keen CL, Bell JG, Lonnerdal B: The effect of age on manganese uptake and retention from milk and infant formulas in rats. J Nutr 116:395, 1986

213. Keen CL, Clegg MS, Lonnerdal B, et al: Whole-blood manganese as an indicator of body manganese (letter). N Engl J Med 308:1230, 1983

214. Keen CL, Gershwin ME: Zinc deficiency and immune function. Ann Rev Nutr 10: 1990

215. Keen CL, Graham TW: Trace elements. *In* Kaneko JJ (ed): Clinical Biochemistry of Domestic Animals, ed 4. San Diego, Academic Press, 1989, p 753

216. Keen CL, Hurley LS: Zinc and reproduction: Effects of deficiency on foetal and postnatal development. *In* Mills CF (ed): Zinc in Human Biology. London, Springer-Verlag, 1989, p 183

217. Keen CL, Lonnerdal B: Manganese toxicity in man and experimental animals. *In* Schramm VL, Wedler FC (eds): Manganese in Metabolism and Enzyme Function. Orlando, Academic Press, 1986, p 35

218. Keen CL, Zidenberg-Cherr S, Lonnerdal B: Dietary manganese toxicity and deficiency: Effects on cellular manganese metabolism. *In* Kies C (ed): Nutritional Bioavailability of Manganese. Washington, DC, American Chemical Society, 1987, p 21

219. Kelly WR: The liver and biliary system. *In* Jubb KVF, Kennedy PC, Palmer N (eds): Pathology of Domestic Animals, ed 3, vol 2. Orlando, Academic Press, 1985, p 239

220. Kendall-Taylor P: Adenyl cyclase activity in the mouse thyroid gland. J Endocrinol 52:533, 1972

221. Kendall-Taylor P: Comparison of the effects of various agents on thyroidal adenyl cyclase activity with their effects on thyroid hormone release. J Endocrinol 54:137, 1972

222. Kennedy S, Rice DA, Davidson WB: Experimental myopathy in vitamin E- and selenium-depleted calves with and without added dietary polyunsaturated fatty acids as a model for nutritional degenerative myopathy in ruminant cattle. Res Vet Sci 43:384, 1987

223. Kennedy S, Rice DA: Selective morphologic alterations of the cardiac conduction system in calves deficient in vitamin E and selenium. Am J Pathol 130:315, 1988

224. Khan AA, Lovejoy D, Sharma AK, et al: Effects of high dietary sulphur on enzyme activities, selenium concentrations and body weights of cattle. Can J Vet Res 51:174, 1987

225. Kirchgessner M, Roth H-P, Schwarz WA: Zur wirkung von zinkmangel auf den serum-insulinspiegel bei milchkühen. Z Tierphysiol, Tierernährg u Futtermittelkde 36:175, 1975

226. Kiremidjian-Schumacher L, Roy M, Wishe HI, et al: Selenium and immune cell functions. I. Effect on lymphocyte proliferation and production of interleukin 1 and interleukin 2. Proc Soc Exp Biol Med 193:136, 1990
227. Korzeniowsky A, Geurink JH, Kemp A: Nitrate poisoning in cattle. 6. Tungsten (wolfram) as a prophylactic against nitrate-nitrate intoxication in ruminants. Neth J Agric Sci 29:37, 1981
228. Korzeniowsky A, Geurink JH, Kemp A: Nitrate poisoning in cattle. 5. The effect of tungsten on nitrite formation by ruminant microbes. Neth J Agric Sci 28:16, 1980
229. Krishnamurti CR, Ramberg CF Jr, Shariff MA: Kinetic modeling of selenium metabolism in nonpregnant ewes. J Nutr 119:1146, 1989
230. Lamand M, Levieux D: Effects of infection on plasma levels of copper and zinc in ewes. Ann Rech Vét 12:133, 1981
231. Lamand M: Copper and zinc deficiencies treatment by intramuscular injections in sheep. Ann Rech Vét 9:495, 1978
232. Langer P, Greer MA: Antithyroid Substances and Naturally Occurring Goitrogens. Basel, S Karger, 1977, p1
233. Larsen HJ, Moksnes K, Overnes G: Influence of selenium on antibody production in sheep. Res Vet Sci 45:4, 1988
234. Larsen HJ, Overnes G, Moksnes K: Effect of selenium on sheep lymphocyte responses to mitogens. Res Vet Sci 45:11, 1988
235. Lassiter JW, Miller WJ, Pate FM, et al: Effect of dietary calcium and phosphorus on 54-Mn metabolism following single tracer intraperitoneal and oral doses in rats (36140). Proc Soc Exp Biol Med 139:345, 1972
236. Leach RM: Mn(II) and glycosyltransferases essential for skeletal development. In Schramm VL, Wedler FC (eds): Manganese in Metabolism and Enzyme Function. Orlando, Academic Press, 1986, p 81
237. Legg SP, Sears L: Zinc sulphate treatment of parakeratosis in cattle. Nature 186:1061, 1960
238. Leung K, Convey EM, Conner GH: Effect of dietary iodide on hypophyseal and thyroid hormone secretions in Holstein-Friesian heifers. Am J Vet Res 41:1402, 1976
239. Levander OA: Selenium. In Mertz W (ed): Trace Elements in Human Health and Disease, vol 2, ed 5. San Diego, Academic Press, 1986, p 209
240. Li ETS, O'Dell BL: Effect of zinc status on the binding of prostaglandins to ovarian membranes and intact platelets of pregnant rats. J Nutr 116:1448, 1986
241. Lilley GW, Hamar DW, Gerlach M, et al: Linking copper and bacteria with abomasal ulcers in beef calves. Vet Med October:85, 1985
242. Lissitzky S: Physiology of the thyroid, iodine metabolism in the thyroid, thyroid hormone formation, and the biosynthesis and structure-function relationship of thyroglobulin. In DeGroot LJ (ed): Endocrinology, vol 1. Philadelphia, WB Saunders Co, 1989, p 512
243. Lohuis JACM, Verheijden JHM, Burvenich C, et al: Pathophysiological effects of endotoxins in ruminants 2. Metabolic aspects. Vet Q 10:117, 1988
244. Long JF, Gilmore LO, Hibbs JW: The effect of different levels of iodide feeding on serum inorganic and protein-bound iodine, with a note on the frequency of administration required to maintain a high level of serum inorganic iodine. J Dairy Sci 39:1323, 1956
245. Lonnerdal B, Keen CL, Bell JG, et al: Manganese Uptake and Retention: Experimental Animal and Human Studies. In Kies C (ed): Nutritional Bioavailability of Manganese. Washington, DC, American Chemical Society, 1987, p 9
246. Lonnerdal B: Vitamin-mineral interactions. In Bodwell CE, Erdman JW (eds): Nutrient Interactions. New York, Marcel Dekker, 1988, p 163
247. Lytton FDC, Bunce GE: Dietary zinc and parturition in the rat I. Uterine pressure cycles. Biol Trace Elem Res 9:151, 1986
248. Maas J, Berg JN, Peterson RG: Serum distribution of iodine after oral administration of ethylenediamine dihydroiodide in cattle. Am J Vet Res 50:1758, 1989
249. Maas J, Davis LE, Hempstead BS, et al: Efficacy of ethylenediamine dihydroiodide in the prevention of naturally occurring foot rot in cattle. Am J Vet Res 45:2347, 1984

250. Maas J, Parish S, Hodgeson D: Nutritional Myodegeneration. *In* Smith BP (ed): Large animal Internal Medicine, Diseases of Horses, Cattle, Sheep, and Goats. St Louis, CV Mosby Co, 1990, p 1352
251. Maas JP: Diagnosis and management of selenium-responsive diseases in cattle. Comp Cont Ed 5:S393, 1983
252. MacDougall LG, Anderson R, McNab GM, et al: The immune response in iron-deficient children: Impaired cellular defense mechanisms with altered humoral components. J Pediatr 86:833, 1975
253. Mace DL, Tucker JA, Bills CB, et al: Reduction in incidence of birth of premature, weak, or dead calves following sodium selenite d-alpha tocopheryl therapy in pregnant cows. California Department of Agriculture Bulletin No 152:21, 1963
254. Machlin LJ, Langseth L: Vitamin-vitamin interactions. *In* Bodwell CE, Erdman JW (eds): Nutrient Interactions. New York, Marcel Dekker, 1988, p 287
255. MacPherson A, Gray D, Mitchell GBB, et al: Ostertagia infections and neutrophil function in cobalt-deficient and cobalt-supplemented cattle. Br Vet J 143:348, 1987
256. MacPherson A, Kelly EF, Chalmers JS, et al: The effect of selenium deficiency on fertility in heifers. *In* Hemphill DD (ed): Trace Substances in Environmental Health — XXI. Proceedings of the University of Missouri's 21st Annual Conference on Trace Substances in Environmental Health, 1987, p 551
257. Mahmoud OM, Bakeit AO, Elsamini F: Treatment of zinc deficiency in sheep by zinc injections. *In* Mills CF, Bremner I, Chesters JK (eds): Trace Elements in Man and Animals — TEMA 5. Farnham Royal, Slough, Commonwealth Agricultural Bureaux, 1985
258. Malthiery Y, Marriq C, Berge-Lefranc J-L, et al: Thyroglobulin structure and function: Recent advances. Biochimie 71:195, 1989
259. Mano MT, Potter BJ, Belling GB, et al: The effect of thyroxine, 3,5-dimethyl-3'-isopropyl-L-thyronine and iodized oil on fetal brain development in the iodine-deficient sheep. Acta Endocrinol (Copenh) 121:7, 1989
260. Maqsood M: Thyroid functions in relation to reproduction of mammals and birds. Biological Review of the Cambridge Philosophical Society 27:281, 1952
261. Mason J, Woods M, Poole DBR: Accumulation of copper on albumin in bovine plasma in vivo after intravenous trithiomolybdate administration. Res Vet Sci 41:108, 1986
262. Masters DG, Fels HE: Effect of zinc supplementation on the reproductive performance of grazing Merino ewes. Biol Trace Elem Res 2:281, 1980
263. Masters DG, Moir RJ: Effect of zinc deficiency on the pregnant ewe and developing foetus. Br J Nutr 49:365, 1983
264. Masters DG, Moir RJ: Provision of zinc to sheep by means of an intraruminal pellet. Aust J Exp Agric Anim Husb 20:547, 1980
265. Matthew A, Thomas AD: Goitre in Afrikander calves. S Afr Vet Med Assoc J 6:123, 1935
266. Maurizi MR, Pinkofsky HB, McFarland PJ, et al: Mg^{2+} is bound to glutamine synthetase extracted from bovine or ovine brain in the presence of 1-methionine-S-sulfoximine phosphate. Arch Biochem Biophys 246:494, 1986
267. Mayland HF, Rosenau RC, Florence AR: Grazing cow and calf responses to zinc supplementation. J Anim Sci 51:966, 1980
268. McAdam PA, O'Dell GD: Mineral profile of blood plasma of lactating dairy cows. J Dairy Sci 65:1219, 1982
269. McCance RA, Widdowson EM: The absorption and excretion of iron following oral and intravenous administration. J Physiol 94:148, 1938
270. McFarlane JM, Morris GL, Curtis SE, et al: Some indicators of welfare of crated veal calves on three dietary iron regimens. J Anim Sci 66:317, 1988
271. McGuire SO, Miller WJ, Gentry RP, et al: Influence of high dietary iron as ferrous carbonate and ferrous sulfate on iron metabolism in young calves. J Dairy Sci 68:2621, 1985
272. McIntosh GH, Baghurst KI, Potter BJ, et al: Foetal thyroidectomy and brain development in the sheep. Neuropathol Appl Neurobiol 5:363, 1979
273. McIntosh GH, Baghurst KI, Potter BJ, et al: Foetal brain development in the sheep. Neuropathol Appl Neurobiol 5:103, 1979

274. McPherson EA, Beattie IS, Young GB: An inherited defect in Friesian calves. Nord Vet-Med 16 (Suppl 1):533, 1964
275. Medici N, Minucci S, Nigro V, et al: Metal binding sites of the estradiol receptor from calf uterus and their possible role in the regulation of receptor function. Biochemistry 28:212, 1989
276. Mendel CM: The free hormone hypothesis: A physiologically based mathematical model. Endocr Rev 10:232, 1989
277. Meydani SN, Dupont J: Effect of zinc deficiency on prostaglandin synthesis in different organs of the rat. J Nutr 112:1098, 1982
278. Miller DS, O'Dell BL: Milk and casein-based diets for the study of brain catecholamines in copper-deficient rats. J Nutr 117:1890, 1987
279. Miller JK: Absorption and gastric secretion of iodine-131 and chlorine-36 in dairy calves. Proc Soc Exp Biol Med 121:291, 1966
280. Miller JK, Chandler PT, Cragle RG, et al: Radioiodine absorption and secretion by the calf abomasum. J Dairy Sci 54:397, 1971
281. Miller JK, Miller WJ: Development of zinc deficiency in Holstein calves fed a purified diet. J Dairy Sci 43:1854, 1960
282. Miller JK, Miller WJ: Experimental zinc deficiency and recovery of calves. J Nutr 76:467, 1962
283. Miller JK, Moss BR, Swanson EW: Effects of 131-I thyroid irradiation damage, thyroxine, and thiocyanate on radioiodine metabolism in dairy cows. J Dairy Sci 52:677, 1969
284. Miller JK, Swanson EW, Aschbacher PW, et al: Iodine transfer and concentration in the prepartum cow, fetus and neonatal calf. J Dairy Sci 50:1301, 1967
285. Miller JK, Swanson EW, Cragle RG: Effect of feeding thiocyanate to dairy cows on absorption and clearance of intramammary iodine. J Dairy Sci 48:1118, 1965
286. Miller JK, Swanson EW, Cragle RG: Effect of feeding thyroxine on secretion of I-131 in milk. J Dairy Sci 46:819, 1963
287. Miller JK, Swanson EW, Hansen SM: Effects of feeding potassium iodide, 3,5-diiodosalicylic acid, or L-thyroxine on iodine metabolism of lactating dairy cows. J Dairy Sci 48:888, 1965
288. Miller JK, Swanson EW, Lyke WA: Iodine concentration in nonthyroid tissues of cows. J Dairy Sci 56:1344, 1973
289. Miller JK, Swanson EW, Spalding GE: Iodine absorption, excretion, recycling and tissue distribution in the dairy cow. J Dairy Sci 58:1578, 1975
290. Miller JK, Swanson EW: Performance and iodine metabolism of dairy cattle with iodine[131] irradiation injury. J Dairy Sci 50:90, 1967
291. Miller WJ: Copper and zinc in ruminant nutrition. In O'Dell B, Miller EA, Miller WJ (eds): Copper and Zinc in Animal Nutrition. Des Moines, National Feed Ingredients Association, 1979, p 1
292. Miller WJ, Amos HE, Gentry RP, et al: Long-term feeding of high zinc sulfate diets to lactating and gestating dairy cows. J Dairy Sci 72:1499, 1989
293. Miller WJ, Neathery MW, Gentry RP, et al: Distribution and turnover rates of radioactive manganese in various tissues after duodenal dosing in Holstein calves fed a practical-type diet. J Anim Sci 34:460, 1972
294. Miller WJ, Neathery MW, Gentry RP, et al: Fecal excretion, tissue accumulation and turnover of 54-manganese after intravenous dosing in Holstein calves fed a practical-type diet. J Anim Sci 37:827, 1973
295. Miller WJ, Stake PE, Neathery MW, et al: Metabolism of manganese in calves as affected by dietary manganese and intravenous or duodenal manganese-54 dosing. J Dairy Sci 70:2085, 1987
296. Mills CF, Dalgarno AC, Wenham G: Biochemical and pathological changes in tissues of Friesian cattle during the experimental induction of copper deficiency. Br J Nutr 35:309, 1976
297. Mills CF, Dalgarno AC, Williams RB, et al: Zinc deficiency and the zinc requirements of calves and lambs. Br J Nutr 21:751, 1967
298. Mills CF, Davis GK: Molybdenum. In Mertz W (ed): Trace Elements in Human Health and Disease, vol 1, ed 5. San Diego, Academic Press, 1987, p 143
299. Mills CF: Biochemical and physiological indicators of mineral status in animals: Copper, cobalt and zinc. J Anim Sci 65:1702, 1987

300. Milos M, Comte M, Schaer J-J, et al: Evidence for four capital and six auxiliary cation-binding sites on calmodulin: Divalent cation interactions monitored by direct binding and microcalorimetry. J Inorg Biochem 36:11, 1989
301. Miyata Y, Furugouri K, Shijimaya K: Developmental changes in serum ferritin concentration of dairy calves. J Dairy Sci 67:1256, 1984
302. Moberg R: Possible influences of supplementary iodine, administered by evaporation, on reproductive performances in cattle. International Congress on Animal Production (Proceedings) 3:682, 1961
303. Mohammed R, Lamand M: Cardiovascular lesions in cobalt-vitamin B_{12} deficient sheep. Ann Rech Vet 17:447, 1986
304. Mollerberg L-LJ, Moreno-Lopez J: The response of normal and iron anemic calves to nasal infection with an attenuated strain of parainfluenza-3 virus. Acta Vet Scand 16:186, 1975
305. Morris ER: Iron. In Mertz W (ed): Trace Elements in Human Health and Disease, vol 1, ed 5. San Diego, Academic Press, 1987, p 79
306. Morris JG, Cripe WS, Chapman HLJ, et al: Selenium deficiency in cattle associated with Heinz bodies and anemia. Science 223:491, 1984
307. Motsenbocker MA, Tappel AL: A selenocysteine-containing selenium-transport protein in rat plasma. Biochim Biophys Acta 719:147, 1982
308. Mulei CM, Daniel RCW: The association of plasma magnesium concentration and thyroid gland activity in young calves. J Vet Med Assoc 35:516, 1988
309. Murakami K, Whiteley MK, Routtenberg A: Regulation of protein kinase C activity by cooperative interaction of Zn^{2+} and Ca^{2+}. J Biol Chem 262:13902, 1987
310. National Research Council, Subcommittee on Zinc: Zinc. Baltimore, University Park Press, 1979, p 1
311. National Research Council: Nutrient requirements of beef cattle, ed 6. Washington, DC, National Academy Press, 1984
312. Nichols CWJJ, Chaikoff IL, Wolff J: The relative growth of the thyroid gland in the bovine fetus. Endocrinology 44:502, 1949
313. Nixon DA, Akasha MA, Anderson RR: Free and total thyroid hormones in serum of Holstein cows. J Dairy Sci 71:1152, 1988
314. Nowak T: Manganese and phosphoenolpyruvate carboxykinase. In Schramm VL, Wedler FC (eds): Manganese in Metabolism and Enzyme Function. Orlando, Academic Press, 1986, p 165
315. O'Dell BL, Browning JD, Reeves PG: Plasma levels of prostaglandin metabolites in zinc-deficient female rats near term. J Nutr 113:760, 1983
316. O'Dell BL, Browning JD, Reeves PG: Zinc deficiency increases the osmotic fragility of rat erythrocytes. J Nutr 117:1883, 1987
317. Odiawo GO: The relationship between selenium deficiency and the development of pulmonary and subcutaneous emphysema in bovine ephemeral fever virus-infected cattle. Onderstepoort J Vet Res 56:123, 1989
318. Olkowski AA, Gooneratne SR, Christensen DA: Effects of diets of high sulphur content and varied concentrations of copper, molybdenum and thiamine on in vitro phagocytic and candidacidal activity of neutrophils in sheep. Res Vet Sci 48:82, 1990
319. Olson OE, Schulte BM, Whitehead EI, et al: Effect of arsenic on selenium metabolism in rats. J Ag Food Chem 11:531, 1963
320. Olson WG, Stevens JB, Anderson J, et al: Iodine toxicosis in six herds of dairy cattle. J Am Vet Med Assoc 184:179, 1984
321. Oteiza PI, Cuellar S, Lönnerdal B, et al: Influence of maternal dietary zinc intake on in vitro tubulin polymerization in fetal rat brain. Teratology 41:97, 1990
322. Ott EA, Smith WH, Stob M, et al: Zinc deficiency syndrome in the young calf. J Anim Sci 24:735, 1965
323. Pallini V, Bacci E: Bull sperm selenium is bound to a structural protein of mitochondria. J Submicrosc Cytol 11:165, 1979
324. Pammenter M, Albrecht C, Liebenberg W, et al: Afrikander cattle congenital goiter: Characteristics of its morphology and iodoprotein pattern. Endocrinology 102:954, 1978
325. Papadopoulous V, Brown AS, Hall PF: Isolation and characterization of calcineurin

from adrenal cytoskeleton: Identification of substrates for Ca^{2+}-calmodulin-dependent phosphatase activity. Mol Cell Endocrinol 63:23, 1989

326. Pastan I, Katzen R: Activation of adenyl cyclase in thyroid homogenates by thyroid-stimulating hormone. Biochem Biophys Res Comm 29:792, 1967

327. Perry TW, Beeson WM, Smith WH, et al: Value of zinc supplementation of natural rations for fattening beef cattle. J Anim Sci 27:1674, 1968

328. Perryman LE, Leach DR, Davis WC, et al: Lymphocyte alterations in zinc-deficient calves with lethal trait A 46. Vet Immunol Immunopathol 21:239, 1989

329. Phillippo M, Arthur JR, Price J, et al: Lack of effect of selenium treatment on pneumonia in housed calves (letter). Vet Rec 122:94, 1988

330. Phillippo M, Arthur JR, Price J, et al: The effects of selenium, housing and management on the incidence of pneumonia in housed calves. Vet Rec 121:509, 1987

331. Phillippo M, Humphries WR, Atkinson T, et al: The effect of dietary molybdenum and iron on copper status, puberty, fertility and oestrous cycles in cattle. J Agric Sci, Camb 109:321, 1987

332. Phillippo M, Humphries WR, Lawrence CB, et al: Investigation of the effect of copper status and therapy on fertility in beef suckler herds. J Agric Sci, Camb 99:359, 1982

333. Phillips DR, Chappel RJ, Hayes J: A possible role of Cu-2+ ions in bovine antibody-antigen interactions. Res Vet Sci 32:221, 1982

334. Pierson RE: Zinc deficiency in young lambs. J Am Vet Med Assoc 149:1279, 1966

335. Pitts WJ, Miller WJ, Fosgate OT, et al: Effect of zinc deficiency and restricted feeding from 2 to 5 months of age on reproduction in Holstein bulls. J Dairy Sci 49:995, 1966

336. Polk DH, Wu SY, Wright C, et al: Ontogeny of thyroid hormone effect on tissue 5'-monodeiodinase activity in fetal sheep. Am J Physiol 254:E337, 1988

337. Potter BJ, Mano MT, Belling GB, et al: Restoration of brain growth in fetal sheep after iodized oil administration to pregnant iodine-deficient ewes. J Neurolog Sci 66:15, 1984

338. Potter BJ, Mano MT, Belling GB, et al: Retarded fetal brain development resulting from severe dietary iodine deficiency in sheep. Neuropathol Appl Neurobiol 8:303, 1982

339. Prasad AS, Oberleas D, Wolf P, et al: Effect of growth hormone on nonhypophysectomized zinc-deficient rats and zinc on hypophysectomized rats. J Lab Clin Med 73:486, 1969

340. Prasad CS, Arora SP: Influence of dietary zinc on β-carotene conversion and on the level of retinol binding protein in the blood serum. Indian J Dairy Sci 32:275, 1979

341. Pratt MAC, Eggo MC, Bachrach L, et al: Regulation of thyroperoxidase, thyroglobulin and iodide levels in sheep thyroid cells by TSH, tumor promoters and epidermal growth factor. Biochimie 71:227, 1989

342. Price J, Humphries WR: Investigation of the effect of supplementary zinc on growth rate of beef cattle on farms in N Scotland. J Agric Sci, Camb 95:135, 1980

343. Prohaska JR, Heller LJ: Mechanical properties of the copper-deficient rat heart. J Nutr 112:2142, 1982

344. Prosser HJ, Wilson AD, Groffman DM, et al: The development of acid-base reaction cements as formulations for the controlled release of trace elements. Biomaterials 7:109, 1986

345. Pryor WJ: The distribution of copper in bovine and ovine foetuses, with reference to their age and maternal liver copper concentrations. Res Vet Sci 5:123, 1964

346. Puls R: Mineral Levels in Animal Health: Diagnostic Data. Clearbrook, Sherpa International, 1988, p 240

347. Reddy CS, Mohammad FK, Ganjam VK, et al: Mobilization of tissue cadmium in mice and calves and reversal of cadmium induced tissue damage in calves by zinc. Bull Environ Contam Toxicol 39:350, 1987

348. Reece WO, Brackelsberg PO, Hotchkiss DK: Erythrocyte changes, serum iron concentration and performance following iron injection in neonatal beef calves. J Anim Sci 61:1387, 1985

349. Reece WO, Self HL, Hotchkiss DK: Injection of iron in newborn beef calves: Erythrocyte variables and weight gains with newborn-dam correlations. Am J Vet Res 45:2119, 1984
350. Reece WO: Acid-base balance and selected hematologic, electrolytic, and blood chemical variables in calves nursing cows: One week through 15 weeks. Am J Vet Res 45:666, 1984
351. Reece WO: Response of anemic calves to exertion. Am J Vet Res 45:437, 1984
352. Refetoff S, Larsen R: Transport, cellular uptake, and metabolism of thyroid hormone. In DeGroot LS (ed): Endocrinology. Philadelphia, WB Saunders Co, 1989, p 541
353. Reffett JK, Spears JW, Brown TTJ: Effect of dietary selenium on the primary and secondary immune response in calves challenged with infectious bovine rhinotracheitis virus. J Nutr 118:229, 1988
354. Reffett-Stabel J, Spears JW, Brown TTJ, et al: Selenium effects on glutathione peroxidase and the immune response of stressed calves challenged with Pasteurella hemolytica. J Anim Sci 67:557, 1989
355. Reffett-Stabel J, Spears JW: Effect of copper on immune function and disease resistance. In Kies C (ed): Copper Bioavailability and Metabolism. New York, Plenum Press, 1990, p 243
356. Reid JT, Ward GM: Mineral metabolism studies in dairy cattle. J Nutr 35:591, 1948
357. Reid RL, Horvath DJ: Soil chemistry and mineral problems in farm livestock: A review. Animal Feed Science and Technology 5:95, 1980
358. Rice DA, McMurray CH, Kennedy S, et al: Lack of effect of selenium supplementation on the incidence of weak calves in dairy herds. Vet Rec 119:571, 1986
359. Rice DA, McMurray CH: Use of sodium hydroxide treated selenium deficient barley to induce vitamin E and selenium deficiency in yearling cattle. Vet Rec 118:173, 1986
360. Rice RW, Nelms GE, Schoonover CO: Effect of injectable iron on blood hematocrit and hemoglobin and weaning weight of beef calves. J Anim Sci 26:613, 1967
361. Ricketts MH, Simons MJ, Parma J, et al: A nonsense mutation causes hereditary goitre in the Afrikander cattle and unmasks alternative splicing of thyroglobulin transcripts. Proc Natl Acad Sci USA 84:3181, 1987
362. Roeser HP, Lee GR, Nacht S, et al: The role of ceruloplasmin in iron metabolism. J Clin Invest 49:2408, 1970
363. Rognstad R: Possible sites of Mn(II) action on carbohydrate metabolism in the liver. In Schramm VL, Wedler FC (eds): Manganese in Metabolism and Enzyme Function. Orlando, Academic Press, 1986, p 133
364. Rojas MA, Dyer IA, Cassatt WA: Manganese deficiency in the bovine. J Anim Sci 24:664, 1964
365. Romero N, Tinker D, Hyde D: Role of plasma and serum proteases in the degradation of elastin. Arch Biochem Biophys 244:161, 1986
366. Root AW, Duckett G, Sweetland M, et al: Effects of zinc deficiency upon pituitary function in sexually mature and immature male rats. J Nutr 109:958, 1979
367. Roth H-P, Kirchgessner M: Zinc and insulin metabolism (review). Biol Trace Element Res 3:13, 1981
368. Roti E, Gnudi A, Braverman LE: The placental transport, synthesis and metabolism of hormones and drugs which affect thyroid function. Endocr Rev 4:131, 1983
369. Rousset B, Selmi S, Alquier C, et al: In vitro studies of the thyroglobulin degradation pathway: Endocytosis and delivery of thyroglobulin to lysosomes, release of thyroglobulin cleavage products—iodotyrosines and iodothyronines. Biochimie 71:247, 1989
370. Roy M, Kiremidjian-Schumacher L, Wishe HI, et al: Selenium and immune cell functions. II. Effect on lymphocyte-mediated cytotoxicity. Proc Soc Exp Biol Med 193:143, 1990
371. Sanders DE, Koestner A: Bovine neonatal ataxia associated with hypocupremia in pregnant cows. J Am Vet Med Assoc 176:728, 1980
372. Sansom BF, Gibbons RA, Dixon SN, et al: Absorption of dietary manganese by dairy cows and the role of plasma proteins and the liver in its homeostasis. In Nuclear Techniques in Animal Production and Health as Related to the Soil-Plant System. Vienna, International Atomic Energy Agency, 1976, p 179

373. Sansom BF, Symonds HW, Vagg MJ: The absorption of dietary manganese by dairy cows. Res Vet Sci 24:366, 1978
374. Saraswat RC, Arora SP: Effect of dietary zinc on the vitamin A level and alkaline phosphatase activity in blood sera of lambs. Indian J Anim Sci 42:358, 1972
375. Sarkozy P, Palfi V, Schultz E, et al: Immune response in anaemic calves. Zbl Vet Med B 32:317, 1985
376. Scheuhammer AM, Cherian MG: Binding of manganese in human and rat plasma. Biochim Biophys Acta 840:163, 1985
377. Schramm VL: Evaluation of Mn(II) in metabolic regulation: Analysis of proposed sites for regulation. In Schramm VL, Wedler FC (eds): Manganese in Metabolism and Enzyme Function. Orlando, Academic Press, 1986, p 109
378. Schubert JR, Muth OH, Oldfield JE, et al: Experimental results with selenium in white muscle disease of lambs and calves. Fed Proc 20:689, 1961
379. Schulz KCA, Groenewald JW: The familial incidence of "grey" Afrikander calves with and without goitre. J South African Vet Assoc 54:147, 1983
380. Schwarz WA, Kirchgessner M: Experimental zinc deficiency in lactating dairy cows Vet Med Rev 1/2:19, 1975
381. Scrutton MC: Manganese and pyruvate carboxylase. In Schramm VL, Wedler FC (eds): Manganese in Metabolism and Enzyme Function. Orlando, Academic Press, 1986, p 147
382. Segel GB, Simon W, Lichtman AH, et al: The activation of lymphocyte plasma membrane (Na,K)-ATPase by EGTA is explained better by zinc than calcium chelation. J Biol Chem 256:6629, 1981
383. Shamberger RJ: Biochemistry of Selenium. In Frieden E (ed): Biochemistry of the Elements, vol 2. New York, Plenum Press, 1983, p 334
384. Shamberger RJ: Selenium: Biochemistry of the Essential Ultratrace Elements. In Frieden E (ed): Biochemistry of the Elements, vol 3. New York, Plenum Press, 1984, p 201
385. Sherman AR, Helyar L: Iron deficiency, immunity and disease resistance in early life. In Chandra RK (ed): Nutrition and Immunology. New York, Alan R Liss, 1988, p 169
386. Smith BL, Embling PP, Towers NR, et al: The protective effect of zinc sulphate in experimental sporidesmin poisoning of sheep. NZ Vet J 25:124, 1977
387. Smith JB, Dwyer SD, Smith L: Cadmium evokes inositol polyphosphate formation and calcium mobilization. J Biol Chem 274:7115, 1989
388. Smith JC, McDaniel EG, Fan FF, et al: Zinc: A trace element essential in vitamin A metabolism. Science 181:954, 1973
389. Smith JE: Iron metabolism and its diseases. In Kaneko JJ (ed): Clinical Biochemistry of Domestic Animals, ed 4. San Diego, Academic Press, 1989, p 256
390. Smith KL, Conrad HR: Vitamin E and selenium supplementation for dairy cows. In Proceedings of the Roche Technical Symposium—"The Role of Vitamins on Animal Performance and Immune Response," Daytona Beach, 1987, p 47
391. Smith KL, Harrison JH, Hancock DD, et al: Effect of vitamin E and selenium supplementation on incidence of clinical mastitis and duration of clinical symptoms. J Dairy Sci 67:1293, 1984
392. Smith RM: Cobalt. In Mertz W (ed): Trace Elements in Human Health and Disease, vol 1, ed 5. San Diego, Academic Press, 1987, p 143
393. Solomons NW: Physiological interaction of minerals. In Bodwell CE, Erdman JW (eds): Nutrient Interactions. New York, Marcel Dekker, 1988, p 115
394. Sorensen PH: Studies of thyroid function in cattle and pigs. In Use of Radioisotopes in Animal Biology and the Medical Sciences, vol 1. New York, Academic Press, 1962, p 455
395. Spais AG, Papasteriadis AA: Zinc deficiency in cattle under Greek conditions. In Hoekstra WG, Suttle JW, Ganther HE, et al (eds): Trace Element Metabolism in Animals-2. Baltimore, University Park Press, 1974, p 628
396. Spaulding SW: Lithium effects on the thyroid gland. In Gaitan E (ed): Environmental Goitrogenesis. Boca Raton, CRC Press, 1989, p 149
397. Srisuchart B, Taylor MJ, Sharma RP: Alteration of humoral and cellular immunity in manganese chloride-treated mice. J Toxicol Environ Health 22:91, 1987
398. Stauber EH: Weak calf syndrome: A continuing enigma. J Am Vet Med Assoc 168:223, 1976

399. Stengel D, Henry D, Tomova S, et al: Purification of the proteolytically solubilized, active catalytic subunit of adenylate cyclase from ram sperm. Eur J Biochem 161:241, 1986

400. Strbak B, Tomsik F: Thyroid hormone levels in cow maternal and fetal sera during last trimester of pregnancy. Endocrinol Exp 22:113, 1988

401. Subcommittee on Mineral Toxicity in Animals: Mineral Tolerance of Domestic Animals. Washington, DC, National Academy Press, 1980

402. Sunde RA, Evenson JK: Serine incorporation into the selenocystein moiety of glutathione peroxidase. J Biol Chem 262:993, 1987

403. Sunde RA: The biochemistry of selenoproteins. JAOCS 61:1891, 1984

404. Surks MI, Ramirez IJ, Shapiro LE, et al: Effect of zinc(II) and other divalent cations on binding of 3,5,3'-triiodo-L-thyronine to nuclear receptors from cultured GC cells. J Biol Chem 264:9820, 1989

405. Suttle NF, Jones DG, Woolliams C, et al: Heinz body anaemia in lambs with deficiencies of copper or selenium. Br J Nutr 58:539, 1987

406. Suttle NF, Jones DG: Recent developments in trace element metabolism and function: Trace elements, disease resistance and immune responsiveness in ruminants. J Nutr 119:1055, 1989

407. Suttle NF, McMurray CH: Use of erythrocyte copper:zinc superoxide dismutase activity and hair or fleece copper concentrations in the diagnosis of hypocuprosis in ruminants. Res Vet Sci 35:47, 1983

408. Suttle NF: Problems in the diagnosis and anticipation of trace element deficiencies in grazing livestock. Vet Rec 119:148, 1986

409. Suttle NF: Safety and effectiveness of cupric oxide particles for increasing liver copper stores in sheep. Res Vet Sci 42:219, 1987

410. Suttle NF: Safety and effectiveness of cupric oxide particles for increasing liver copper stores in cattle. Res Vet Sci 42:224, 1987

411. Suttle NF: The role of comparative pathology in the study of copper and cobalt deficiencies in ruminants. J Comp Pathol 99:241, 1988

412. Symonds HW, Mather DL, Vagg MJ: The excretion of selenium in bile and urine of steers: The influence of form and amount of Se salt. Br J Nutr 46:487, 1981

413. Symonds HW, Sansom BF, Mather DL, et al: Selenium metabolism in the dairy cow: The influence of the liver and the effect of the form of Se salt. Br J Nutr 45:117, 1981

414. Taurog A: Thyroid peroxidase and thyroxine biosynthesis. Recent Prog Horm Res 26:189, 1970

415. Taylor RF, Puls R, MacDonald KR: Bovine abortions associated with selenium deficiency in Western Canada. Am Assn Veterinary Laboratory Diagnosticians 22:77, 1979

416. Tennant B, Harrold D, Reina-Guerra M, et al: Hematology of the neonatal calf. III. Frequency of congenital iron deficiency anemia. Cornell Vet 65:543, 1975

417. Thomas DG, Linton HJ, Garvey JS: Fluorometric ELISA for the detection and quantitation of metallothionein. J Immunol Methods 89:239, 1986

418. Thomson ABR, Oltaunbosun D, Valberg LS: Interrelation of intestinal transport system for manganese and iron. J Lab Clin Med 78:642, 1971

419. Thomson ABR, Valberg LS, Sinclair DG: Competitive nature of the intestinal transport mechanism for cobalt and iron in the rat. J Clin Invest 50:2384, 1971

420. Thomson CD, Robinson MF, Campbell DR, et al: Effect of prolonged supplementation with daily supplements of selenomethionine and sodium selenite on glutathione peroxidase activity in blood of New Zealand residents. Am J Clin Nutr 36:24, 1982

421. Torresani J, DeGroot LJ: Triiodothyronine binding to liver nuclear solubilized proteins in vitro. Endocrinology 96:1201, 1975

422. Towers NR, Smith BL: The protective effect of zinc sulphate in experimental sporidesmin intoxication of lactating dairy cows. NZ Vet J 26:199, 1978

423. Trinder N, Hall RJ, Renton CP: The relationship between the intake of selenium and vitamin E on the incidence of retained placentae in dairy cows. Vet Rec 93:641, 1973

424. Trinder N, Woodhouse CD, Renton CP: The effect of vitamin E and selenium on the incidence of retained placentae in dairy cows. Vet Rec 85:550, 1969

425. Ullrey DE: Biochemical and physiological indicators of selenium status in animals. J Anim Sci 65:1712, 1987
426. Underwood EJ: The Mineral Nutrition of Livestock. Farnham Royal, Slough, Commonwealth Agricultural Beureaux, 1981, p 1
427. Van Saun RJ, Herdt TH, Stowe HD: Maternal and fetal selenium concentrations and their interrelationships in dairy cattle. J Nutr 119:1128, 1989
428. Van Saun RJ, Herdt TH, Stowe HD: Maternal and fetal vitamin E concentrations and selenium-vitamin E interrelationships in dairy cattle. J Nutr 119:1156, 1989
429. Vogt DW, Carlton CG, Miller RB: Hereditary parakeratosis in Shorthorn beef calves. Am J Vet Res 49:120, 1988
430. Wada LL, Rosyner-Cohen H, King JC: Effect of low zinc intakes on thyroid hormones and basal energy expenditure (BEE). Fed Proc 42:390, 1983
431. Wang ZY, Poole D, Mason J: The uptake and intracellular distribution of ^{35}S trithiomolybdate in bovine liver in vivo. J Inorg Biochem 31:85, 1987
432. Wang ZY, Poole DBR, Mason J: The effects of supplementation of the diet of young steers with Mo and S on the intracellular distribution of copper in liver and on copper fractions in blood. Br Vet J 144:543, 1988
433. Waschulewski IH, Sunde RA: Effect of dietary methionine on utilization of tissue selenium from dietary selenomethionine for glutathione peroxidase in the rat. J Nutr 118:367, 1988
434. Watson LT, Ammerman CB, Feaster JP, et al: Influence of manganese intake on metabolism of manganese and other minerals in sheep. J Anim Sci 36:131, 1973
435. Wedler FC, Toms R: Interactions of Mn(II) with mammalian glutamine synthetase. In Schramm VL, Wedler FC (eds): Manganese in Metabolism and Enzyme Function. Orlando, Academic Press, 1986, p 221
436. Welch H: Goiter in Farm Animals. Bull Mont Agr Exp Sta 214:1, 1928
437. Welch H: Hairlessness and goiter in new-born domestic animals. Bul Mont Agr Exp Sta 119:83, 1917
438. Welchman DdeB, Whelehan OP, Webster AJF: Haematology of veal calves reared in different husbandry systems and the assessment of iron deficiency. Vet Rec 123:505, 1988
439. West TS: Soil as the source of trace elements. In Fowden L, Garton GA, Mills CF (eds): Trace Element Deficiency: Metabolic and Physiological Consequences. London, The Royal Society, 1981, p 19
440. Wheatley LE, Beck NFG: The influence of season and husbandry on the selenium status of sheep in a deficient area. Br Vet J 144:246, 1988
441. White CL, Cadwalader TK, Hoekstra WG, et al: The metabolism of 75-Se-selenomethionine in sheep given supplementary copper and molybdenum. J Anim Sci 67:2400, 1989
442. White IG, Vishwanath R, Swan MA, et al: Studies of the mechanism of action of gossypol as a male antifertility agent. Contraception 37:269, 1988
443. Widdowson EM, McCance RA: The absorption and excretion of iron before, during and after a period of very high intake. Biochem J 31:2029, 1937
444. Williams DM, Kennedy FS, Green BG: The effect of iron substrate on mitochondrial haem synthesis in copper deficiency. Br J Nutr 53:131, 1985
445. Williams DM, Loukopoulos D, Lee GR, et al: Role of copper in mitochondrial iron metabolism. Blood 48:77, 1976
446. Wilson JG: Bovine functional infertility in Devon and Cornwall: Response to manganese therapy. Vet Rec 79:562, 1966
447. Wiltbank MC, Diskin MG, Flores JA, et al: Regulation of the corpus luteum by protein kinase C II inhibition of lipoprotein-stimulated steroidogenesis by postaglandin F2α. Biol Reprod 42:239, 1990
448. Winge DR, Gray WR, Zelazowski Z, et al: Sequence and antigenicity of calf metallothionein II. Arch Biochem Biophys 245:254, 1986
449. Wolff J, Chaikoff IL, Nichols CW: The accumulation of thyroxine-like and other iodine compounds in the fetal bovine thyroid. Endocrinology 44:510, 1949
450. Wolffram S, Stingelin Y, Scharrer E: Inhibition of sulphate and selenate transport in sheep jejunum by oxalate and other dicarboxylate anions. J Vet Med 34:679, 1987

451. Wong-Valle J, Henry PR, Ammerman CB, et al: Estimation of the relative bioavailability of manganese sources for sheep. J Anim Sci 67:2409, 1989
452. Woods M, Mason J: Spectral and kinetic studies on the binding of trithiomolybdate to bovine and canine serum albumin in vitro: The interaction with copper. J Inorg Chem 30:261, 1987
453. Wright DE, Towers NR, Hamilton PB, et al: Intake of zinc sulphate in drinking water by grazing beef cattle. NZ J Agr Res 21:215, 1978
454. Wright PL, Bell MC: Comparative metabolism of selenium and tellurium in sheep and swine. Am J Physiol 211:6, 1966
455. Yang J-G, Hill KE, Burk RF: Dietary selenium intake controls rat plasma selenoprotein P concentration. J Nutr 119:1010, 1989

Address reprint requests to

Dr. Thomas W. Graham
Department of Nutrition
University of California, Davis
Davis, CA 95616

Vitamin Deficiencies in Cattle

T.M. Frye, PhD,* Scot N. Williams, PhD,†
and Thomas W. Graham, DVM, MPVM‡

This article focuses on the vitamin deficiencies most likely to occur in beef cattle. A companion article, describing trace element deficiencies, discusses how interactions among nutrients can affect availability and retention of specific nutrients. It is more likely that fat-soluble rather than water-soluble vitamins will become limiting factors in beef production. In particular, deficiencies of vitamins A and E can severely impair reproduction and development in range and feedlot environments. Properties, metabolism and function of vitamin A/β carotene, vitamins E, D, K, thiamin, and niacin are discussed. Vitamin B_{12} is discussed with cobalt in the article describing trace element deficiencies. Each nutrient discussed has typical clinical parameters associated with deficiency, how to diagnose adequacy/status, and forms of dietary and parenteral therapy addressed.

VITAMIN A

Properties and Metabolism

Preformed vitamin A itself does not occur in plant products, but its precursors, carotenes, do occur in several forms. These compounds (carotenoids) are commonly referred to as provitamin A, because the body can transform them into the active vitamin.

The combined potency of a feed, represented by its vitamin A and carotene content, is referred to as its vitamin A value. Retinol is the alcohol form of vitamin A. Replacement of the alcohol group (-OH) by

*Group Leader, Technical Services, Department of Animal Health and Nutrition, Roche Vitamins and Fine Chemicals, Nutley, New Jersey
†Senior, Technical Services Manager, Department of Animal Health and Nutrition, Roche Vitamins and Fine Chemicals, Nutley, New Jersey
‡Assistant Veterinarian, Department of Nutrition, University of California, Davis, Davis, California

an aldehyde group (-CHO) gives retinal, and replacement by an acid group (-COOH) gives retinoic acid. Vitamin A is used in the feed industry as the ester forms of acetate, propionate, or palmitate.

Vitamin A is a nearly colorless, fat soluble, long-chain, unsaturated alcohol with five double bonds. Since it contains double bonds, vitamin A can exist in different isomeric forms. Only two isomers are of practical importance, namely all-trans-vitamin A, the form with highest biological and the 13-cis isomer with a relative biologic activity of 50%[211] for chicks. Vitamin A and the precursor carotenoids are rapidly destroyed by oxygen, heat, light, and acids. Presence of moisture and trace minerals reduces vitamin A activity in feeds.[159]

Precursors of vitamin A, the carotenes, occur as orange-yellow pigments in green leaves and, to a lesser extent, in corn. Four of these carotenoids, α-carotene, β-carotene, γ-carotene, and cryptoxanthin (the main carotenoid of corn), are of particular importance because of their provitamin A activity. Vitamin A activity of β-carotene is substantially greater than that of other carotenoids. However, biological tests have consistently shown that pure vitamin A has twice the potency of β-carotene on a weight to weight basis. Thus, only one molecule of vitamin A is formed from one molecule of β-carotene. Efficiency of conversion of carotenoids to retinol is variable in breeds of cattle and generally lower than that for nonruminants. The rat is quite efficient in converting carotene to vitamin A, whereas this process is limited in the cat. There is also a within-species variation. For example, Holsteins convert carotene efficiently, while Guernseys are much less efficient.[164] The reasons for these breed differences have not been elucidated. Some factors that influence the rate at which carotenoids are converted to vitamin A are type of carotenoid, class and production level of animal, individual genetic difference in animals, and level of carotene intake.[153] Efficiency of vitamin A conversion from β-carotene is decreased with higher levels of intake; as β-carotene level is increased, conversion drops from a ratio of $2:1$ to $5:1$ for the chicken and from $8:1$ to $16:1$ for the calf.[11] The conversion rate of the rat has been used as the standard value, with 1 mg of β-carotene equal to 1667 IU of vitamin A. Based on this standard, the comparative efficiency of various species were listed by McDowell.[137] For beef cattle, one mg of β-carotene is assigned a value of 400 IU of vitamin A (2.5 μg β-carotene per IU).[153]

Beta-carotene present in feed is cleaved in the intestinal mucosa by an enzyme to retinal, which is then reduced to retinol (vitamin A). The absorption of vitamin A in the intestine is believed to be 80% to 90%, while that of β-carotene is about 50 to 60%.[159] Efficiency of vitamin A of absorption decreases somewhat with very high doses.

The main site of vitamin A and carotenoid absorption is the mucosa of the proximal jejunum. Carotenoids are normally converted to retinol in the intestinal mucosa, but may also be converted in the liver and other organs, especially in yellow fat species.[141] In cattle, significant amounts of carotene can be absorbed. Absorbed carotene can be stored in the liver and fatty tissues. However, cattle breeds that have yellow body fat and milk fat (Guernsey) absorb significantly more carotene than cattle with white fat such as the Holstein breed. Either dietary

retinol or retinol resulting from conversion of carotenoids is then ester-
ified with a long-chain fatty acid, usually palmitate. Dietary retinyl
esters are hydrolyzed to retinol in the intestine; they are absorbed as
the free alcohol and then re-esterified in the mucosa. In cattle, the
retinyl esters are transported mainly in association with lymph chylo-
microns to the liver where they are hydrolyzed to retinol and re-esterified for storage. Hydrolysis of the ester storage form mobilizes vitamin
A from the liver as retinol.

Retinol is released from the hepatocyte as a complex with retinol-
binding protein (RBP) and thyroxide binding prealbumin; it is transported in this form to the tissues. When the RBP-retinol complex
reaches the target cells, the retinol is released at a RBP receptor site on
the cell surface. Once the retinol passes through the cell membrane it
combines with a cellular retinol binding protein (CRBP). The CRBP is
believed to carry the retinol to its intracellular site of action.[159] The
main excretory pathway for vitamin A is by elimination as glucuronide
conjugates in the bile prior to fecal excretion.

Liver normally contains about 90% of total body vitamin A. The
remainder is stored in the kidneys, lungs, adrenals, and blood, with
small amounts also found in other organs and tissues. Several studies
have shown that the liver can store enough vitamin A to protect the
animal from long periods of dietary scarcity. This large storage capacity
must be considered in studies of vitamin A requirements; intakes that
appear adequate for a given function may deplete reserves stored prior
to the period of observation. Measurement of the liver store of vitamin
A at slaughter is a useful technique in studies of vitamin A status and
requirements.

Functions

Vitamin A is necessary for support of growth, reproduction, and
maintenance of higher animals. In the absence of vitamin A, animals
will cease to grow and eventually die. The metabolic function of vitamin A, explained in biochemical terms, is still incompletely known.
Vitamin A deficiency causes at least four different lesions: loss of vision
due to a failure of rhodopsin formation in the retina; defects in bone
growth; defects in reproduction (i.e., failure of spermatogenesis in the
male and resorption of the fetus in the female); and defects in growth
and differentiation of epithelial tissues, frequently resulting in keratinization. Keratinization of these tissues results in loss of function; this
occurs in the alimentary, genital, reproductive, respiratory, and urinary tracts. Such altered characteristics make the affected tissue more
susceptible to infection. Thus, diarrhea and pneumonia are typical
secondary effects of vitamin A deficiency. Greater than optimal intake
of vitamin A, however, will not aid in preventing infections.

More is known about the role of vitamin A in vision than any of its
other functions. Retinal is utilized (transformed to 11-cis-retinal) in the
retina as the prosthetic group in rhodopsin for dim light vision (rods)
and as the prosthetic group in iodopsin for bright light and color vision
(cones). It has been found that retinoic acid, another form of vitamin A
present in the body, will support growth and tissue differentiation, but

not vision or reproduction.[186] Vitamin A deficient rats fed retinoic acid were healthy in every respect, with normal estrus and conception, but failed to give birth and resorbed their fetuses. When retinol was given even at a late stage in pregnancy, fetuses survived through parturition. Male rats given retinoic acid were healthy but produced no sperm, and without vitamin A both sexes were blind.[5]

Recently, it was suggested that β-carotene plays a role, independent of vitamin A, in bovine health and reproduction.[118,34,18] These studies indicate a deficiency of carotene in the diet was associated with altered estrous in cows and heifers. The possible protective effects of vitamin A and β-carotene against mastitis in Holsteins has been reported.[34] Supplementing dairy cows with 53,000 IU vitamin A and 300 mg β-carotene, starting 30 days prepartum, reduced milk somatic cell counts during lactation. Higher levels of supplemental vitamin A (173,000 IU) also reduced somatic cell counts compared with lower levels (53,000 IU). These findings are perhaps more important in dairy cattle nutrition compared with beef cows, considering the tendency of the latter to have greater access to pasture and for the farmer to see a higher incidence of mastitis. Diets containing stored roughages such as wheat straw, corn silage, and dried beet pulp are low in β-carotene.[18] Except for its role in vision, the function of vitamin A at the cellular level is not yet clear. It is thought that retinyl phosphate may act to regulate cell differentiation.

Vitamin A is required for normal disease resistance, and this is related to maintenance of mucous membranes and normal function of the adrenal gland. An animal's ability to resist disease also depends on a normally responsive immune system, with vitamin A deficiency causing a reduced immune response. In many experiments with laboratory and domestic animals, the effects of both clinical and subclinical deficiencies of vitamin A on the production of antibodies and on the resistance of the different tissues against microbial infection or parasitic infestation have frequently been demonstrated.[106]

Assessment of Status

Deficiencies. The classic sign of vitamin A deficiency in ruminants is night blindness, with total and permanent blindness in younger animals resulting from stenosis of the optic nerve. Excessive lacrimation in cattle (rather than xerophthalmia) usually occurs; the corners of the eyes become keratinized and, with infection, may develop ulceration.

Signs of vitamin A deficiency in cattle include reduced feed intake, rough hair coat, edema of the joints and brisket, lacrimation, xerophthalmia, night blindness, slow growth, diarrhea, convulsive seizures, improper bone growth, blindness, low conception rates, abortion, stillbirths, blind calves, abnormal semen, reduced libido, and increased susceptibility to respiratory and other infections.[153]

Adequate vitamin A is necessary for fertility in cows and bulls.[31,146,176,178] Increased semen volume and sperm count, and reduced incidence of abnormal sperm occurred in breeding bulls receiving supplemental vitamin A that was added to rations containing normal amounts of carotene[178] (Table 1). Recent studies suggest that β-caro-

Table 1. *Influence of Vitamin A Supplementation on Semen Production*

SEMEN CHARACTERISTICS	CONTROL	45,000 IU VITAMIN A/ HEAD/DAY
Volume (ml)	5.4	5.9
Sperm concentration (10^6)	963	1010
Methylene blue reduction time, minute	4.8	4.5
Abnormal sperm, %	11.8	9.7

(*Adapted from* Roussel JD, Patrick TE, Kellgren HC et al: Influence of high levels of vitamin A supplementation on semen characteristics and blood composition of breeding bulls. J Dairy Sci 46:583, 1963; with permission.)

tene influences reproductive performance in cows independent of the vitamin A activity (Tables 2 and 3).

Clinical Parameters. In the calf, elevated cerebrospinal fluid pressure is the earliest change specific to vitamin A deficiency. When a vitamin A free diet is fed to calves, cerebrospinal fluid pressure will become elevated. The length of time for this change in cerebrospinal fluid pressure depends upon the initial body vitamin A reserve. Eaton reported the effects of feeding a diet either deficient in carotene or vitamin A or carotene and vitamin A to Holstein calves.[56] Growth was continuous and insignificantly affected by withdrawal of carotene from the diet. Plasma vitamin A concentration increased slightly in the calves fed carotene but decreased to a very low concentration in calves fed no carotene. Cerebrospinal fluid pressure increased slightly (27mm) over a 25 week period in calves fed carotene and increased markedly (276 mm) in calves fed no carotene (Table 4).

In feedlot cattle, signs of vitamin A deficiency developed in crossbred beef steers, heifers, and bulls fed a diet consisting of barley and chopped barley straw without vitamin or mineral supplementation.[19] In these animals, serum vitamin A was moderate to extremely low, ranging from 2.01 to 18.05 μg/dL. The plasma vitamin A correlated with the severity of clinical signs of deficiency. Cattle with plasma concentrations of 2.01 to 4.87 μg/dL appeared blind and had fixed, dilated pupils, severe ataxia and poor weight gain. Another group in the same herd, with plasma concentrations between 4.87 and 8.88 μg/dL,

Table 2. *Influence of Vitamin A on Conception Rate*

AGE GROUP	CONTROL GROUP		VITAMIN A* TREATED GROUP	
	NO. ANIMALS	% PREGNANT	NO. ANIMALS	% PREGNANT
Mature cows	582	70.1	1097	84.5
First-calf heifer	129	74.9	241	83.0
Replacement heifers	107	64.5	261	79.3

(*Adapted from* Bradfield D, Behrens WC: Effect of vitamin ADE injection on conception rates in cows and heifers. *In* Proceedings of Western Sec American Society of Animal Science. 19:1, 1968; with permission.)
*2 M.U., IM Injection

Table 3. *Effect of Supplemental β-Carotene on Conception Rate and Services Per Conception in Dairy Cows Fed Adequate Vitamin A*

PER COW	VITAMIN A 220 iu/kg bw	β-CAROTENE PLUS VITAMIN A 0.3 mg plus 100 iu/kg bw	IMPROVEMENT FROM β-CAROTENE PLUS VITAMIN A VS. VITAMIN A ALONE
Average conception rate from:			
First service	40%	68.4%	28.4% difference
Second service	15%	21.1%	6.1% difference
Average no. of services/ conception	20 ± 0.91	1.42 ± 0.69	29% reduction

(*Adapted from* Lotthammer KH, Ahlswede HL, Meyer H: Untersuchungen uber eine spezifiche vitamin A uhabhangige wirkung des β-carotenes aus die fertilitat des Rindes Z. mitt. Weitere Klinische betunde und Besamungsenge bnisse. Dtsch Tieraertzl Wochenschr 83:353, 1976, with permission.)

appeared blind and had varying degrees of ataxia and poor weight gain. Yet another group in the herd, with plasma vitamin A concentrations that were greater than 8.88 μg/dL, only had poor weight gains.

Histologic lesions in deficient animals include optic papilledema, retinal degeneration with focal loss of rod and cone layers and degeneration of the optic nerves. Macrophages that had ingested axonal and myelin debris were also found.[19] Additionally, Divers et al reported blindness and convulsions in feedlot steers associated with vitamin A deficiency. Serum vitamin A concentrations ranged from no detectable vitamin A to 4.25 μg/dL.[51]

Retinol is the major vitamin A metabolite in plasma and ovarian

Table 4. *Live Weight, Plasma Vitamin A and Cerebrospinal Fluid Pressure of Calves Fed Adequate Carotene (+) or No Carotene (−)[a]*

CRITERIA	CAROTENE INTAKE	WEEKS 0	5	10	15	20	25
Live weight, kg	+	158	185	211	240	269	299
	−	160	189	216	244	270	296
	SED[b]	6	6	7	8	9	10
Plasma vitamin A, μg/100 mL	+	31	31	32	36	39	40
	−	33	20	18*	14*	9*	6*
	SED	5	6	4	4	4	4
Cerebrospinal fluid pressure, mm saline Actual	+	67	65	65[c]	102	79	94
	−	72[c]	75	98	127	178	348

[a]Average of five calves fed 660 μg of carotene/kg live wt per day and average of five calves fed no carotene.

[b]Standard erıor of the difference between the averages of the + and − calves.

[c]Average of four calves.

*Significantly different at P≤0.05 from calves (+) fed carotene.

(*Adapted from* Eaton HD: Chronic bovine hypo- and hypervitaminosis A and cerebrospinal fluid pressure. Am J Clin Nutr 22:1070, 1969; with permission.)

follicular fluid (58% and 67%, respectively, of total vitamin A). Retinyl ester (apparently palmitate) is the major constituent in bovine liver and corpora lutea (94% and 75%, respectively, of total vitamin A). β-Carotene concentrations are high in bovine plasma, follicular fluid, and corpora lutea, whereas the liver contained low concentrations of this provitamin. These metabolite concentrations are quite variable in all tissues possibly due to the varied nutritional background and stage of growth or maturity status of cattle.[35]

Normal serum vitamin A concentrations in the bovine range from 25 to 60 μg/dL (83.3 to 200 IU/dL). Increases in cerebrospinal fluid pressure can be observed when concentrations approach 15 μg/dL (50 IU/dL). Slow weight gain and night blindness are reported at serum vitamin A concentrations around 8 to 10 μg/dL (27 to 33 IU/dL). Optic nerve damage and convulsions, in growing cattle, are expected as serum vitamin A concentrations decrease to less than 5 μg/dL (16.6 IU/dL).[194]

The diagnosis of vitamin A deficiency can be aided, by ophthalmoscopic examination, liver biopsy, blood vitamin A quantitation, measurement of cerebrospinal fluid pressure, and response to vitamin A supplementation.

Dietary Sources and Fortification

Concentrations of vitamin A in feedstuffs are highly variable. The richest natural sources of vitamin A are fish oils and liver. Among the common foods of animal origin, milk fat, egg yolk, and liver are rich sources of vitamin A, unless the animals had been fed a vitamin A deficient diet for an extended period.

Provitamin A carotenoids, mainly β-carotene in green feeds, are principal natural sources of vitamin A for beef cattle. All green parts of growing plants are rich in carotene and, therefore, have a high vitamin A value. In fact, the degree of green color in a roughage is a good index of its carotene content. Of the grains, only yellow corn has significant quantities of carotene. However, corn often has only one-fifth to one-tenth the carotene value of a green dehydrated forage such as alfalfa meal. Average values for carotene in feedstuffs are presented in Table 5.

Sources of supplemental vitamin A are primarily synthetic. Before the era of chemical production of vitamin A, the principal sources of vitamin A concentrates were the liver and/or body oils of marine fish and the carotene present in forages and grains. Since chemical synthesis was developed in 1949, the synthesized form has become the major source of the vitamin for domestic animals.

The major source of vitamin A used in beef cattle feed is trans retinyl acetate.[141] The acetate, like the propionate and palmitate esters, is chemically synthesized coated, and made into a beadlet form to be used in mash and pelleted feeds. The beadlet generally contains carbohydrates, gelatin, and antioxidants that are incorporated to stabilize the vitamin A by providing physical and chemical protection against adverse factors normally present in feed. The most popular vitamin A acetate product used in cattle feed contains 650,000 IU or United States Pharmacopoeia Units (USP) per gram of product. IU and USP

Table 5. *Carotene Content of Feedstuffs*

FEEDSTUFFS	CAROTENE (MG/LB)	
	AVERAGE	RANGE
Grains:		
Corn	1.5	0.1–6.0
Corn dent #2	0.9	–NPRA[a]
Corn gluten meal	15.0	–NPRA[a]
Sorghum (milo)	0.2	–NPRA[a]
Dry Roughages:		
Alfalfa hay	27.7	0–321.2
Alfalfa hay, sun cured (S.C.)	17.2	1.1–65.0
Alfalfa dehy. 17%	70.0	0–288.4
Brome hay	16.7	1.0–84.0
Clover hay	30.7	0.5–149.1
Alfalfa-timothy hay	6.0	1.5–16.7
Alfalfa-brome hay	8.9	4.8–16.0
Grass-legume	12.5	0.5–127.3
Green Roughages:		
Alfalfa	90.2	33.1–177.5
Blue stem	53.7	0.3–173.7
Brome	141.0	30–264.4
Clover	128.6	34.5–253.1
Fescue	153.1	36.3–285.8
Timothy	101.6	34.0–215.0
Wheat	184.7	81.5–433.2
Silages:		
Alfalfa	40.7	0.2–133.3
Brome	32.3	12.2–47.6
Clover	49.8	14.5–213.2
Corn	7.1	3.6–10.5
Corn dent	23.6	2.1–25.6
Sorghum	15.3	0.3–65.1
Alfalfa-brome	6.2	5.1–7.3

[a]No published range available.
(*Adapted from* National Research Council guidelines.)

units are equal in value, and one unit equals the activity of 0.3 μg of all-trans retinol or 0.344 μg of all-trans retinyl acetate.

The vitamin A activity contained in ingredients of typical beef cattle rations is very unpredictable. Therefore, the total requirement is usually added to the diet as a commercially synthesized, stabilized, vitamin A product. Available means of supplementing with vitamin A are as part of a concentrate or liquid supplement or in drinking water preparations. The most convenient and often most effective means to provide vitamin A to cattle is inclusion in concentrate mixtures that will provide uniform consumption of the vitamin.

Because Vitamin A is unstable, particularly when exposure to oxygen, trace minerals, pelleting, feed storage, and other factors, the feed industry has readily accepted the dry stabilized forms of the vitamin. Stabilized and protectively coated (or beadlet) forms of vitamin A slow destruction of the vitamin, but for highest potency, fresh supplies of the mixture should be available on a regular basis. Practical considerations that affect vitamin A stability are listed in Table 6.

Table 6. *Practical Factors That Affect the Stability of Vitamin A**

Factors detrimental to stability:
  Prolonged storage of the vitamin products or premixes prior to mixing or of the final feed product.
  Vitamin premixes containing trace minerals.
  High environmental temperature and humidity.
  Pelleting, blocking, and extrusion.
  Hot feed bins that sweat inside upon cooling.
  Rancid fat in the feed.
  Moisture leakage into feed bins or storage facilities.
Factors promoting stability:
  Minimizing time between manufacture of the vitamin product and consumption by the animal.
  Storage of vitamins in a cool, dark, dry area in closed containers.
  Do not mix vitamins and trace minerals in the same premix until ready to mix the feed.
  Control the premix to maintain pH within a range of 4.5 to 6.5 to avoid extreme acidic or alkaline pH.
  Use good quality feed ingredients and vitamins.
  Use appropriate antioxidant systems in the vitamin A product forms.
  Proper maintenance of storage bins and other equipment.
  Minimize time between purchase and use.

---

*(Adapted from Hoffmann-La Roche: Vitamin Fortification Guidelines. Update 2; 1989; with permission.)

The stability of vitamin A in feeds and premixes has been improved in recent years by chemical stabilization as an ester and by physical protection using antioxidants, emulsifying agents, and stabilized materials, including gelatin, crosslinked gelatin, and sugar in spray-dried, beadlet, or prilled products.[13,95,189] These vitamin A product forms result in enhanced chemical and physical stability, as well as excellent biologic availability. Nevertheless, vitamin A supplements should not be stored for prolonged periods prior to use and feeding.

Several factors can influence the loss of vitamin A activity from feedstuffs during storage. The trace minerals in feeds and supplements, particularly copper (Cu), are detrimental to vitamin A stability. Dash and Mitchell reported the vitamin A content of 1293 commercial feeds over a 3 year period.[45] The loss of vitamin A was over 50% in 1 year's time.[45] Vitamin A loss in commercial feeds was evident even if the commercial feeds contained stabilized vitamin A supplements.[45]

There is evidence that yellow corn may lose carotene rapidly during storage. For instance, a hybrid corn, high in carotene, lost about half of its carotene in 8 months' storage at 25C° and approximately 75% in 3 years. Less carotene was lost during storage at 7°C (Quackenbush, 1963). Because of vitamin A variability in feeds and losses during processing and storage, most animal nutritionists tend to ignore vitamin A activity in feedstuffs and rely exclusively on dietary fortification to arrive at vitamin allowances for beef cattle.

Vitamin A and carotene destruction also occurs from processing of feeds with steam and pressure. Pelleting effects on vitamin A in feed are caused by die thickness and hole size, which produce frictional heat and a shearing effect that can expose the vitamin to destructive processes. In addition, steam application exposes feed to heat and moisture.

Diseases and mycotoxins increase the need for supplemental vitamin A. It should be noted that diseases can interfere with the absorption and utilization of vitamin A (i.e., enteric diseases such as malabsorption syndrome, mycotoxins, diarrhea, etc.). The effect of mycotoxins in the feed should also be considered, since aflatoxin is known to interfere with protein synthesis.[52] Thus, mycotoxins might interfere with RBP synthesis and transport of vitamin A.

Short term administration of vitamin A in drinking water or by injection is recommended to support any specific measures used in correction of vitamin A deficiency and convalescent animals. This is particularly true for cattle in which vitamin A stores may have been depleted due to fever or in animals suffering from intestinal disorders when vitamin A absorption is seriously impaired.

The decision to supplement vitamin A should be based mainly on whether or not a deficiency could be a practical problem. As with most nutrients, a borderline deficiency is much more likely to occur than a severe deficiency. Likewise, a marginal deficiency adversely affecting performance by a few percentage points is not easily detected. Based on the positive results that may be derived and taking into account that vitamin A supplementation is inexpensive and no toxicity problems have been reported when given at recommended levels, it seems beneficial to supplement vitamin A for cattle and to increase the supplementation amounts substantially for cattle that are diseased or under stress. Cattle on good quality pasture consume significant amounts of β-carotene there is a greater safety factor from deficiency than when animals are fed diets of stored and processed grains and forages.

The amount of vitamin A added to cattle diets is usually in excess of the requirements contained in the NRC publication because no safety factors are built into the NRC values. Additional vitamin A is added to allow for loss of activity due to oxidative destruction of the vitamin A ester during feed processing and storage, variability of carotenes in feedstuffs, changes in feed consumption, genetic differences in animals, and stress due to disease and other environmental factors.

In the early 1940s, the vitamin A requirement of cattle was determined based on vitamin A activity from β-carotene.[147] Test results have shown that carotene is not efficiently converted to vitamin A activity in cattle.[80] An optimum vitamin A recommendation of 2000 IU per 100 pounds of body weight was suggested for beef cattle. The vitamin A requirement of breeding, growing, and finishing beef cattle can be met by (1) provitamin A (carotene) in feedstuffs, or (2) by supplementary vitamin A, either by intramuscular injection or orally, or (3) by combinations of (1) and (2).

The minimum vitamin A requirement for normal growth may be lower than that required for higher rates of gain, resistance to various diseases, and normal bone development and nervous system function in cattle.[218] It was suggested that (a) calves born with low vitamin A liver stores should receive a minimum injection of 7500 IU of vitamin A per

100 lb of body weight and (b) three to five times this level — 22,500 to 37,500 IU per 100 lbs. of body weight — may be necessary for adequate vitamin A liver stores in calves during the critical first few months of life. Minimum vitamin A requirements as defined by the NRC are given in (Table 7).

Test results showed that the vitamin A requirement of calves was increased by as much as seven-fold, depending on the criteria used to determine it.[115] The vitamin A requirement values (IU per 100 lb of body weight) were 1200 for adequate weight gains, 2400 for increased weight gains, and 8000 for optimum weight gains and vitamin A liver stores.

In a 168 day experiment, moderate to extremely high vitamin A levels were fed to fattening cattle; 40,000 IU per head daily was needed to maintain initial vitamin A liver stores.[82] Cattle fed 2.5 million IU of vitamin A per head daily, which totalled 420 million IU per head for 168 days, showed no evidence of vitamin A toxicity. Vitamin A toxicosis in ruminant animals is not well established and the presumed safe level is 30 times the optimum level (Table 8). This presumed upper safe level is considered conservative since there is a lack of reported toxicity in most functioning ruminants. In one reported long term study, steers were fed for 168 days, a daily intake of 2.56 million IU per head, and no gross evidence of toxicosis was reported.[82]

Carotene absorption and utilization among and within species is genetically controlled (Table 9). High intake of carotenoids from natural feedstuffs does not produce vitamin A toxicity and is not a practical problem in animals. In normal ranges, blood levels are poorly correlated with either intakes or liver stores. Blood levels of 5 to around 20 μg/dL of retinol are indicative of depleted liver stores and deficiency. Blood levels persistently above 100 μg/dL are indicative of vitamin A toxicity.[56]

VITAMIN D

Properties and Metabolism

Vitamin D designates a group of closely related compounds that possess antirachitic activity. It may be supplied through the diet or by irradiation of the body. The two most prominent forms of vitamin D are ergocalciferol (vitamin D_2) and cholecalciferol (vitamin D_3). Ergocalciferol is derived from a common plant steroid, ergosterol, whereas cholecalciferol is produced from the precursor 7-dehydrocholesterol and exclusively from animal products. 7-Dehydrocholesterol, which is derived from cholesterol or squalene, is synthesized in the body and present in large amounts in skin, intestinal wall, and other tissues. Vitamin D precursors have no antirachitic activity.

Vitamin D, in the pure form, occurs as colorless crystals that are insoluble in water but readily soluble in alcohol and other organic solvents. Vitamin D can be destroyed by ultraviolet light (UV) and by peroxidation in the presence of rancidifying polyunsaturated fatty acids (PUFA). Like vitamins A and E, unless vitamin D_3 is stabilized, it is

Table 7. *Minimum Requirements and Suggested Vitamin Supplementation for Beef Cattle*

	GROWING AND FINISHING STEERS AND HEIFERS		PREGNANT COWS AND HEIFERS		BREEDING BULLS AND LACTATING COWS		RUMINANT STRESS FORMULATION[d]
	NRC[a]	SUGGESTED SUPPLEMENTATION	NRC[b]	SUGGESTED SUPPLEMENTATION	NRC[c]	SUGGESTED SUPPLEMENTATION	
Vitamin A, TIU	18	50–70	25.4	50–100	46.0	50–100	375
Vitamin D_3, TIU	2.2	5–7	2.5	5–7	3.2	5–7	1600
Vitamin E[d] IU	122–490	200–500	136–544	150–340	177–708	150–340	550
Niacin, mg[e]	—	500–1000	—	—	—	—	200
Thiamin, mg[e]	—	60–250	—	—	—	—	
d-Pantothenic Acid, mg	—	—	—	—	—	—	
Vitamin B_{12}, mg	—	—	—	—	—	—	0.40
Folic Acid, mg	—	—	—	—	—	—	40
Pyridoxine, mg	—	—	—	—	—	—	800

[a]Based on 700 lbs body weight and daily feed consumption of 18 lbs, estimated from NRC (1984).[153]
[b]Based on 1100 lbs body weight and daily feed consumption of 20 lbs, estimated from NRC (1984).[153]
[c]Based on bull weighing 1400 lbs and lactating cow weighing 1100 lbs each consuming 26 lbs of feed daily, estimated from NRC.
[d]Requirement not determined but estimated from the minimum requirement for young calves.
[e]For cattle on high concentrate rations first 28–35 days on feed.
(*Adapted from* Hoffman-LaRoche: Vitamin Fortification Guidelines: Update 2, Nutley, New Jersey, 1989; with permission and Johnson AB, Krautman BA: Water soluble vitamins for ruminants. *In* Proceedings of the 24th Pacific Northwest Animal Nutrition Conference, Boise, 1989, p 81; with permission.)

Table 8. *Apparent Vitamin Toxicity Potential (AVTP)*

VITAMIN	AVTP	THEORETICAL INTOXICATION LEVEL (TIMES REQUIREMENT)	SIGNS
A	Greatest	Nonruminants, 10× req. Ruminants, 30× req.	Nervous dysfunction; liver dysfunction; skin disorders; anorexia; gastrointestinal distress; hypercalcemia; polyuria; calcinosis
D	Greatest	>60 days, 4–10× req. <60 days, 1000× req.	
Choline (as chloride)	Greatest	2–4× req.	Depressed growth
Niacin	Moderate	Nicotinamide, 10–20× req. Nicotinic acid, 40–80× req.	Depressed growth; altered lipid Metabolism; nervous dysfunction
Riboflavin	Moderate	10–20× req.	Reproductive disorders
Pantothenic acid	Moderate	20× req.	Liver dysfunction
Vitamin E	Least	1000× req.	Depressed growth; hepatic dysfunction; hypoprothrombinemia; bone demineralization
Vitamin K	Least	Menadione, 1000× req.	Renal dysfunction
Ascorbic acid	Least	5–10 g/kg diet fish, 10–20× req.	Oxaluria; uriosuria; hypoglycemia; hyperabsorption of iron; allergic reactions; anemia; gastrointestinal distress
Thiamin	Least	1000× req.	Nervous dysfunction
Pyridoxine	Least	1000× req.	Nervous dysfunction
Folic acid	Least	1000× req.	Nervous dysfunction; renal hypertrophy
Biotin	Least	(Probably very high)	Unknown
Vitamin B_{12}	Least	(Probably very high)	Unknown

(*Adapted from* Combs GF Jr: Vitamin tolerance of livestock. *In* Proceedings of 1988 Cornell Nutrition Conference for Feed Manufacturers. Syracuse, 1988, p 35; with permission.)

Table 9. *Conversion of β-Carotene to Vitamin A by Different Animals**

ANIMALS	CONVERSION OF MG OF β-CAROTENE TO IU OF VITAMIN A (MG) = (IU)	IU OF VITAMIN A ACTIVITY (CALCULATED AS PERCENT OF STANDARD)
Standard (rat)	1 = 1667	100
Beef cattle	1 = 400	24
Dairy cattle	1 = 400	24
Sheep	1 = 400–450	24–30
Swine	1 = 500	30
Horse		
Growth	1 = 555	33.3
Pregnancy	1 = 333	20
Poultry	1 = 1667	100
Dog	1 = 833	50
Rat	1 = 1667	100
Fox	1 = 278	16.7
Cat	Carotene not utilized	—
Mink	Carotene not utilized	—
Human	1 = 556	33.3

(*Modified from* McDowell LR: Vitamin A. *In* Vitamins and Animal Nutrition: Comparative Aspects to Human Nutrition. San Diego, Academic Press, 1989, p 10; with permission.)

destroyed by oxidation unless it is stabilized. Its oxidative destruction is increased by heat, moisture and trace minerals.

Dietary vitamin D is absorbed from the intestinal tract and is more likely to be absorbed in the ileal portion due to longer retention time of food in the distal portion of the intestine.[158] Vitamin D is absorbed from the intestinal tract in association with fats, as are all the fat-soluble vitamins. Like the others, it requires the presence of bile salts for absorption[21] and is absorbed with other neutral lipids via chylomicron into the lymphatic system of mammals. It has been reported that only 50% of an oral dose of vitamin D is absorbed. It is also clear that absorption of vitamin D can take place through the skin as topical application can be used to treat ricketts.

Presence of the provitamin, 7-dehydrocholesterol, in the epidermis of the skin and sebaceous secretions is well recognized. The cholecalciferol formed by UV irradiation of the 7-dehydrocholesterol in the skin is transported by the blood, primarily bound to an α-globulin, and becomes immediately available for further metabolism.[100]

Prior to 1968, it was almost universally thought that vitamin D_3 and D_2 were the circulating antirachitic agents in animals. Starting in 1968 DeLuca and others demonstrated that vitamin D_3 undergoes a multiple series of transformations and multisite interactions.[48]

In the microsomal fraction of the liver a 25 hydroxylase hydroxylates the 25 carbon in the side chain of cholecalciferol to produce 25-hydroxyvitamin D (25-(OH)D_3). This metabolite is the major circulating form of vitamin D both under normal conditions and during vitamin D excess.[116] The 25-(OH)D_3 is then transported on the vitamin D transport globulin, to the kidney where it can be converted in the proximal convoluted tabule cells to a variety of compounds. The most important metabolites appear to be 1,25 dihydroxyvitamin D_3 (1,25-$(OH)_2D_3$).[47] Once formed in the kidney, 1,25-$(OH)_2D_3$ is transported to the intestine, bones, and elsewhere in the body, where it is involved in the metabolism of calcium and phosphorus. From studies of vitamin D metabolism, it has been found that the vitamin functions as a hormone. The hormonal form, 1,25-$(OH)_2D_3$, is the metabolically active form of the vitamin that functions in intestine and bone, whereas 25-$(OH)D_3$ and vitamin D_3 do not function at these specific sites under physiologic conditions.[47]

Production of 1,25-$(OH)_2D_3$ is regulated by parathyroid hormone (PTH) in response to serum calcium and phosphate concentrations. It is now known that the most important point of regulation of the vitamin D endocrine system occurs through the stringent control of the activity of the renal 1 alpha-hydroxylase. In this way, the production of the hormone 1,25-$(OH)_2D_3$ can be modulated according to the calcium needs of the organism.[144] Concentrations of calcium parathyroid hormone, and vitamin D status affect the activity of the 1-hydroxylase.

In most mammals, vitamin D_3, 25-$(OH)D_3$, and possibly 24,25-$(OH)_2D_3$ and 1,25-$(OH)_2D_3$ are transported on the same protein, transcalciferin, or vitamin D-binding protein. While aquatic species store significant amounts of vitamin D in liver, land animals do not store appreciable amounts of the vitamin. The body has some ability to store the vitamin, although to a much lesser extent than is the case for vitamin A. Principal stores of vitamin D occur in blood and liver, but it is also found in lungs, kidneys, and other organs. Excretion of absorbed vitamin D and its metabolites occurs primarily in feces, with the aid of bile salts.

Functions

The general function of vitamin D is to elevate plasma calcium and phosphorus to a level that will support normal mineralization of bone and other body functions. Recent, evidence suggests a regulatory role of vitamin D_3 (1,25-$(OH)_2D_3$) in immune cell functions.[173] The possible use of vitamin D analogs to induce differentiation of myelocytic-type leukemias has been an important new development.[48]

Two hormones, thyrocalcitonin (calcitonin) and PTH, function with 1,25-$(OH)_2D_3$ to control blood calcium and phosphorus levels.[62] Production rate of 1,25-$(OH)_2D_3$ is under physiologic, as well as dietary control. Calcitonin, contrary to the other two, regulates high serum calcium levels by (1) depressing gut absorption of calcium, (2) halting bone demineralization, and (3) depressing reabsorption of calcium in the kidney. Vitamin D brings about an elevation of plasma calcium and phosphorus by stimulating specific pump mechanisms in the intestine, bone, and kidney. These three sources of calcium and phosphorus provide reservoirs that enable vitamin D to elevate blood calcium and phosphorus to levels necessary for normal bone mineralization and other functions.

Vitamin D stimulates active transport of Ca and P across intestinal epithelium. This stimulation does not involve PTH directly, but involves 1,25-$(OH)_2D_3$. Parathyroid hormone indirectly stimulates intestinal Ca absorption by stimulating production of 1,25-$(OH)_2D_3$ under conditions of hypocalcemia.

During bone formation, minerals are deposited on the protein matrix in young animals. This is accompanied by vascular invasion of epiphyseal and metaphyseal bone that gives rise to trabecular bone. This process causes bones to elongate. During vitamin D deficiency, this organic matrix fails to mineralize, causing rickets in the young and osteomalacia in adults. The active metabolite, 1,25-$(OH)_2D_3$, brings about mineralization of the bone matrix. Additionally, there is some indication that 24,25-$(OH)_2D_3$ and possibly 25-$(OH)D_3$ may have unique actions on bone. The 24,25-$(OH)_2D_3$ appears to accumulate in bone, where it promotes normal development.[7]

Vitamin D is also involved in the mobilization of Ca from bone to the extracellular fluid compartment. This function is shared by PTH.[69] It is an active process requiring energy. Presumably vitamin D stimulates Ca and P transport by acting on osteocytes and osteoclasts. In addition to its involvement in bone mineralization, it has been proposed that vitamin D is involved in the biosynthesis of collagen in preparation for mineralization.[75]

Assessment of Status

Deficiencies. Vitamin D deficiency, combined with unbalanced Ca and P uptake, leads to rickets in the young, and to osteomalacia in the adult. Rickets is characterized by reduced deposition of Ca in the growing bone, and osteomalacia is characterized by a loss of Ca from the fully developed bone.

Clinical signs of vitamin D deficiency in ruminants are decreased appetite and growth rate, digestive disturbances, stiffness in gait, labored breathing, irritability, weakness, and, occasionally, tetany and convulsions. There is enlargement of joints, slight arching of the back, and bowing of legs, and erosion of joint surfaces causing difficulty in locomotion.[153] Young ruminants may be born dead, weak or deformed.

Clinical signs involving bones begin with the thickening and swelling of the metacarpal or metatarsal bones. As the disease progresses, the forelegs bend forward or sideways. In severe or prolonged vitamin D deficiency, tension of the muscles will cause a bending and twisting of long bones to give the characteristic deformity of bone. There is enlargement at ends of bones with excess cartilage, giving the characteristic "beading" effect along the sternum where ribs attach. The mandible becomes thick and soft; in the worst cases eating is then difficult. In calves so affected there can be slobbering, inability to close the mouth, and protrusion of the tongue. Joints (particularly the knee and hock) become swollen and stiff, the pastern straight, and the back humped. In more severe cases, synovial fluid accumulates in the joints.[152] In older animals with a vitamin D deficiency, bones become weak and fracture easily, and posterior paralysis may accompany vertebral fractures.

Vitamin D deficiency in beef cattle is very unlikely, unless a deficient diet is fed, and animals are kept away from sunlight. Cows fed a vitamin D deficient diet and kept out of direct sunlight showed definite symptoms of vitamin D deficiency within 6 to 10 months.[217] Functions that deplete vitamin D are high milk production and advancing pregnancy, especially during the last few months before calving. The visible signs of vitamin D deficiency in dairy cows are similar to those of rickets in calves. The animals begin to show stiffness in its limbs and joints, which makes it difficult to walk, lie down and get up. The knees, hocks, and other joints become swollen, tender, and stiff. The knees often spring forward, the posterior joints straighten, and the animal is tilted on its toes. The hair becomes coarse and rough and there is an overall appearance of unthriftiness.[217] As the deficiency becomes advanced, the back often becomes stiff, humped, and is bent or flexed as little as possible. In deficient herds, calving rates are lower and calves have been born dead or weak. Calves may die shortly after birth.

Clinical Parameters. Methods for assessing the vitamin D status of beef cattle are very limited and often not specific. Poor bone development and bone abnormalities are evident in severely deficient animals. Incomplete skeletal development is detectable by radiographs, but abnormalities may not be different from those caused by simple calcium or phosphorus deficiency or other nutritional inadequacies.

Low serum calcium levels, in the range of 5 to 7 mg/dL, and high serum alkaline phosphatase activity can be used to help diagnose rickets and osteomalacia. Sturen reported serum concentration of approximately 10.82, 6.89 and 3.82 for calcium, inorganic phosphorus, and magnesium, respectively, in vitamin D_3 deficient dairy cows.[198] In the same study, none of the animals had detectable levels of 25-hydroxy-vitamin D_3 in serum because of their limited access to solar radiation and the lack of vitamin D_3 supplementation.[198] Further, suspected vitamin D deficient beef animals of various breeds between the ages of 3 and 12 months had undetectable serum levels of 25-hydroxy-vitamin D_3 compared with normal animals, having values of about 36 ng/mL (least square mean).[198] In this case vitamin D deficiency was described as skeletal disorders including achilles tendon rupture, stiffness, difficulty in moving, and visibly enlarged growth zones of the long bones.[198] Several investigators have used 25-hydroxyvitamin D_3 as a measure of vitamin D status in ruminants. Dietary vitamin D_3 intake, exposure to sunlight and blood parameters of calcium, phosphorus and 25-hydroxyvitamin D_3 as well as skeletal abnormalities should all be evaluated in assessing vitamin D status in beef cattle.

Dietary Sources and Fortification

Vitamin D can be provided to beef cattle by natural vitamin D_2 available in sun-cured forms, by injectable vitamin D_3 and by feed supplementation. In summer months animals on pasture may receive sufficient exposure to sunlight. During winter months, when daylight hours are reduced and animals may be housed, it is unsafe to rely on exposure to sunlight to provide the antirachitic factor. Sun-cured forage is the best natural source of vitamin D, even though 1 to 4 hours per day of sunlight is thought to provide adequate vitamin D for calves.

Newlander measured vitamin D activity in field and barn-cured hay. Concentrations varied with season and hay cuttings, ranging from 0.47 to over 2.4 U.S.P. units per gram of hay.[155] Calves fed this hay from birth to 6 months of age consumed from 90 to 750 I.U. of vitamin D per day. Hay, when partially dried in the sun to between 53 to 63 percent dry matter and then flue-cured in storage, contained sufficient vitamin D for the growth requirement of dairy animals.[155] However, intensively raised calves are increasingly showing skeletal disorders, and standardized vitamin D sources may be necessary to ensure sufficiency.

A commercially available product containing vitamin D_3 with appropriate stability should be used for vitamin D_3 fortification of ruminant feeds. Cattle fed poor quality stored forages and confined from sunlight should be supplemented daily. Deficient animals will achieve normal status more quickly when injected with high potency aqueous suspensions, than with oily solutions given orally.[145] Cattle fed concentrated diets need to be adequately supplemented with vitamin D, since livestock feeds composed of grain, roots and oilseeds, as well as their numerous by-products, contain insufficient amounts of vitamin D. Green fodders are equally poor sources. The principal source of the antirachitic factor in the diets of farm animals is sunlight irradiating ergosterol in forages. Legume hay that is cured to preserve most of its leaves and green color contains considerable amounts of vitamin D activity. Alfalfa, for example, will range from 650 to 2200 IU per kg (295 to 1000 IU per lb).[133] Cattle that are fed sun cured alfalfa leaf meal receive a limited amount of vitamin D from this source. However, fewer commercial cattle operations use alfalfa leaf meal than in the past.

Due to lack of vitamin D in feeds and management systems without direct sunlight, modern cattle operations must provide a supplemental source of the vitamin. Vitamin D_3 is the principal source of supplemental vitamin D for livestock. Vitamin D_3 is commercially available as a resin or crystal, usually containing 24 to 40 million IU per gram. Vitamin D_3 products for feed include gelatin beadlets (as with vitamin A), oil dilutions, oil adsorbates, emulsions, and spray- and drum-dried powders. Incorporating vitamins D_3 and A in the beadlet form provides physical protection from oxidation, and the antioxidants included in the beadlets afford chemical protection.

In addition to providing supplemental vitamin D in feed and water, injectable sources are available. Parenteral vitamin D_3 treatment of sows before parturition provided an effective means of supplementing piglets with vitamin D_3 (via the sow's milk) and its dihydroxy metabolites by placental transport.[73]

Cost of vitamin D supplementation to livestock diets is nominal.[179] In contrast, the potential losses from vitamin D deficiency are very high. Supplemental levels of vitamin D_3, administered to cattle through the feed, should be adjusted to provide the margin-of-safety needed to offset factors which can increase the vitamin D requirement. This is important to prevent deficiency and allow optimum performance. Factors that increase the amount of vitamin D needed to maximize productive and reproductive responses may not be reflected in NRC minimum requirements. Consequently, nutritionists often use more than the minimum levels of vitamin D in feeds. Successful nutrition programs may greatly exceed the NRC minimum requirement for vitamin D. Importantly, no amount of vitamin D can make up for an imbalance of Ca or P in the diet.

Besides inadequate quantities of dietary vitamin D, deficiencies may result from (1) errors in vitamin addition to diets, (2) inadequate mixing and distribution in feed, (3) separation of vitamin D particles after mixing, (4) instability of the vitamin content of the supplement, or (5) excessive duration of storage under environmental conditions causing vitamin D loss.[92]

Supplementation considerations are dependent on other dietary ingredients. The requirements for vitamin D are increased several fold by inadequate levels of Ca and/or P or by improper ratios of these two elements in the diet. A number of reports have indicated that molds in feeds interfere with vitamin D. For example, when corn contains the mold *Fusarium roseum*, a metabolite of this mold prevents intestinal vitamin D_3 from being absorbed by monogastrics.[43] A similar deleterious effect on vitamin D metabolism would be expected in cattle.

Other factors that influence vitamin D status are diseases of the endocrine system, intestinal disorders, liver malfunction, kidney disorders and drugs. Hepatic and renal disease can limit production of the active forms of the vitamin, while intestinal disorders reduce absorption. The possibility exists that cattle with certain diseases or heavy infestation of internal parasites might be unable to synthesize the metabolically active forms of vitamin D, as a result of liver or kidney damage.

Following vitamin A, vitamin D is the next most likely vitamin to be consumed in concentrations toxic to livestock. Although vitamin D is toxic at high concentrations, short-term administration of as much as 100 times the required level may be tolerated. For most species, including cattle, the presumed maximal safe level of vitamin D_3 for long-term feeding conditions (more than 60 days) is 4 to 10 times the dietary requirement. For the cow, the upper safe dietary level for short time exposure is 25,000 IU per kg (3364 IU per lb) and, for over 60 days, 2200 IU per kg (1000 IU per lb) of diet.[154]

Excessive intake of vitamin D produces a variety of effects, all associated with abnormal elevation of blood Ca. Elevated blood Ca is caused by greatly stimulated bone resorption, as well as increased intestinal Ca absorption. The main pathological effect of massive doses of vitamin D is widespread calcification of soft tissues. In cattle, signs of toxicity are anorexia, cardiovascular mineralization and cardiac irregularity. Death was reported in 30 days when pregnant cattle were injected with a single IM dose of 15,000,000 IU of vitamin D_3. Studies in a number of species, including cattle, indicate that vitamin D_3 is 10 to 20 times more toxic than vitamin D_2 when provided in excessive amounts.

VITAMIN E

Properties and Metabolism

Vitamin E activity in feed is derived from a series of compounds of plant origin, the tocopherols and tocotrienols. The term vitamin E, according to the International Union of Pure and Applied Chemistry-International Union of Biochemistry (IUPAC-IUB) Commission on Biochemical Nomenclature, is used as a generic descriptor for all tocol and tocotrienol derivatives which qualitatively exhibit biologic activity of α-tocopherol.[101] Both the tocols (tocopherols) and tocotrienols consist of a hydroquinone nucleus and an isoprenoid side chain. Characteristically, tocols have a saturated side chain, whereas, the tocotrienols have an unsaturated side chain containing three double bonds. Four isomers of each of these two classes of vitamin E exist (α, β, γ, δ), differentiated by the presence of methyl-groups at positions 5, 7 or 8 of the chroman ring. Alpha-tocopherol, the most biologically active of these compounds, is the predominant compound in feedstuffs with vitamin E activity, and the biological activity of the other tocols is limited (Table 10).

Alpha-tocopherol is a yellow oil that is insoluble in water, but soluble in organic solvents. Tocopherols are extremely resistant to heat,

Table 10. *Relative Biological Activities of Various Tocopherols and Tocotrienols**

	FETAL RESORPTION (RAT)	HEMOLYSIS (RAT)	MUSCLE DYSTROPHY (CHICKEN)
Alpha-tocopherol (5,7,8-trimethyl tocol)	100	100	100
Beta-tocopherol (5,8-dimethyl tocol)	25–40	15–27	12
Gamma-tocopherol (7,8-dimethyl tocol)	1–11	3–20	5
Delta-tocopherol (8-methyl tocol)	1	0.3–2	—
Alpha-tocotrienol-3	29	17–25	—
Beta-tocotrienol-3 (5,8-dimethyl tocotrienol)	5	1–5	—

(*Adapted from* Machlin LJ: Vitamin E. *In* Handbook of Vitamins: Nutritional, Biochemical and Clinical Aspects. New York, Marcel Dekker, 1984, p 99; with permission.)

but readily oxidized. Natural vitamin E is subject to destruction by oxidation, and this is accelerated by heat, moisture, rancid fat, copper and iron. Alpha-tocopherol is an excellent natural antioxidant that protects carotene and other oxidizable materials in feed and in the body. However, while acting as an antioxidant it is destroyed.

Animals do not synthesize vitamin E and require an external source of the nutrient, generally green pasture, to meet their dietary requirements. Absorption, as with vitamins A and D, is dependent on normal fat digestion, and facilitated by bile and pancreatic lipase in the small intestine. Esters are largely hydrolyzed in the gut wall and free alcohol enters the intestinal lacteals where it is transported via lymph to the general circulation. In people, 20 to 30% of small doses of vitamin E is recovered using lymphatic cannulation techniques. A marked decrease in intestinal absorption is seen with larger doses.

There appears to be little or no preintestinal absorption of dietary tocopherol, although preintestinal destruction has been reported.[2] It has been reported that vitamin E absorption is related to vitamin E status with vitamin E deficient ruminants absorbing 50 to 75% of dietary tocopherol intake. Vitamin E adequate animals absorb 20 to 30% and animals receiving excess dietary vitamin E only 1 to 5%. Hidiroglou et al. reported no correlation between vitamin E status and tocopherol absorption.[90] Vitamin E absorption may be impaired by a variety of disorders associated with fat malabsorption.[39] The animal appears to have preference for tocopherol versus other tocols.[142] Rumenal microbial destruction of tocopherol has also been reported.

Alpha-tocopherol is best absorbed, with γ-tocopherol absorption 85% of α-forms, but with a more rapid excretion. One can generally assume that most of the vitamin E activity within plasma and other animal tissues is α-tocopherol.[212] Vitamin E in plasma is mainly attached to lipoproteins in the globulin fraction. Intracellular vitamin E is localized mainly in membrane fractions of mitochondria and microsomes.

The fetus obtains its tocopherol through placental transfer, but levels in the neonate are generally lower than in the dam.[90] This is probably due to inefficient transfer from the placenta to the fetus, as there appears to be no barrier to the entry of tocopherol into the placenta.[127] Less than 1% of the dam's tocopherol intake is excreted in the milk,[143] with values of about 2 mg/1 have been reported for cow's milk.[143] Levels in the colostrum are higher than in the milk (Table 11).

The detailed mechanism of tocopherol uptake and retention by tissues is unknown, but relatively little storage occurs: the liver is not a storage organ for vitamin E. Liver contains only a small fraction of total body stores, in contrast to vitamin A, for which about 95% of the body reserves are in the liver. Small amounts of vitamin E will persist tenaciously in the body for a long time. However, stores are exhausted rapidly by polyunsaturated fatty acids (PUFA) in the tissues, the rate of disappearance being proportional to the intake of PUFA. A major excretory route of absorbed vitamin E is bile, in which tocopherol

Table 11. Levels of Various Vitamins in Colostrum and Whole Milk[a]

VITAMIN	UNITS	COLOSTRUM (MILKINGS AFTER CALVING)						MILK
		1ST	2ND	3RD	4TH	5TH	6TH	
A	I.U./100 ml	982	633	376	253	246[b]	—	113
D	I.U./g fat	0.89–1.81[c]	—	—	—	—	—	0.41
E	I.U. g fat	0.125	0.113	0.083	0.066	0.046[b]	—	0.022
Thiamine (B$_1$)	mcg/ml	0.58	—	0.59	—	0.59	—	0.38
Riboflavin (B$_2$)	mcg/ml	4.83	2.71	1.85	1.80	1.76	1.73	1.47
Nicotinic	mcg/ml	0.74–0.097[c]	—	—	—	—	—	0.80
d-Pantothenic Acid	mcg/ml	1.73	—	3.20	—	3.96	—	3.82
d-Biotin	mcg/100 ml	11.0–2.7[c]	—	2.5	—	2.4	—	2.0
Vitamin B$_{12}$	mcg/100 ml	4.9	—	0.2	—	0.1	—	0.6
Folic Acid	mcg/100 ml	0.8	—	—	—	—	—	0.2
Choline	mg/ml	0.70	0.34	0.23	0.19	0.16	0.15	0.13
C (Ascorbic Acid)	mg/100 ml	2.5	—	2.3	—	2.0	—	2.2

[a]Analyses of colostrum and milk primarily from Holstein cows.
[b]Composite of fifth and sixth milkings after calving.
[c]Composite of first through sixth milkings after calving.
(*Adapted from* Foley JA, Otterby DE: Availability, storage, treatment, composition, and feeding value of surplus colostrom: A review. J Dairy Sci 61:1033, 1978; with permission.)

appears mostly in the free form. Tocopherol entering the circulatory system becomes distributed throughout the body with the majority localizing in the fatty tissues.[94] Subcellular fractions from different tissues vary considerably in their tocopherol content,[201] with the highest levels found in membranous organelles, such as microsomes and mitochondria, that contain highly active redox systems.[134,201]

Function

Vitamin E has been shown to be essential for integrity and optimum function of reproductive, muscular, circulatory, nervous and immune systems.[16,93,138,188] One of the most important functions of vitamin E is as a chain-breaking *in vivo* antioxidant, both inter- and intracellularly.

Vitamin E is now recognized as being part of the body's intracellular defense against the adverse effects of reactive oxygen and free radicals that initiate oxidation of unsaturated phospholipids[36] and critical sulphydryl groups.[26] Burton and Ingold have shown that α-tocopherol is the most reactive chain-breaking phenolic antioxidant known and that previous discrepancies between in vitro antioxidant activity and *in vivo* vitamin E activity are attributable to inappropriate experimental techniques.[27]

Oxidation of vitamin E prevents oxidation of other lipid materials to free radicals and peroxides within cells, thus protecting the cell membrane from damage.[55] This function is closely related to and synergistic with the role of selenium. Selenium has been shown to act in aqueous cell media (cytosol and mitochondrial matrix) by destroying hydrogen peroxide and hydroperoxides via the enzyme glutathione peroxidase of, which it is a co-factor.

If lipid hydroperoxides are allowed to form in the absence of adequate vitamin E compounds, direct cellular damage may result. Oxidation of lipids, proteins and nucleic acids results in alteration of the structural integrity of the cell and metabolic derangements. Myodegeneration is common in cases of vitamin E-selenium deficiency. Increased membrane permeability results in leakage of cellular compounds, such as creatine kinase and various transaminases, and elevation of serum creatine kinase is indicative of vitamin E deficiency. The more active the cell (e.g., cells of skeletal and involuntary muscles), the greater the influx of lipids for energy, enhancing the risk of tissue damage when vitamin E is limiting.

Primary defenses against the production of singlet oxygen and hydroxyl radicals act in the aqueous phase of the cell. The swelling and lysis of mitochondrial membranes is thought to be caused by lipid peroxidation.[96] The lipid soluble tocopherol is able to function in the hydrophobic environment and quenches singlet oxygen and free radicals that may be present.[109,134] Burton et al. reported that tocopherol is the major, and probably only, lipid-soluble, chain-breaking (peroxyl-radical trapping) antioxidant in plasma and in erythrocyte ghost membranes.[29] Tocopherol appears to be aligned, through its phytyl side-chain, with the prevailing direction of the acyl chains of the polyunsaturated phospholipids.[70,130] Tocopherol is well-placed to protect the membrane against the harmful effects of singlet oxygen on membranal phospholipids, and of hydroxyl radicals on the critical sulphydryl groups.

Other functions attributed to vitamin E include involvement in arachidonic acid and prostaglandin metabolism,[50,112] immunocompetency,[60,156,202] blood clotting,[160] as well as electron transport and deoxyribonucleic acid (DNA) synthesis.[139]

Assessment of Status

Deficiencies. Feed deficient in vitamin E is the principal cause of vitamin E deficiency in ruminants. Most unsupplemented ruminant rations containing stored and(or) processed feedstuffs are relatively poor sources of vitamin E.[197] Generally, pasture cattle would not require supplemental vitamin E if adequate green forage is available.[132,197] However, cattle consuming dormant or drought stricken pasture, hay, haylage or silage during winter months may be at risk.[120,139,185] Other factors influencing the vitamin E requirement of ruminants include the use of preservatives (e.g., propionic acid or sodium hydroxide) which destroy the alpha-tocopherol content of feedstuffs,[174] ruminal microbial destruction,[2] nitrate ingestion,[12] excessively high dietary vitamin A intake,[49] and high dietary polyunsaturated fatty acid intake.[156] The need for vitamin E may be additionally increased if antioxidants such as carotenoids and vitamin C, which could spare vitamin E, are deficient.[28]

With respect to neonatal ruminants, several investigators have reported limited placental transport of alpha-tocopherol, making neonates highly susceptible to vitamin E deficiency.[89,126,163,213] This may be related to either a decreasing efficiency in placental vitamin E transfer as gestation proceeds, a dilution effect as a result of rapid fetal growth, or possibly a decrease in available maternal vitamin E. With limited placental transfer of vitamin E neonatal ruminants must rely heavily on ingestion of colostrum as a source of vitamin E.[89,163,220] Van Saun et al. reported decreased fetal serum vitamin E concentrations with increasing fetal age and increased fetal vitamin E status with greater maternal vitamin E concentration in dairy calves and cows.[213] Additionally, these authors reported less of a decline in fetal serum vitamin E concentration during gestation in fetuses from vitamin E adequate dams.[213] Adequacy of vitamin E was defined as dams with serum alpha-tocopherol concentrations >2 μg/ml (0.2 mg/dL).

Nutritional myodegeneration (NMD; also known as white muscle disease) is the most widely recognized syndrome associated with vitamin E deficiency in ruminants. In ruminants, NMD is characterized by degeneration of both skeletal and cardiac muscle. The biochemical processes causing the myodegeneration are only partially understood. However, increased lipid peroxidation in muscle before and during development of the visible lesions has been reported.[3] Lipid peroxidation occurs through the activity of free radicals generated in a wide variety of metabolic reactions.

Young nursing and rapidly growing ruminants (calves, lambs, kids) are most frequently affected with NMD, but NMD can develop *in utero*.[138] However, older animals have also been reported to be affected.[3,99,148,168] Investigators have reported white muscle lesions in suckling and weanling lambs with adequate selenium status, but deficient in vitamin E. This suggests inadequate colostrum intake, low colostrum vitamin E concentrations or inadequate postnatal vitamin E supplementation.[121,196] These findings are consistent with reports of NMD in goat kids associated with low alpha-tocopherol tissue concentrations; supplementation with selenium alone may not be sufficient.[168] There is a tendency in NMD for lesions to be localized in those muscles which are most actively exercised, with evidence that free radical production is higher in such muscles.[6,20] Typically, the disease is characterized by generalized leg weakness, stiffness and myodegeneration. Affected animals have difficulty standing and exhibit crossover walking, and impaired suckling ability, which can be attributed to affected tongue muscles, heart failure and paralysis.[150,195] Secondary infections such as pneumonia are frequently observed.[102] Polypnea may develop in these animals, which is the only respiratory manifestation of this syndrome. It is accompanied by cardiac disorders which are characterized by a pendulum rhythm and a reduction in heart sounds upon auscultation, the characteristic signs of myocarditis.

Clinical Parameters. Adams reported that plasma tocopherol concentrations between 0.06 and 0.16 mg/dL (0.60 to 1.6 μg/ml) were associated with NMD in calves. Serum alpha-tocopherol concentrations of 1.0 to 1.5 μg/ml (0.10 to 0.15 mg/dL) have been associated with clinical lesions of white muscle disease, with values <2 μg/ml (0.2 mg/dl) considered severely deficient.[1,142] Serum alpha-tocopherol concentrations >4.0 μg/ml (0.4 mg/dL) have been considered to indicate adequacy in adult cattle.[14] Similarly, marginal vitamin E status in adult cattle was associated with plasma tocopherol concentrations between 0.20 and 0.30 mg/dl (2.0 to 3.0 μg/ml). In a survey of 14 feedlots in nine states, plasma alpha-tocopherol levels and dietary vitamin E were measured in 286 cattle. The average plasma alpha-tocopherol value was 0.26 mg/100 ml, but the range was from 0.1 to 2.2 mg/100 ml. Sixty percent of the cattle sampled had plasma alpha-tocopherol values that were below 0.3 mg/100 ml. Vitamin E supplied in the feed varied in these feedlots, but generally, the vitamin E intake was considered inadequate to maintain plasma values above the suggested normal range of 0.40 mg/100 ml.[1] Incidences of nutritional myodegeneration in lambs and yearling ewes receiving selenium supplementation, and considered selenium adequate, have been reported.[121] The mean plasma alpha-tocopherol concentration in these animals was 0.65 μg/ml (.065 mg/dl).

The use of blood serum (or plasma) alpha-tocopherol concentration as an indicator of an animal's vitamin E status should be critically interpreted in each individual case. The use of this parameter as an indicator of status is related to the ease in obtaining the sample tissue, as well as the fact that vitamin E is not stored in appreciable concentrations in the body.[67] However, blood serum (or plasma) alpha-tocopherol concentration is most likely reflective of recent dietary intake of vitamin E. Rousseau et al. and Frye[66] indicated that plasma vitamin E concentration may not reflect vitamin E status, while others indicate that it may have limited value for diagnosing vitamin E deficiency.[38,157]

Dietary Sources and Fortification

Feedstuffs are the principal sources of vitamin E for ruminants, principally as alpha-tocopherol. Differences in the overall content and biologic activity between alpha and other naturally occurring tocopherols,[42] as well as instability of these compounds in the presence of moisture, heat, oxygen, acids, unsaturated fats and minerals, contribute to the wide variation in their vitamin E activity.[12] Other factors which affect vitamin E activity in feedstuffs include losses due to processing, storage,[185] poor inherent feedstuff quality, and varietal differences in vitamin E activity.[40]

Although feedstuffs contain a wide variety of tocopherols and tocotrienols, only alpha-tocopherol appears in appreciable levels in blood and tissues of animals. Naturally occurring vitamin E activity of feedstuffs cannot be accurately estimated from earlier published vitamin E or tocopherol values. Table 10 presents the alpha-tocopherol content of various feedstuffs. Cort, utilizing HPLC procedures, which allows separation of alpha and nonalpha forms of both tocopherol and tocotrienols, determined that corn, corn gluten meal, oats, barley and wheat contained significant amounts of alpha-tocotrienol which has minimal biological activity.[42]

HPLC methodology enables nutritionists to more accurately determine the vitamin E activity contributed by feedstuffs. Adams surveyed feedlots and determined the alpha-tocopherol content of feedstuffs and complete rations. It was observed that the alpha-tocopherol content of shelled, rolled, and high moisture corn ranged from 36 to 63% lower than published values.[1,153] These results are in agreement with those of Cort.[42]

Recently, it was reported that variability in forage vitamin E content is so great, both between and within farms, that one must have current results of representative samples to ensure proper vitamin E fortification programs.[86] These authors indicated that previously published values on vitamin E content of forages are unacceptable for use in feed formulations.[86]

Commercially available sources of vitamin E activity are shown in Table 12. Differences in biopotency of the stereoisomers of alphatocopherol can be seen from the definition of International Unit (IU). According to The United States Pharmacopeia, dl-alpha-tocopheryl acetate is the International Standard of vitamin E activity, with one IU equivalent to one milligram of dl-alpha-tocopheryl acetate (see Table

Table 12. *Commercially Available Sources of Vitamin E Activity*

SOURCE	I.U. OF VITAMIN E ACTIVITY PER MG
dl-Alpha Tocopheryl Acetate	1.0
dl-Alpha Tocopherol	1.10
d-Alpha Tocopheryl Acetate	1.36
d-Alpha Tocopherol	1.49

(*Adapted from* The United States Pharmacopoeia, 20th ed, Easton, Mack Publishing Company, 1980; with permission.)

12).[204] This is the most widely available source of vitamin E for animal feed supplementation. The acetate ester of d- or dl-alpha-tocopherol is synthesized to stabilize the compound from oxidation and maintain vitamin E activity.

Compared with vitamin A and vitamin D, both acute and chronic studies with animals have shown that vitamin E is relatively non-toxic, but not entirely devoid of undesirable effects. Hypervitaminosis E studies in rats, chicks, and humans indicate maximum tolerable levels in the range of 1000 to 2000 IU per kg of diet.[154] Vitamin E toxicity has not been demonstrated in cattle.

Dietary vitamin E requirements of young beef and dairy cattle have not been clearly defined, as evidenced by a requirement range of 15 to 60 IU per kg diet dry matter,[153] and no requirement has been defined for adult cattle.

Results of early studies on the effects of low level vitamin E supplementation on performance of cattle were inconsistent.[197] Recently, trials involving high level vitamin E supplementation in cattle have been evaluated. Results of these studies would suggest that criteria for determining minimum dietary requirements should not be based entirely on growth rates or amounts necessary to prevent overt deficiencies, but should also consider optimal health and immunocompetency.

Supplementing vitamin E in well balanced diets has been shown to increase humoral immunity against a wide variety of particulate and soluble antigens in chickens, mice, turkeys, guinea pigs and rabbits.[202] The effects of vitamin E supplementation on protection against infection by several types of pathogenic organisms, as well as antibody titers and phagocytosis of the pathogens in various species, has been reviewed.[37,84,156,161,202,203]

When animals are in a stressed or disease state, there is an increased production of glucocorticoids, epinephrine, and eicosanoids, as well as elevated phagocytic activity.[157] Synthesis of these compounds leads to production of free radicals, which challenge the animal's antioxidant system, including vitamin E. The protective effects of vitamin E on animal health may be involved with its role in reduction of glucocorticoids,[17] which are known to be immunosuppressive.[74] Vitamin E most likely has an immunoenhancing effect by altering arachidonic acid metabolism and subsequent synthesis of prostaglandins, thromboxanes and leukotrienes. Under stress conditions, increased levels of some of these compounds may adversely affect immune function.[81] The effects of oral vitamin E supplementation in young calves was evaluated.[38] Calves were fed skimmed colostrum and supplemented with either 0 or 1000 mg dl-alpha-tocopheryl acetate for 6 weeks in a vitamin E deficient ration. Conventionally managed calves were included as positive controls. Vitamin E supplemented calves had greater plasma alpha-tocopherol concentrations at 6 weeks, as well as mean lymphocyte blastogenesis response to phytohemagglutinin (PHA) that was expressed as mean lymphocyte stimulation indices (LSI). These authors suggested that the enhancing effect of vitamin E on the immune response of cattle could have been partially masked in this study by feeding diets high in emulsified fats.

Reddy et al. supplemented calves with 0, 1400, or 2800 mg of vitamin E (as dl-alpha-tocopheryl acetate) orally at weekly intervals, or as weekly injections of 1400 mg (as dl-alpha-tocopheryl acetate) over a 12 week period.[170] Mean LSI were significantly higher in calves given injections at weeks four and eight; overall means across all weeks were greater for calves given 2800 mg orally or 1400 mg vitamin E by injection.[170] Subsequently, calves were supplemented with 0, 125, 250 or 500 IU vitamin E per calf per day (as dl-alpha-tocopherol) over a 24 week period. Overall mean LSI for concalvalin A (a T-cell mitogen) were 29.2, 37.2, 34.5 and 36.3, respectively.[171] With lipopolysaccharide (a B-cell mitogen) LSI values were 3.7, 5.8, 5.0 and 5.9, respectively. In both cases, values were greater for calves supplemented with 125 or 500 IU vitamin E than control calves, suggesting that vitamin E plays an important role in both cell-mediated and humoral immunity in calves. Additionally, vitamin E administration to calves enhanced immune response and weight gain, while the presence of enzymes of muscle origin (e.g., creatine kinase and serum gluten oxaloacetic transaminase) and plasma cortisol concentration were decreased.[171,172] Vitamin E also positively influenced neutrophil-mediated antibody dependent cellular cytotoxicity, phagocytosis and lymphocyte stimulation in calves fed milk replacer supplemented with 57 IU vitamin E per kg for an eight week period, versus controls.[165] In a series of 28 day feedlot receiving trials, improvement in early performance of newly arrived growing cattle (250 kg) was noted in calves supplemented with 450 IU vitamin E (as dl-alpha-tocopheryl acetate) per head per day. These calves were stressed by long distance shipment and changes in diet from green forages to high grain feedlot rations.[114] Depression of circulating cortisol concentrations may explain the improved gain and feed efficiency in this trial. Carrica et al. reported no improvement in performance, when compared to controls, in heavy weight steers (366 kg) entering the feedlot and supplemented with 200 IU vitamin E (as dl-alpha-tocopheryl acetate) per head per day.[32] These authors concluded that vitamin E supplementation was more critical in lightweight calves, or cattle that have undergone stress due to shipment and handling. Hutchinson and Cole reported increased average daily gains in yearling cattle supplemented with either 100 or 300 IU vitamin E (as dl-alpha-tocopheryl acetate) per head per day and 0.10 mg/kg selenium.[98] Plasma alpha-tocopherol levels were not influenced by vitamin E supplementation up to 300 IU vitamin E.[98] Increased body weight, altered absorptive efficiency or ruminal destruction may partially explain this response, suggesting that supplementation should be increased with increased age, and recommendations should be based on a body weight basis.

Gill et al. supplemented newly received feedlot cattle with 1600 IU vitamin E (as dl-alpha-tocopheryl acetate) per head per day for the first 21 days and 800 IU vitamin E for the remaining 7 days of a 28 day trial.[72] Average daily gain and gain to feed ratios were improved by 23.2 and 28.6%, respectively for vitamin E supplemented stressed cattle. The number of sick pen days per head was reduced by 15.6%, and morbidity was reduced by 13.4% with vitamin E supplementation.[72] The growth response to vitamin E could be related to the fact that young, rapidly growing animals are in a metabolically demanding state resulting from overall tissue growth, which has a high energy demand. Vitamin E is an integral part of this response via its ability to quench free radicals, which are generated during the course of metabolism.

Three 28 day feedlot receiving trials were conducted to evaluate the effect of vitamin E supplementation on performance of steers and heifers. In trial one, 230 heifers were injected intramuscularly (i.m.) with either 0, 1250 or 2500 IU of vitamin E (as dl-alpha-tocopherol) at processing; 192 steers in trial two were injected I.M. with either 0, or 1250 IU vitamin E on day 0, and received 800 IU vitamin E (as dl-alpha-tocopheryl acetate) per head per day orally. An additional 360 steers in trial three received either 0 or 800 IU vitamin E per head per day orally.[132] Animals in trials one and two moved from wheat pasture to the feedlot, and those utilized in trial three were moved from native grass pastures. An initial single injection of vitamin E had no effect on 28 day performance in all three trials.[132] Plasma alpha-tocopherol concentration at 28 days was not influenced by injection, but was increased by oral vitamin E supplementation in both trials two and three.

Two trials were conducted with newly arrived feedlot cattle to evaluate the effects of oral vitamin E supplementation on growth and performance.[91] Steers were subjected to mild stress associated with abruptly moving animals from pasture to a slatted floor feedlot. In trial one, either 0 or 200 IU vitamin E (as dl-alpha-tocopheryl acetate) per head per day was fed for 130 days. Steers in trial two received either 0, 500 or 1000 IU per head per day for 84 days. Vitamin E supplementation had no effect on average daily gain or feed conversion in trial one. However, both average daily gain and feed conversion were improved in trial two during the first 28 days, regardless of vitamin E supplementation level, as compared to controls.[91] Both vitamin E treatments in trial two tended to improve average daily gain throughout the trial. Vitamin E supplementation in trial one resulted in higher plasma alpha-tocopherol concentration at 56 and 112 days than controls. However, vitamin E concentration decreased over time across all treatments.[91] The decrease in plasma alpha-tocopherol concentration may be related to change in diet (i.e., fresh forage based to high grain) and depletion of body stores of vitamin E as the trial progressed.[216] This is similar to the results obtained by May et al.[132]

Droke and Lerch conducted five trials with newly arrived feedlot steers to determine the effects of one or two I.M. injections of selenium and (or) vitamin E (as dl-alpha-tocopheryl acetate) on performance, health status and serum antibody response to *Pasteurella hemolytica* vaccination.[54] Steers were treated with selenium and vitamin E 14 days prior to shipment and again on arrival, 25 mg selenium, 340 IU vitamin E, or 25 mg plus 340 IU. No improvement in health or performance was noted in treated steers compared to controls.[54] However, serum IgG antibody titers to *P. hemolytica* vaccination was enhanced with the combination of selenium and vitamin E.[54]

Lightweight Holstein steers (111 kg initially) were fed a basal diet containing 90% high-moisture corn plus supplement and 10% corn silage for approximately 10 months. Calves were supplemented with either 0 or 370 IU vitamin E (as dl-alpha-tocopheryl acetate) per head per day to determine the effects of dietary vitamin E supplementation on health, growth, rumen papillae and liver and carcass characteristics.[182,183] Supplemental vitamin E had no effect on dry matter intake, growth rate, feed efficiency or carcass traits. Vitamin E reduced the ulceration score of the ventral rumen wall, but had no effect on other ruminal locations studied.[182,183] Dramatic effects of vitamin E supplementation on the stability of beef color were observed, although color score and pigmentation intensity were unaffected. Loin steaks of control steers discolored two to three days sooner than those supplemented with vitamin E. Supplemental dietary vitamin E extended the color shelflife of loin steaks from 3.7 to 6.3 days. This was most likely due to the increased alpha-tocopherol content of the loin tissue of the supplemented animals, which was approximately 4-fold greater than controls.[63] Color is an extremely critical component of fresh red meat appearance and greatly influences customers' perceptions of meat quality. In a subsequent report, Faustman et al. observed that vitamin E stabilized the pigments and lipids of meat from the supplemented steers.[64] Marusich et al. showed that both tocopherol and its acetate ester were equivalent as dietary sources of tissue antioxidants.[129] Perhaps the vitamin E supplemented steers were able to incorporate a greater amount of vitamin E into cellular membranes where it can perform its antioxidant function.[63,183] The effects of vitamin E as an *in vivo* lipid stabilizer and its effect on flavor and storage properties of various meats and milk have been reviewed.[128]

The influence of vitamin E and selenium on mastitis was first reported by Smith. Diets of multiparous dairy cows were supplemented with either 0 or 100 IU vitamin E (as dl-alpha-tocopheryl acetate) during the dry period.[192] Cows were additionally administered selenium at the rate of 0 or 0.1 mg/kg body weight by i.m. injection, 21 days prepartum.[192] No vitamin E or selenium was supplemented during lactation. Incidence of new clinical cases of mastitis was reduced by 37% in both groups receiving vitamin E, compared to control. The reduction in clinical mastitis was only 12% when cows were injected with selenium but not supplemented with dietary vitamin E. These authors also reported that clinical cases in the vitamin E supplemented-selenium injected cows were consistently of shorter duration than those occurring in all other groups.

In a follow-up study, 55 first lactation Holstein and Jersey heifers were assigned to either vitamin E and selenium supplementation or to an unsupplemented control group 60 days prior to parturition. Supplemented heifers received 2 IU vitamin E (as dl-alpha-tocopheryl acetate) and 2 µg selenium per kg body weight per day prepartum.[191] These heifers were also injected subcutaneously with 0.1 mg selenium per kg body weight 21 days prepartum.[191] During lactation the supplemented group received 88 IU vitamin E and 0.3 mg selenium per kg of concentrate.[191] Regardless of treatment group, plasma alpha-tocopherol concentration decreased from day 60 prepartum to calving, although the decrease was greater for unsupplemented heifers.[191] The high initial plasma alpha-tocopherol values are most likely associated with the fact that the majority of heifers were on pasture up to this time. Weiss et al. reported that plasma alpha-tocopherol concentrations are consistent from drying off until 7 days prepartum, and then drop by about 50% until 20 to 30 days postpartum. Plasma alpha-tocopherol concentrations return to baseline levels by 60 days postpartum.[219] They speculate that this profile may be related to differences in absorptive efficiency for vitamin E between dry and lactating cows, loss of vitamin E in milk and products of conception, or differences in feed intake between dry and lactating cows.[219]

Smith and Conrad reported that intrammary infection was reduced 42.2% in vitamin E-selenium supplemented cows versus unsupplemented controls.[191] The duration of all intrammary infections in lactation was reduced 40 to 50% in supplemented heifers.[191] Mean somatic cell count was lower in supplemented heifers throughout lactation. Supplemented and unsupplemented heifers, with a lactation mean somatic cell count greater than 200,000 cells per ml, were compared; supplemented heifers had a 68% lower mean somatic cell count.[191] Clinical mastitis during the first 4 days of lactation was reduced by 57% in supplemented heifers. Incidence of clinical cases of mastitis throughout lactation was reduced by 32% in supplemented heifers, compared to controls. The specific mode of action of vitamin E in enhancing mammary gland health remains to be elucidated. However, possible mechanisms may involve improvement in phagocytic cell function and improved mammary gland immunocompetence, as well as altered arachidonic acid metabolism.[191]

Studies have been conducted to evaluate the effects of vitamin E and selenium on the incidence of retained placenta in dairy cows. Cows injected with vitamin E and selenium at one month,[210] or 20 days prior to calving,[105] had lower incidence of retained placenta than cows not supplemented. Other workers supplemented a practical diet based on legume-grass haylage with 1000 IU vitamin E per animal per day, beginning 21 days prepartum. All cows were injected with 0.1 mg selenium/kg body weight 21 days prepartum.[85] Similarly, this work indicated that vitamin E and selenium alone had no effect on the incidence of retained placenta, but the combination of the two nutrients proved to be very effective.

The efficacy of vitamin E supplementation in ruminant animals is no longer questioned. The ability of this essential nutrient to affect animals' growth, health and reproductive capabilities are well documented. The requirements for supplementation of vitamin E to ruminants depend on many factors. These factors must be considered when a vitamin E supplementation program is implemented, as it is critical to assure proper vitamin E status in the animal. Based on currently available data, a vitamin E supplementation program utilizing either parenteral or oral vitamin E should be considered when fresh green pasture is lacking.

VITAMIN K

Properties and Metabolism

The general term vitamin K is now used to describe not a single chemical entity, but a group of quinone compounds that have characteristic antihemorrhagic effects. Vitamin K is a generic term for a homologous group of fat-soluble, antihemorrhagic compounds. The basic molecule is a naphthoquinone, and the various isomers differ in the nature and length of the side chain. Vitamin K, extracted from plant material, was named phylloquinone or vitamin K_1. Vitamin K-active compounds from material that had undergone bacterial fermentation were named menaquinones or vitamin K_2. The simplest form of vitamin K is the synthetic menadione (K_3), which has no side chain. Menaquinone is synthesized in the liver from ingested menadione or changed to a biologically active menaquinone by intestinal microorganisms. Microorganisms in the rumen synthesize vitamin K, and milk from cattle is reported to contain one-tenth the amount of vitamin K as in human milk.[124]

Vitamin K_1 is a golden, yellow, viscous oil. Natural sources of vitamin K are fat soluble, stable to heat, and labile to oxidation, alkali, strong acids, light and irradiation. Vitamin K_1 is slowly degraded by atmospheric oxygen, but fairly rapidly destroyed by light. In contrast to natural sources of vitamin K, vitamin K_3 salts of menadione are water-soluble.

A number of vitamin K antagonists exist that increase the need for this vitamin. A deficiency of vitamin K is brought about by ingestion of dicumarol, an antagonist of vitamin K, or by the feeding of sulfonamides (in monogastric species) at levels sufficient to inhibit intestinal synthesis of vitamin K. Dicumarol serves as an anticoagulant to inhibit thrombosis, by inhibiting the synthesis of coagulation factors, in people afflicted with cardiovascular disease. Thus, additional vitamin K will overcome this action by dicumarol. Mycotoxins are also antagonists that may cause a vitamin K deficiency.

Like all fat-soluble vitamins, vitamin K is absorbed in association with dietary fats and requires the presence of bile salts and pancreatic juice for adequate uptake from the alimentary tract. Absorption of vitamin K depends on its incorporation into mixed micelles, and optimal formation of these micellar structures requires the presence of both bile and pancreatic juice. Thus, any malfunction of the fat absorption mechanism, for example, biliary obstruction, will reduce availability of vitamin K. Unlike phylloquinone and the menaquinones, menadione salts are relatively water soluble and, therefore, are absorbed satisfactorily from low-fat diets. The lymphatic system is the major route of transport of absorbed phylloquinone from the intestine. Shearer et al. demonstrated the association of phylloquinone with serum lipoproteins, but little is known of the existence of specific carrier proteins.[187] Ingested phylloquinone is absorbed by an energy dependent process from the proximal portion of the small intestine.[97] In contrast to the active transport of phylloquinone, menaquinone is absorbed from the small intestine by a passive noncarrier-mediated process.

Efficiency of vitamin K absorption has been measured to be from 10 to 70%, depending on the form in which the vitamin is administered. Some reports have indicated menadione to be completely absorbed, but phylloquinone is absorbed only at a rate of 50%. Speculation is that the aqueous solubility of the menadione salts is responsible for the high absorption of menadione. Rats were found to excrete about 60% of ingested phylloquinone in the feces within 24 hours of ingestion, but only 11% of ingested menadione.[77,78] However, 38% of ingested menadione, but only a small amount of phylloquinone, were excreted via the kidneys in the same period of time. The conclusion was that although menadione is well absorbed, it is poorly retained, while just the opposite was true for phylloquinone.

Griminger and Brubacher showed that a major portion of phylloquinone fed to chicks was absorbed and deposited intact in the liver. Phylloquinone and menaquinone were equally effective in stimulating prothrombin synthesis. Menaquinone was found in the chick's liver following feeding of menadione.[79] Therefore, menaquinone is most likely produced if menadione is fed or if the intestinal microorganisms degrade dietary K_1 or K_2 to menadione. Formation of menaquinone is not obligatory for metabolic activity, since phylloquinone is equally active in bringing about synthesis of the vitamin K-dependent blood-clotting proteins.[186]

Coagulation of blood is prolonged when vitamin K is deficient because the vitamin is required for the synthesis of prothrombin (factor II) and factors VII (proconvertin), IX (Christmas factor), and X (Stuart-

Prower factor). These four blood-clotting proteins are synthesized in the liver in inactive precursor forms and then converted to biologically active proteins by the action of vitamin K.[199] Administration of vitamin K promptly restores synthesis and conversion of factors II, VII, IX, X in 4 to 6 hours. This occurs in the liver.

The action of converting inactive precursor proteins to biological activity involves the carboxylation of glutamic acid residues in the inactive molecules. The end product of vitamin K dependent carboxylation is the formation of gamma-carboxyglutamic acid residues. Vitamin K-dependent carboxylase enzyme systems may have other roles, in addition to blood clotting, such as in bone formation. Osteocalcin is a vitamin K-dependent protein found in bone, and it appears in embryonic chick bone and rat bone matrix at the beginning of mineralization of bone.[68] A vitamin K-dependent carboxylase system has been identified in skin, which may be related to calcium (Ca) metabolism in skin.[46] Although much is unknown about the function of vitamin K, apart from blood coagulation, it is apparent that a reasonably large number of proteins may be involved.

The blood clotting mechanism can be stimulated by either an intrinsic system, in which all the factors are in the plasma, or an extrinsic system. The common factor in both the intrinsic and extrinsic systems is Stuart factor, which in turn leads to activation of prothrombin. A variety of stimuli activates the intrinsic system, which contains factor IX. In the extrinsic system of coagulation, injury to the skin or other tissue frees tissue thromboplastin, which activates factor VII. Factor VII stimulates the activation of factor X, which, in the presence of phospholipid, factor V and Ca, stimulates the activation of prothrombin to thrombin. The enzyme thrombin facilitates the conversion of the soluble fibrinogen into insoluble fibrin. Fibrin polymerizes into strands and enmeshes the formed elements of the blood, especially the red blood cells, to form the blood clot.[78]

Assessment of Status

Deficiencies. In ruminants, vitamin K deficiency can result from lack of rumen synthesis and dietary deficiency, inadequate absorption or inability of the liver to use the available K activity.

Vitamin K responsive sweet clover hay poisoning (hemorrhagic sweet clover disease) has been produced experimentally in calves. Baled sweet clover containing a minimum dicumarol content of 90 ppm and an average of 132 ppm was fed to calves weighing 205 to 250 kg. Early signs of dicumarol were detectable within 21 days after calves were allowed access to the contaminated hay. Early signs of sweet clover poisoning included hematomas in tissues of the ventral cervical area, ventricle abdominal wall and muscles of the hindlimb, and hemorrhage in carpal or tarsal joints.[4]

Dicumarol leads to prolonged blood clotting times and can result in death from uncontrolled hemorrhage. Dicumarol passes through the placenta in pregnant animals and newborn animals may become affected immediately after birth. Clinical signs of hemorrhagic sweet clover disease are related to the hemorrhages caused by blood coagulation failure and varies with age of animal and the content of dicumarol content of spoiled sweet clover. If dicumarol content is low, animals may be consuming it long before signs of the disease appears. The coumarin derivatives in hay are antagonists of vitamin K. They are not active in the fresh plant because they are bound to glycosides, but are active when sweet clover is improperly cured.[215] Another common cause of vitamin K deficiency in veterinary practice is the accidental poisoning of animals with warfarin. Vitamin K functions in blood clotting via the carboxylation of vitamin K-dependent coagulation proteins. Vitamin K is suspected to be involved in other carboxylation reactions involved in bone development and in sperm cell production in testes. The significance of these proteins is not fully understood.[215]

Clinical Parameters. Measurement of clotting time has been used to evaluate the body status of vitamin K and is considered a fairly good measure of vitamin K deficiency. However a more accurate measure of deficiency is obtained by determining the "prothombin time." A determination of prothombin time measures activity of factors VII, X, V, II and fibrinogen. In experimentally induced dicumarol poisoning, "hemorrhagic sweet clover disease," Alstad et al. reported that normal prothrombin time is equal to or less than 20 seconds. Deficiency of vitamin K is characterized by prothrombin times greater than 40 to 60 seconds, with a packed cell volume (PCV) of 20% or less.[4] With severe deficiency, prothrombin time can be as long as 5 to 6 minutes.

In deficient calves normal prothrombin time is achieved within 6 to 8 days after injection (IM) with phylloquinone (vitamin K_1) at 0.22 to 1.1 mg per kg body weight. Vitamin K_1 dosages of 1.1, 2.2 and 3.3 mg per kg administered IM were effective in lowering prothrombin times to approximately normal values within 24 hours.[4] Goplen and Bece have shown that vitamin K_1 is much more potent than is vitamin K_3 in cattle.[76]

Dietary Sources and Fortification

There are two major natural sources of vitamin K, phylloquinones (vitamin K_1) in plant sources and menaquinones (vitamin K_2) produced by bacterial flora.

Vitamin K is present in fresh dark-green vegetables. Alfalfa leaf meal contains a small amount of vitamin K, while liver and fish meal are good animal sources of the vitamin. All by-product feedstuffs of animal origin, including fish meal and fish liver oils, are much higher in vitamin K after they have undergone extensive bacterial putrefaction.

The menaquinones (vitamin K_2) are produced by the bacterial flora in animals and are especially important in providing the vitamin K requirements of mammals. In nonruminants, site of synthesis is in the lower gut, an area of poor absorption, and availability. Animals which practice coprophagy ingest a highly available source of vitamin K.

Early data indicated that rumen contents were a good source of

vitamin K when animals were fed diets practically devoid of this vitamin. Recent data suggest that adequate amounts of this vitamin are
synthesized in the rumen and/or lower gut, except in situations in
which excessive dicumarol is found in the diet. Vitamin K production in
the rumen and subsequent passage along sites of active absorption
in the small intestine make such synthesized vitamins highly available
to the host animal.

Vitamin K_1 is not utilized by the feed industry, due to cost and lack
of a stabilized form. Instead, water-soluble menadione (vitamin K_3)
salts are used to provide vitamin K activity in feeds. Because of poor
stability, menadione is not used as the pure vitamin, but is produced as
water soluble salts. Water-soluble derivatives of menadione, including
menadione sodium bisulfite (MSB), menadione sodium bisulfite complex (MSBG), and menadione dimethyl-pyrimidinol bisulfite (MPB), are
the principal forms of vitamin K included in commercial diets.

The vitamin K requirement of mammals is met by a combination of
dietary intake and microbial biosynthesis in the rumen and gut, which
may involve intestinal microorganisms such as *Escherichia coli*. Because
of rumen and gut microbial synthesis, a precise expression of vitamin K
requirements is not feasible. Rapid rate of food passage through the
digestive tract may also influence vitamin K synthesis in cattle. The
daily requirement for most species falls in a range of 2 to 200 μg
vitamin K per kg (0.91 to 91 μg per lb) body weight. Schendel and
Johnson established a daily dietary vitamin K requirement of 5 μg of
menadione sodium phosphate per kg (2.3 μg per lb) body weight in
young pigs fed a purified diet containing a high level of sulfathiazole to
preclude gut synthesis of vitamin K_2.[184] It should be remembered that
requirements can be altered by age, sex, strain, anti-vitamin K factors,
disease conditions and any condition influencing lipid absorption or
altering the intestinal flora. Dicumarol leads to prolonged blood clotting times and can be responsible for animal deaths from uncontrolled
hemorrhage. Most cases of deficiency are expected to be treatable with
appropriate injectable and dietary sources of vitamin K.

Toxic effects of the vitamin K family are manifested mainly as
hematological and circulatory derangements. Not only are species variation encountered, but profound differences are observed in the ability
of the various vitamin K compounds to evoke a toxic response.[8] The
natural forms of vitamin K, phylloquinone and menaquinone, are non-
toxic at very high dosage levels. The synthetic menadione compounds,
however, have shown to be toxic when fed to humans, rabbits, dogs and
mice in excessive amounts. The toxic dietary level of menadione is at
least 100 times the dietary requirement.[154] Menadione compounds can
safely be used at low levels to prevent the development of a deficiency,
but should not be used as a pharmacological treatment. Menadione or
its derivatives, when administered parenterally, have an LD_{50} in the
range of a few hundred mg per kg of BW in some species and dosages of
2 to 8 mg per kg BW have been reported to be lethal in horses. This
data is not available for cattle.[154]

THIAMIN

Properties and Metabolism

Thiamin consists of a molecule of pyrimidine and a molecule of thiazole linked by a methylene bridge; it contains both nitrogen and sulfur atoms. Thiamin is isolated in pure form as the white thiamin hydrochloride. The vitamin has a characteristic sulfurous odor and a slightly bitter taste. Thiamin is very soluble in water, sparingly so in alcohol, and insoluble in fat solvents. It is very sensitive to alkali, in which the thiazole ring opens at room temperature when pH is above 7. In a dry state, thiamin is stable at 100 C for several hours, but moisture greatly accelerates destruction, making it is much less stable to heat in fresh than in dry foods. Under ordinary conditions, thiamin hydrochloride is more hygroscopic than the mononitrate form. However, both products should be kept in sealed containers.

Substances with an antithiamin activity are fairly common in nature and include structurally similar antagonists, as well as structure altering antagonists. The synthetic compounds pyrithiamin, oxythiamin and amprolium (an anticoccidial) are structurally similar antagonists; their mode of action is competitive inhibition with the biologically active compound, interfering with thiamin at different points in metabolism. Pyrithiamin chiefly blocks the esterification of thiamin with phosphoric acid, resulting in inhibition of the thiamin coenzyme cocarboxylase. Likewise, oxythiamin displaces cocarboxylase from important metabolic reactions. Amprolium inhibits the absorption of thiamin from the intestine and also blocks the phosphorylation of the vitamin.[139]

Thiaminase activity destroys thiamin activity by altering the structure of the vitamin, and certain microorganisms and plants have been shown to produce thiaminases. The disease of "Chastek paralysis," in foxes and other animals fed certain types of raw fish, results from a thiaminase that splits the thiamin molecule into two components, rendering it inactive. Since thiaminase is heat labile, the problem can be avoided by cooking the fish at 83 C for at least 5 minutes.

Thiamin appears to be readily digested and released from natural sources. A precondition for normal absorption of thiamin is sufficient production of gastric hydrochloric acid. Phosphoric acid esters of thiamin are split in the intestine. Free thiamin is water soluble and easily absorbed, especially in the duodenum. The mechanism of thiamin absorption is not yet fully understood, but apparently both active transport and simple diffusion are involved.[22] At low concentrations there is an active sodium-dependent transport against the electrochemical potential, whereas at high concentrations it diffuses passively through the intestinal wall. Absorbed thiamin is transported via the portal vein to the liver via a carrier plasma protein.

Thiamin phosphorylation can take place in most tissues, particularly in the liver. Four-fifths of thiamin in animals is ATP phosphorylated in the liver to the metabolically active enzyme form, thiamin pyrophosphate (TPP or cocarboxylase). Of total body thiamin, about 80% is TTP, about 10% is thiamin triphosphate (TTP) and the remainder is thiamin monophosphate (TMP) and free thiamin.

Although thiamin is readily absorbed and transported to cells throughout the body, it is not stored to any great extent. Thiamin content in individual organs varies considerably, with the vitamin preferentially retained in organs with a high metabolic activity. During deficiencies, thiamin is retained in greatest quantities in important organs such as heart, brain, liver and kidney. Intakes in excess of current needs are rapidly excreted. The principal storage organ is the liver[44]. However, approximately one-half of total thiamin is present in muscle.[200]

Absorbed thiamin is excreted in both urine and feces, with small quantities excreted in sweat. Fecal thiamin may originate from feed, synthesis by microorganisms or endogenous origin (e.g., via bile or excretion through the mucosa of the large intestine). When thiamin is administered in large doses, urinary excretion first increases then reaches a saturation level, and with additional thiamin the fecal concentration increases considerably.[22]

Function

A principal function of thiamin in all cells is as the coenzyme cocarboxylase or TPP. The vitamins riboflavin and niacin, as well as thiamin, play roles in the Tricarboxylic Acid (TCA) cycle. Thiamin is the coenzyme for all enzymatic carboxylations of α-keto acids. Thus, it functions in the oxidative decarboxylation of pyruvate to acetate, which is combined with coenzyme A for (CoA) entrance into the TCA cycle.

Thiamin is essential in two oxidative decarboxylation reactions which occur in the mitochondria and one reaction in the cytoplasm. These are essential reactions for utilization of carbohydrates to provide energy. Decarboxylation in the mitochondrial TCA cycle removes carbon dioxide and the substrate is converted into the compound having the next lower number of carbon atoms:

$$\text{Pyruvate} \rightarrow \text{acetyl-CoA} + CO_2$$
$$\alpha\text{-Ketoglutaric acid} \rightarrow \text{succinyl-CoA} + CO_2$$

Thiamin pyrophosphate is a cytoplasmic coenzyme in the transketolase reaction that is part of the pentose phosphate cycle. This oxidative pathway for glucose occurs primarily in liver, brain, adrenal cortex and kidney, but not skeletal muscle. Transketolase catalyzes transfer of two carbon (C_2) fragments, hence with ribulose 5-phosphate as donor and ribose 5-phosphate as acceptor, sedoheptulose 7-phosphate and triose phosphate are formed. This is the only mechanism known for synthesis of ribose, which is needed for nucleotide formation and also results in formation of nicotinamide adenine dinucleotide phosphate (NADPH). NADPH is essential for reducing intermediates from carbohydrate metabolism to form fatty acids.

Little is known of thiamin function in nervous tissue. However, there is evidence for a specific role of thiamin in neurophysiology, independent of its coenzyme function. Possible mechanisms of action of thiamin in nervous tissue include the following: (a) synthesis of acetylcholine, (b) passive transport of Na in excitable membranes (important for transmission of impulses at the membrane of ganglionic cells) and (c) reduction in transketolase activity in the pentose phosphate pathway. Reduction of transketolase activity follows a thiamin deficiency, which reduces the synthesis of fatty acids and the metabolism of energy in the nervous system.[41,149]

Assessment of Status

Deficiencies. Ruminant nutritionists have generally assumed that rumen microorganisms produce adequate quantities of B-complex vitamins to meet requirements. Despite the fact that rumen microbes synthesize thiamin, deficiencies do develop in ruminants. Polioencephalomalacia (PEM), or cerebrocortical necrosis (CCN), is a thiamin responsive disease, that has been reported worldwide and occurs sporadically in cattle, sheep and goats. The term PEM refers to a laminar softening or degeneration of the cerebrocortical gray matter. However, it is commonly used to describe a central nervous system (CNS) condition in ruminants. Calves and young cattle (4 months to 2 years of age), as well as young sheep and goats (2 months to 7 months of age) are generally the animals most severely affected.

Clinical signs associated with thiamin deficiency include scouring (which is often perfuse but transient),[58,61] depressed growth rate, weight loss and anorexia.[151] Clinical signs of CNS disorders associated with PEM are more readily recognized. However, these signs are exhibited at later stages of thiamin deficiency.[167] Thornber et al. reported that animals on thiamin deficient diets may not show clinical signs of a CNS disorder for three to five weeks or longer, although depressed blood thiamin levels and other clinical signs may be observed.[208]

Thiamin levels in most body tissues, including blood, may fluctuate widely as diet varies. Brain thiamin levels are relatively stable and fall significantly only in severe depletion. Blood transketolase levels fall much faster than brain levels of the enzyme.[53,136] Irreversible pathological changes are thought to occur only when brain transketolase activity and thiamin levels fall below 50 and 20% of normal, respectively.[53]

Rapid onset, hyperexcitability, incoordination, listlessness, circling, rigid stance, opisthotonos, recumbency, nystagmus, apparent blindness, convulsions and coma are typical signs of PEM.[58] The most severe cases result in death. Seasonal trends have been associated with PEM, which may be due to increased metabolic demands of gestation, lactation and growth. Additionally, feeding of high concentrate diets may induce PEM.

Several researchers report that most field cases of PEM result from a progressive thiamin deficiency, likely a result of gut and ruminal bacterial thiaminases.[23,57,58,61] The precise role of the thiaminases in this regard has been difficult to establish because ruminal thiaminase is often present without overt clinical signs.

Edwin et al. first proposed the involvement of a thiaminase enzyme with PEM.[57] Two types of thiaminase were described. Thiaminase II simply cleaves the vitamin at the methylene bridge between the thiazole and the pyrimidine rings, yielding free thiazole and free pyrimidine. Thiaminase I substitutes a new base for the thiazole ring. This leads to less thiamin, but it also gives rise to thiamin analogs composed of the pyrimidine ring of the original thiamin, and another ring from the 'cosubstrate.' This thiamin analog may then be absorbed and possibly inhibit thiamin-requiring reactions.

A working hypothesis for PEM proposed by Bartley and Brent is: Thiaminase I, in the presence of a cosubstrate, produces a thiamin analog, which in turn, blocks thiamin reactions. Because the brain depends on glucose utilization via glycolysis, and because thiamin pyrophosphate is a cofactor in decarboxylation, it is possible that the CNS would be first to show symptoms.[9,23] Lusby was able to induce PEM in 3 to 4 days, using a continuously infused, liquid high-carbohydrate diet. This work supports the thiaminase I hypothesis, as it would seem unlikely that animals develop primary thiamin deficiency in such a short period of time.[119] There is a complex balance between thiamin production and thiamin destruction in the rumen, which depends upon the rumen microflora. Presumably, PEM occurs when the rate of thiamin destruction exceeds the rate of synthesis or dietary contributions, thus depleting body reserves.[23,167] Thomas has suggested that normal body reserves are sufficient for approximately three weeks prior to the onset of PEM.

Bacterial thiaminase is often described as an exoenzyme. That is, it is bound to the surface of the cell. Sapienza found that if rumen fluid is taken from normal animals, adjusted to pH 6.8, and assayed for thiaminase, little, if any activity is found.[180] More thiamin may be recovered than is added due to thiamin synthesis. However, if samples were "acid shocked" to approximately pH 4.5, then adjusted to pH 6.8 before assay, thiaminase activity was present.[180] Apparently, the thiaminase had been separated from the bacterial cell. In rumen fluid from PEM cases, the enzyme is found in the supernatant, and no additional enzyme is released by acid shocking. In field cases of PEM, rumen acidosis has already accomplished the acid-shock procedure.

Both *Clostridium sporogenes* and *Bacillus thiaminolyticus* have been isolated from the rumen of PEM cases. Both organisms produce thiaminase I. However, that does not mean that these organisms are the source of thiaminase I, especially since no one has been able to establish populations of those organisms in the rumen of cattle. Also, several workers have reported that the characteristics of thiaminase from those organisms are not like those found in spontaneous PEM. Spontaneously occurring thiaminase has two pH optima and that from *Cl. sporogenes* and *B. thiaminolyticus* has only one.

Thiaminase I can also come from a number of plant species. This has been a special problem in Australia, where PEM occurs under pasture conditions, apparently being derived from some of the fern species. In the U.S., PEM generally occurs in feedlot cattle, frequently about 3 weeks after a ration change. If PEM is seen in pasture cattle, thiaminase I from a plant source should receive serious consideration.

The sulfite ion will also cleave thiamin at the methylene bridge and analytically, will mimic thiaminase. Several cases of PEM have occurred when gypsum has been used as a feed intake limiter. It would appear that the sulfate ion of gypsum, during its conversion to sulfide, must pass through sulfite, which may destroy thiamin.[9] There may be a whole series of specific thiaminase I enzymes. The preferred cosubstrate for thiaminase I from spontaneous cases of PEM is aniline.

Amprolium's mode of action as a coccidiostat is apparently through inhibition of thiamin phosphorylation. Lowe and Dunlap found that high levels of amprolium (considerably above the levels needed to prevent coccidiosis) could produce the physical signs and the histological lesions of PEM. It is doubtful that thiaminase I produces amprolium, but amprolium's ability to induce PEM adds credence to the idea that a thiamin antagonist is involved in the disease.[117]

Clinical Parameters. Diagnosis of thiamin deficiency initially depended upon recognition of the clinical signs in live animals, followed by confirmatory brain histopathology or clinical response to thiamin administration.[167] These techniques remain essential for diagnosis. However, they are of limited value in subclinical thiamin deficiencies or in the study and preventive control of thiamin deficiencies.

The best transketolase (TK) assay for assessing thiamin deficiency is based on the so-called TPP effect, which is the percentage increase in TK activity following addition of excess TPP to the sample. This assay has the advantage of having an internal control (sample without added TPP) which tends to eliminate intra- and inter-species variations in normal TK levels. Increases in TPP effect have been detected before clinical signs of thiamin have appeared.[122,209] A TPP effect of over 25% can indicate significant thiamin deficiency in humans,[25] but 95% confidence limits of 2 to 114% have been reported for apparently normal cattle and sheep.[59] Values of 120 to 250% have been reported for animals diagnosed as having PEM.[59] Higher values, sometimes found in apparently normal animals, may reflect differential balance between microbial thiamin synthesis and destruction, and the animal's thiamin requirement. Therefore, animals may often be subclinically deficient. Overt thiamin deficiency occurrs only when thiamin is severely depleted (TPP effects are very high) and PEM manifests itself suddenly.

Blood thiamin may now be analyzed routinely using HPLC. This methodology can measure both individual thiamin phosphate esters,[87,107] as well as total thiamin, after enzymatic hydrolysis of the esters.[108,221] Only the di- and tri-phosphate esters appear to be biologically active.[87] Thornber et al. reported that the di-phosphate ester may be the best indicator of deficiency. However, insufficient data are currently available to justify the routine analysis of diagnostic samples for the individual esters.[207] The usefulness of thiamin determinations to diagnose deficiency, has been questioned, partly because thiamin analogues can induce deficiency, even when thiamin levels are normal.[117,181] However, this consideration applies only when thiamin levels appear normal, it does not influence the interpretation when levels are low.

There are few reference values for the total thiamin content of blood from clinically normal animals. Non-specific analytical techniques have led to wide variation in thiamin values and these may not be reliable. Based on routine diagnostic submissions, some have arbitrarily set a normal reference range of 50 to 150 nmol/l for pasture cattle.[167] However, these researchers indicate that only low thiamin levels (<50 nmol/l) are significant and report levels as low as 6–12 nmol/l in suspected cases of PEM.[167]

Thomas reported various clinical parameters from comatose sheep with histologically confirmed PEM (Table 13). Additionally, other sheep displaying similar clinical signs were sampled and treated for PEM.[206] The results of tests for thiamin activities and biochemical tests for thiamin deficiency are shown in Table 13.

Biochemical changes indicating that PEM is associated with thiamin deficiency include reduced tissue thiamin contents, dramatic ele-

Table 13. *Thiaminase and Thiamin Status of Comatose Sheep With Histologically Confirmed PEM[a]*

TEST PERFORMED		ANIMAL NUMBER 1	ANIMAL NUMBER 2	REFERENCE RANGE
Examination of brain:				
Presence of CCN		Seen	Seen	Normally not seen
Presence of cortical fluorescence under UV light		Seen	Seen	Normally not seen
Thiaminase activity:				
Ruminal	—actual (mU/ml)	0.05	0.04	0–0.01
	—potential (mU/ml)	7.12	2.93	0–0.50
Abomasal	—actual (mU/g)	1.14	1.3	0
	—potential (mU/g)	42.63	17.2	0
Cecal	—actual (mU/g)	0.19	0.3	0–0.01
	—potential (mU/g)	15.10	22.1	0–0.50
Fecal	—actual (mU/g)	0.00	0.7	0–0.10
	—potental (mU/g)	0.00	26.4	0–1.00
Thiamin	—brain (μg/g WM)	0.4	0.2	0.8–2.3
	—liver (μg/g WM)	0.3	0.2	1.5–7.0
Erythrocyte TK (IU)		2	9	24–32
	TK+ (IU)	4	13	25–37
	TPP effect (%)	100	54	2–16
Plasma glucose (mmol/l)		15	ND	2–6

(*Adapted from* Thomas KW: Oral treatment of polioencephomalacia and subclinical thiamine deficiency with thiamine propyl disulphide and thiamine hydrochloride. J Vet Pharmacol Therap 9:402, 1986; with permission.)

vation of blood pyruvate and lactate, and markedly reduced transketolase activity.[22] Moreover, sick animals react so promptly to treatment with thiamin (sometimes within hours) that early treatment is often used to confirm the diagnosis of PEM.

Zintzen suggested that PEM can be positively diagnosed if the following conditions exist:[223]

1. Case history-animals have been maintained on high-energy feeds rich in carbohydrates, and other animals on the same farm have died after exhibiting central nervous system disorders.

2. Biochemical evidence-blood pyruvate has steeply increased and the activity of erythrocyte-transketolase has been reduced.

3. Diagnostic therapy-animals thought to be suffering from PEM respond promptly to treatment with thiamin, provided they are treated in the early stages of the disease.

4. Pathological changes-necropsy shows typical bilateral cerebral cortical necrosis.

Thiamin concentrations in blood and urine are decreased with a deficiency. Urinary excretion of thiamin reflects thiamin saturation or depletion because the vitamin is excreted promptly when ingested in excess of needs. Both blood levels and urinary excretion of thiamin reflect the immediately preceding dietary intake. Other factors can influence blood and urinary thiamin which may not reflect tissue stores, distribution, or actual biochemical function. Thus, blood thiamin and urinary thiamin excretion are of limited value for interpretation of actual thiamin status.

Thiamin is needed for pyruvate metabolism and, with a deficiency, abnormally high concentrations of pyruvic and lactic acid accumulate in the blood (Table 14). For a calf on a deficient diet, urinary excretion of thiamin drops to very low levels in 20 to 25 days, and increased pyruvate excretion follows. Blood pyruvate and lactate levels increase suddenly to 400 and 500% above normal, as the deficiency develops.[152] However, the measurements of these levels often cannot be used to detect mild deficiencies of thiamin. Also these tests are not entirely specific, because toxicity by minerals such as arsenic (As) and antimony (Sb) will inhibit the utilization of pyruvate. Increased pyruvate can result from a number of other pathological conditions, such as those arising from increased adrenal gland activity.

Dietary Sources and Fortification

Cereal grains and their by-products, soybean meal, cottonseed meal and peanut meal are relatively rich sources of thiamin. Brewer's yeast is the richest known natural source of thiamin. Since the vitamin is present primarily in the germ and seed coats, by-products containing the latter are richer than the whole kernel, while highly milled flour is very deficient. Whole rice may contain 5 mg per kg thiamin, with much lower concentrations for polished rice (0.3 mg per kg) and higher concentrations rice bran (23 mg per kg).[124] Wheat germ ranks next to yeast in thiamin concentration. Reddy and Pushpamma studied the

Table 14. Biochemical Responses to Treatment of Sheep With Thiamin Deficiency by Drenching With Thiamin Propyl Disulphid[a]

PERIOD POST-TREATMENT	FECAL THIAMINASE		RUMINAL THIAMINASE		BLOOD GLUCOSE (MMOL/L)	BLOOD PYRUVATE (µMOL/L)	BLOOD LACTATE (MMOL/L)	ERYTHROCYTE		MEAN TPI INCREASE (%)
	ACT (MU/G DM)	POT	ACT (MU/ML)	POT				TK (IU)	TK+ (IU)	
0 h	0.1	8.3	0.014	1.9	8.3	170	4.2	4	7	95
2 h	0.1	8.5	0.005	0.4	9.2	86	2.4	9	13	49
1 d	0.2	18.0	0.007	0.6	6.0	74	3.6	17	22	30
3 d	6.10	72.7	0.001	0.9	4.6	42	3.7	22	27	23
1 week or longer	1.9	66.4	0.006	0.40	4.3	25	1.9	26	29	10
Normal reference values	<0.1	<1.0	<0.012	<0.5	2–6	30–140	0.9–2.4	24–32	25–37	2–16

[a]Values are means of five treated cases of early PEM except that values for 1 week or longer are for four animals only.
(Adapted from Thomas KW: Oral treatment of polioencephomalacia and subclinical thiamine deficiency with thiamine propyl disulphine and thiamin hydrochloride. J Vet Pharmacol Therap 9:402, 1986; with permission.)

effects of one year's storage and insect infestation on thiamin content of feeds.[170] Thiamin losses were high in different varieties of sorghum and pigeonpea (40 to 70%) and lower in rice and chickpea (10 to 40%), with insect infestation causing further loss.[170]

The level of thiamin in grain rises as the level of protein rises; content being dependent on species, strain and use of nitrogenous fertilizers.[223] Since thiamin is water soluble, as well as heat labile, large losses can occur in certain cooking operations.[139]

Thiamin sources available for addition to feed are the hydrochloride and mononitrate forms. Because of its lower solubility in water, the mononitrate form has somewhat better stability characteristics in dry products than the hydrochloride.[10]

Stability of thiamin (hydrochloride and mononitrate forms) can be a problem. More than 50% of the thiamin was destroyed in premixes with trace minerals, after one month at room temperature.[214] When thiamin stability was evaluated in premixes without trace minerals, no losses were encountered when stored at room temperature for 6 months. The thiamin content of most common feeds should be three to four times greater than requirements, for most species.[24]

Subclinical deficiencies of thiamin can result in reduced synthesis of other B-vitamins, since some rumen bacteria require thiamin to grow. Mathison reported on one feedlot trial where a significant response to supplemental thiamin was observed. In this trial, transketolase was numerically reduced in the controls.[131] Thiamin did not increase gain in two subsequent trials, although there appeared to be a reduction in bloat in one trial.[131] A concomitant field survey, conducted in Alberta, showed 2.7% of 645 cattle that were sampled to be marginal in TPP. In acute PEM, 1 g per day of injected thiamin is indicated until the animals are eating, then 500 mg/day can be supplemented in the diet for 7 to 14 days.[131] Mathison suggested 4 to 6 mg per kg diet, in high grain diets, to help prevent subclinical deficiency.[131]

Animals with clinical signs of thiamin deficiency and/or other indicators of thiamin insufficiency (i.e., transketolase activity) should be provided thiamin at therapeutic doses. Since thiamin deficiency causes anorexia, injection of the vitamin is preferred to oral doses, when a severe deficiency exists. Clinical signs in calves weighing less than 50 kg were prevented with 0.65 mg thiamin-HCL per kilogram of liquid diet, fed at 10% of liveweight (65 μg/kg liveweight).[104] Animals with PEM need to be rapidly provided with supplemental thiamin. Levels of thiamin to be administered intravenously or intramuscularly for 3 days have been recommended for lambs and calves (100 to 400 mg/day) and for sheep and cattle (500 to 2000 mg/day).[223]

For general maintenance following the treatment of mild cases (or as a prophylactic measure when a herd is at risk), 5 to 10 mg of thiamin should be added to 1 kg of dry feed. Feeds should be enriched with thiamin in a concentrate such that each animal will receive 100 to 500 mg daily. For therapeutic purposes, a dosage of 6.6 to 11 mg/kg body weight, repeated every 6 hr for 24 hr, has been suggested for goats.[193]

The administration of thiamin to PEM patients generally produces rapid results, sometimes in a matter of hours. Where recognition of the disease has been delayed and irreversible necrosis has developed in the brain, treatment with the vitamin may be useless. Prospects for achieving satisfactory responses to thiamin treatment in animals already incapable of standing is limited. Although treatment improves the condition of such animals, relapses and permanent damage are probable. Without doubt, PEM is the most important disease arising from a deficiency of thiamin in ruminants. It is important to note that thiamin can be used effectively as a support in the treatment of rumen acidosis and ketosis. Even though treatment with thiamin can be therapeutically successful, it does not follow that a deficiency of thiamin contributes to the etiology of these two diseases.[223]

Preliminary investigations from various universities, as well as field reports, indicate thiamin may ameliorate the toxic effects sometimes seen in cattle grazing fescue pasture.[113] Johnson and Krautmann reported that 500 mg of thiamin per head per day, for the first 30 days that cattle are in the feedyard, has reduced the effects of thermal stress.[103]

Large oral amounts of thiamin are not toxic, and usually the same is true of parenteral doses. Dietary intake of thiamin up to 1000 times the requirement is apparently safe for most animal species.[154] The effects of excessive thiamin intake have not been studied in cattle.[154]

NIACIN

Properties and Metabolism

Chemically, niacin is one of the simplest vitamins, having the empirical formula $C_6H_5O_2N$. Nicotinic acid and nicotinamide correspond to 3-pyridine carboxylic acid and its amide, respectively. There are antivitamins or antagonists for niacin. These compounds have the basic pyridine structure, with two of the important antagonists of nicotinic acid being 3-acetyl pyridine and pyridine sulfonic acid. Nicotinic acid and nicotinamide (niacinamide) possess the same vitamin activity; the free acid is converted to the amide in the body. Nicotinamide functions as a component of two coenzymes: nicotinamide adenine dinucleotide (NAD) and nicotinamide adenine dinucleotide phosphate (NADP).

Both nicotinic acid and nicotinamide are white, odorless, crystalline solids soluble in water and alcohol. They are very resistant to heat, air, light and alkali, and are stable in feeds. Niacin is also stable in the presence of the usual oxidizing agents. However, it will undergo decarboxylation at a high temperature, when in an alkaline medium.

Nicotinic acid and its amide are readily and very efficiently absorbed by diffusion at either physiological or pharmacologic doses. By employing the gastrointestinal tube technique, niacin was shown to be equally well-absorbed from both the stomach and the upper small intestine in humans.[15] In a steady-state situation, approximately 85% of a 3 g per day dose of niacin was recovered from the urine of humans. Absorption was considered almost complete. However, the mechanism by which nicotinamide nucleotides, present in animal foods, are absorbed is not known.

Blood transport of niacin is associated mainly with the red blood cells. Niacin rapidly leaves the blood stream and enters kidney, liver and adipose tissues. Evidence indicates that absorbed niacin is actively cycled through the NAD pathway to nicotinamide in the intestinal mucosa.[88] Absorbed nicotinamide is taken up by tissues and incorporated into its coenzymes.

The tissue content of niacin and its analogs, NAD and NADP, is variable and dependent on diet, breed, sex, age and treatment of animals.[83] Although niacin coenzymes are widely distributed in the body, no true storage occurs. The liver is the site of greatest niacin concentration in the body, but the amount stored is minimal.

Urine is the primary pathway of excretion of absorbed niacin and its metabolites. At high dosages the half-life of both nicotinic acid and nicotinamide is determined mainly by rate of excretion of the unchanged compound in urine and not by metabolic change. When low dosages were used, both compounds were excreted principally as metabolites, rather than as unchanged compounds.

Compared to the dog, in which 100% of the niacin is excreted as n'-methyl nicotinamide, herbivores excrete about 30–50% to nicotinyl glycine (nicotinuric acid).

The amino acid tryptophan is a precursor for the synthesis of niacin. There is considerable evidence that synthesis can take place in the intestine. There is also evidence that synthesis can take place elsewhere within the body. The extent to which the metabolic requirement for niacin can be met from tryptophan will depend, firstly, on the amount of tryptophan in the diet and, secondly, on the efficiency of the conversion of tryptophan to niacin.

Animal species differ widely in their ability to synthesize niacin from tryptophan, but all are relatively inefficient. From a variety of experiments, approximately 60 mg of tryptophan is equivalent to 1 mg of niacin in humans. The rat is more efficient, requiring only 35 to 50 mg tryptophan to synthesize 1 mg of niacin. Conversion efficiency is probably due to inherent differences in liver levels of picolinic acid carboxylase, the enzyme which diverts one of the intermediates (2-amino, 3-acroleylfumaric acid) toward the glutaryl-CoA pathway, instead of allowing this compound to condense to quinolinic acid, the immediate precursor of nicotinic acid. Picolinic acid carboxylase, in livers of various species, has a very close inverse relationship to experimentally determined niacin requirements. The cat has so much of this enzyme, that it cannot convert any of its dietary tryptophan to niacin. The cat has an absolute requirement for niacin. Conversely, the rat diverts very little of its dietary tryptophan to carbon dioxide and water, and thus, is relatively efficient in converting tryptophan to niacin. The cow has approximately six-fold greater liver picolinic acid carboxylase activity than the rat and is thus a poor converter of typtophan to niacin.[186]

The major function of niacin is in the coenzyme forms of nicotin-amide, NAD and NADP. Enzymes containing NAD and NADP are important links in a series of reactions associated with carbohydrate, protein, and lipid metabolism. They are especially important in the metabolic reactions which furnish energy to the animal. More than 40 biochemical reactions have been identified involving these coenzymes. The biochemical functions are of paramount importance for normal tissue integrity, and particularly for maintaining the skin, gastrointesti-nal tract and nervous system.

Like the riboflavin coenzymes, the NAD and NADP-containing enzymes play an important role in biological oxidation-reduction sys-tems by virtue of their capacity to serve as hydrogen-transfer agents. Hydrogen is effectively transferred from the oxidizable substrate to oxygen through a series of graded enzymatic hydrogen transfers. Nico-tinamide-containing enzyme systems constitute one such group of hy-drogen transfer agents.

Important metabolic reactions catalyzed by NAD and NADP are summarized as follows: (a) Carbohydrate metabolism: (1) Glycolysis (anaerobic and aerobic oxidation of glucose), (2) TCA (Krebs) cycle; (b) Lipid metabolism: (1) Glycerol synthesis and breakdown, (2) Fatty acid oxidation and synthesis, (3) Steroid synthesis; (c) Protein metabo-lism: (1) Degradation and synthesis of amino acids, (2) Oxidation of carbon chains via the TCA cycle; (d) Photosynthesis; (e) Rhodopsin synthesis.

Rumen microorganisms can synthesize niacin, and for many years rumen microbial synthesis has been considered adequate for optimum animal performance. However, recent evidence suggests that this is not true for all diets, and niacin may be a limiting nutrient in high-concen-trate, low-roughage rations. This limiting factor is considered to be due to the poor bioavailability of niacin in cereal grains.[175] In the ruminant, supplemental niacin increases the concentration of rumen bacterial protein, ammonia and propionic acid. Ruminal concentration of urea nitrogen is decreased in animals fed exogenous niacin. Ruminant mi-crobial synthesis of niacin appears to be limited and generally is not of great importance to cattle. It appears that ruminal niacin synthesis ceases when feedstuffs contain sufficient niacin levels to meet usual bacterial metabolism. However, as in the monogastric animal, bound or unavailable niacin of feedstuffs is not nutritionally available to the ruminant. Metabolically, systemic requirements of ruminants may be even greater than those of other animals, because of the occurrence of ketosis and the need for ammonia detoxification.[30]

Assessment of Status

Deficiencies. Niacin has been reported to enhance protein syn-thesis, but responses to additional dietary niacin in beef animals have been variable.[153]

Preruminant calves are expected to become deficient in B-vitamins, including niacin, if the diet has insufficient amounts of niacin.[140] Although tryptophan conversion to niacin is not considered important in ruminants, the ability to produce niacin deficiency is dependent on the use of a low tryptophan milk diet. Studies in calves fed a low tryptophan and niacin deficient diet showed deficiency signs of sudden anorexia, severe diarrhea and dehydration, followed by sudden death.[140] In growing cattle, niacin supplementation results in production responses including improvements in feed efficiency, growth and better adaptation to high-grain diets.[30,140]

Fronk and Schultz reported that niacin administration at 12 grams per head per day was beneficial in the treatment of subclinical and clinical ketosis in lactating dairy cows.[65] In addition, Kung, Gubert and Huber reported that lactation persistency was higher in dairy cows fed niacin at 6 g per head per day. Soybean meal protein or non protein nitrogen (20% of total nitrogen from non-protein nitrogen) were the sources of protein for this trial.[111]

Clinical Parameters. As with most of the B-vitamins, the determination of cellular or blood serum levels of niacin or niacin-dependent enzymes has not proven to be a reliable or acceptable method for evaluating niacin status.[140]

Riddell, Bartley and Dayton reported on the effects of feeding niacin to rumen fistulated cattle; they noted increased bacterial protein production in the rumen and an increased percentage of rumen propionate.[175]

Dietary Sources and Fortification

Niacin is widely distributed in feedstuffs of both plant and animal origin. Distiller's grains, yeast, various distillation and fermentation solubles, and certain oilseed meals are good sources. Most species can use the essential amino acid tryptophan and synthesize niacin from it. Many animal feedstuffs contain low concentrations of tryptophan, and absorbed tryptophan is preferentially used for protein synthesis.[110] Therefore, it is unlikely that tryptophan conversion greatly contributes to the niacin supply.

Oilseeds contain about 40% of their total niacin in bound form, while only a small proportion of the niacin in pulses, yeast, crustacea, fish, animal tissue, or milk is bound. By use of a rat assay procedure, Carter and Carpenter showed that for eight samples of mature cooked cereals (corn, wheat, rice, and milo) only about 35% of the total niacin was available.[33] Much of the niacin in grains and their mill by-products is in a bound form, which is not totally available to animals.[123,222] Thus, although the bioavailability of niacin is 100% in soybean meal, it is zero in wheat and sorghum and varies from 0 to 30% in corn. In calculating the niacin content of formulated diets, probably all niacin from cereal grain sources should be ignored or at least given a value no greater than one-third of the total niacin.

Niacin is commercially available in two forms, niacinamide and nicotinic acid, with both forms providing about the same biological activity. Crystalline products are used in feeds and pharmaceuticals or as dry dilutions in feeds.

Niacin is produced by microbial synthesis in the rumen, and ruminants can synthesize niacin from tryptophan. However, investigations into these two sources suggest that only enough niacin is produced to cover the animals requirement. Studies with starting and growing feedlot cattle supplemented with niacin, indicate improved performance.[30] Similarly improved milk production in dairy cows suggests that niacin requirements have increased in recent years and that demands can be pushed even higher when the ruminant is subjected to stress conditions.[9]

Niacin supplementation should be considered for calves fed milk replacer, starting feedlot cattle and for the management of cattle fed high energy rations, especially dairy cattle in heavy milk production and cows, whose metabolism is placed under great strain.

Byers reviewed niacin supplementation trials in beef cattle in which niacin was supplemented from 50 to 500 ppm in the diet.[30] This author concluded that 50 ppm was ineffective and that 500 ppm was excessive, as it appeared to reduce performance. However, the 100 ppm level generally enhanced daily gain and efficiency by 3.6 and 3.7%, respectively.[30]

In dairy cows 12 grams niacin per day was effective in overcoming subclinical and clinical ketosis.[65] Further, supplementation of 3 to 6 g niacin per day to cows in their first 100 days of lactation resulted in increased milk yield, increase milk protein and improvement in persistence.[190]

SUMMARY

Deficiencies of vitamins A, D, K, E and thiamin can cause severe limitations in beef production. In particular, vitamin A and E can be common causes of lost profit, secondary to limitations of reproductive and growth potential. Prolonged dry periods will reduce available A and E in pasture forage, as can ensiling and prolonged storage of harvested feedstuffs. Polioencephalomalacia is a thiamin responsive disorder, associated with high concentrate feeding and lush pastures. Antimetabolites, such as amprolium, will cause thiamine deficiency when fed in excess. Recent information has shown improved performance with supplemental β carotene and niacin. The positive responses in reproductive performance, noted with cattle fed supplemental β carotene, was independent of vitamin A. Supplementation of vitamins above National Research Council recommendations can be justified. However, proper evaluation of feed and animal status, and documentation of a response to supplementation is necessary before diagnosing deficiencies of specific nutrients.

REFERENCES

1. Adams CR: Feedlot cattle need supplemental vitamin E. Feedstuffs 54(18):24, 1982
2. Alderson NE, Mitchell GE, Little CO, et al: Preintestinal disappearance of vitamin E in ruminants. J Nutr 101:655, 1971
3. Allen WM, Bradley R, Berrett S, et al: Degenerative myopathy with myoglobinuria in yearling calves. Br Vet J 131:292, 1975
4. Alstad AD, Casper HH, Johnson LJ: Vitamin K treatment of sweet clover poisoning in calves. JAVMA 187:729, 1985
5. Anonymous: Vitamin A and retinal-binding protein in fetal growth and development of the rat. Nutr Rev 35:305, 1977
6. Arthur JR: Nutritional inter-relationships between selenium and vitamin E. Rowett Research Institute Ann Rep 38:124, 1982
7. Bar A, Edelstein S, Eisner I, et al: Cholecalciferol requirements of growing turkeys under normal conditions and during recovery from rickets. J Nutr 112:1779, 1982
8. Barash PG: Nutrient toxicities of vitamin K. In Rechigl M (ed): Handbook Series in Nutrition Food, Section E: Nutrition Disorders, vol 1. West Palm Beach, CRC Press, 1978, p 97
9. Bartley EE, Brent EB: B-vitamins for ruminants. In Proceedings of the 43rd Minnesota Nutrition Conference, Bloomington, 1982, p 66
10. Bauernfeind JC: Vitamins and carotenoids in modern feeds and animal applications. World Rev Anim Prod 21:20, 1969
11. Bauernfeind JC: Carotenoid vitamin A precursor and analysis in foods and feeds. J Agric Food Chem 20:456, 1972
12. Bauernfeind JC: Tocopherols in Foods. In Machlin LJ (ed): Vitamin E: A Comprehensive Treatise. Marcel Dekker, New York, 1980, p 99
13. Bauernfeind JC, DeRitter E: Synthetic vitamin A in animal applications. Feedstuffs 44(36):34, 1972
14. Bayfield RF, Mylrea PJ: Carotenoids and tocopherols in serum of apparently healthy dairy cattle. J Dairy Sci 36:137, 1969
15. Bechgaard H, Jespersen S: GI absorption of niacin in humans. J Pharm Sci 66:871, 1977
16. Bendich A: Role of antioxidant vitamins on immune function. In Proceedings Roche Technical Symposium: The Role of Vitamins on Animal Performance and Immune Response, Daytona Beach, 1987, p 1
17. Bonnette ED, Kornegay ET: Influence of supplemental vitamin E on weaning age and performance, humeral antibody production and serum cortisol levels of pigs. Virginia Tech Livestock Anim Sci Res Rep No 6, 1987
18. Bonsembiante M, Brittante G, Andrighetto I: Effects of B-carotene on fertility of cows fed diets supplemented with vitamin A. Zoot Nutr Anim 6:47, 1980
19. Booth A, Reid M, Clark T: Hypovitaminosis A in feedlot cattle. J Am Vet Med Assoc 190:1305, 1987
19a. Bradfield D, Behrens WC: Effect of vitamin ADE injection on conception rates in cows and heifers. In Proc West Sec Am Soc Anim Sci 19:1, 1968
20. Brady PS, Brady LT, Ullrey DE: Selenium, vitamin E and response to swimming stress in the rat. J Nutr 109:1103, 1979
21. Braun F: The effect of bile or intestinal absorption of calcium and vitamin D. Wiener Klinische Wochenschrift 98 Suppl. 166:23, 1986
22. Bräunlich K, Zintzen H: Vitamin B_1. Basel, F Hoffmann-La Roche Co Ltd, 1976
23. Brent BE, Bartley EE: Thiamin and niacin in the rumen. J Anim Sci 59:813, 1984
24. Brent BE: Is supplementation necessary? Feed Management 36(12):8, 1985
25. Brin M, Tai M, Ostashever AS: Effect of thiamine-deficiency on activity of erythrocyte hemolysate transketolase. J Nutr 71:273, 1960
26. Brownlee NR, Huttner JJ, Panganamala RV, et al: Role of vitamin E and glutathione-induced oxidant stress: methaemoglobin, lipid peroxidation and hemolysis. J Lipid Res 18:635, 1977
27. Burton GW, Ingold KU: Autoxidation of biological molecules. I. The antioxidant

activity of vitamin E and related chain-breaking phenolic antioxidants in vitro. J Am Chem Soc 103:6472, 1981

28. Burton GW and Ingold KU. Beta-carotene: An unusual type of lipid antioxidant. Science 224:569, 1984

29. Burton GW, Joyce A, Ingold KU: First proof that vitamin E is major lipid-soluble chain-breaking antioxidant in human blood plasma. Lancet 11:327, 1982

30. Byers FM: Niacin and beef cattle performance: B vitamin enhances energy efficiency and adaptation to urea. Anim Nutr Health, Nov-Dec:21, 1979

31. Byers JH, Jones IR, Bones JF: Carotene in the ration of dairy cattle. J Dairy Sci 39:1556, 1956

32. Carrica JM, Brandt RT, Lee RW: Influence of vitamin E on feedlot performance and carcass traits of beef steers fed either lasalocid or monensin. J Anim Sci 63 (Suppl 1):432, 1986

33. Carter EGA, Carpenter KJ: The available niacin values of foods for rats and their relation to analytical values. J Nutr 112:2091, 1982

34. Chew BP: Vitamin A and B-carotene: A nutritional approach to bovine mastitis control. Anim Nutr Health, Nov–Dec: 22, 1983

35. Chew BP, Holpach DM, O'Fallon JV: Vitamin A and beta-carotene in bovine and porcine plasma, liver, corpora lutea and follicular fluid. J Dairy Sci 67:1316, 1984

36. Chow CK: Nutritional influence on cellular antioxidant defense systems. Am J Clin Nutr 32:1066, 1979

37. Chow CK: Vitamin E and blood. In Bourne GH (ed): World Nutritional Determinants. Basel, Karger, 1985, p 133

38. Cipriano JE, Morrill JL, Anderson NV: Effect of dietary vitamin E on immune responses of calves. J Dairy Sci 65:2357, 1982

39. Combs GF: Assessment of vitamin E status in animals and man. Proc Nutr Soc 40:187, 1981

40. Combs SB, Combs GF Jr. Varietal Differences in the Vitamin E Content of Corn. In Proceedings of the 1984 Cornell Nutrition Conference for Feed Manufacturers, Ithaca, 1987, p 45

40a. Combs GF Jr: Vitamin tolerance of livestock. In Proceedings 1988 Cornell Nutrition Conference for Feed Manufacturers, Syracuse, 1988, p 35

41. Cooper JR, Roth RH, Kini MM: Biochemical and physiological function of thiamin in nervous tissue. Nature 199:609, 1963

42. Cort WM, Vincente TS, Waysek EH, et al: Vitamin E content of feedstuffs determined by high-performance liquid chromatographic fluorescence. J Agric Food Chem 31:1330, 1983

43. Cunha TJ: Vitamin requirements of the pig. In Swine Feeding and Nutrition. New York, Academic Press Inc, 1977, p 75

44. Dancy M, Evans G, Galitonde MK, et al: Blood thiamine and thiamine phosphate ester concentrations in alcoholic and non-alcoholic liver diseases. Br Med J 289:79, 1984

45. Dash SK, Mitchell DJ: Storage, processing reduce vitamin A. Anim Nutr Health 31(7):16, 1976

46. de Boer-Van den Berg MAG, Verstijnen PHJ, Vermeer C: Vitamin K-dependent carboxylase in skin. J Inves Dermatol 87:377, 1986

47. DeLuca HF: Vitamin D: Not just for bones. In Proceedings of the 1990 National Feed Ingredient Association Nutrition Institute: Developments in Vitamin Nutrition and Health Applications. Des Moines. National Feed Ingredients Association, 1990

48. DeLuca HF: The Vitamin D Story: A collaborative effort of basic science and clinical medicine. J Fed Am Soc Exp Biol 2:224, 1988

49. Dicks MW, Rousseau JE, Eaton HD, et al: Some interrelationships between vitamin E and vitamin A in Holstein calves. J Dairy Sci 42:501, 1959

50. Diplock AT: The role of vitamin E and selenium in the prevention of oxygen-induced tissue damage. In Spallholz JE, Martin JL, Ganther HE (ed): Selenium in Biology and Medicine. New York, AVI Pub Co, 1981, p 303

51. Divers TJ, Blackmon DM, Martin CL, et al: Blindness and convulsions associated with vitamin A deficiency in feedlot steers. J Am Vet Med Assoc 189:1579, 1986

VITAMIN DEFICIENCIES IN CATTLE

269

52. Doerr JA: Influence of aflatoxin on broiler nutrition: Where do we go from here? In Proc 1987 Arkansas Nutrition Conference. North Little Rock, 1987, p 48
53. Dreyfus PM: The regional distribution of transketolase in the normal and the thiamine deficient nervous system. J Neuropath Exp Neurol 24:119, 1965
54. Droke EA, Loerch SC: Effect of parenteral selenium and vitamin E on performance, health and humeral immune response of steers new to the feedlot environment. J Anim Sci 67:1350, 1989
55. Drouchner W: Current status of vitamin E research presented on the example of the vitamin E requirements and supply status of the pig. Ubers Terernahrung 4:93, 1976
56. Eaton HD: Chronic bovine hypo- and hypervitaminosis A and cerebrospinal fluid pressure. Am J Clin Nutr 22:1070, 1969
57. Edwin EE, Lewis G, Allcroft R: Cerebrocortical necrosis: A hypothesis for the possible role of thiaminase in its pathogenesis. Vet Rec 83:176, 1968
58. Edwin EE, Jackman R: Ruminal thiaminase and tissue thiamine in cerebrocortical necrosis. Vet Rec 92:640, 1973
59. Edwin EE, Markson LM, Shreeve J, et al: Diagnostic aspects of cerebrocortical necrosis. Vet Rec 104:4, 1979
60. Ellis RP, Vorhies MW: Effect of supplemental dietary vitamin E on the serologic response of swine to an Escherichia coli bacteria. J Am Vet Med Assoc 168:231, 1976
61. Evans WC, Evans IA, Humphreys DJ, et al: Induction of thiamine deficiency in sheep with lesions similar to those of cerebrocortical necrosis. J Comp Path 85:253, 1975
62. Engstrom GW, Littledike ET: Vitamin D metabolism in the pig. In Tumbleson ME (ed): Swine in Biomedical Research. New York, Plenum Press, 1986, p 1091
63. Faustman C, Cassens RG, Schaefer DM, et al: Improvement of pigment and lipid stability in Holstein steer beef by dietary supplementation with vitamin E. J Food Sci 54(4):858, 1989a
64. Faustman C, Cassens RG, Schaefer DM, et al: Vitamin E supplementation of Holstein steer diets improves sirloin steak color. J Food Sci 54(2):485, 1989b
64a. Foley JA, Otterby DE: Availability, storage, treatment, composition and feeding value of surplus colostrum: A review. J Dairy Sci 61:1033, 1978
65. Fronk TJ, Schultz LH: Oral nicotinic acid as a treatment for ketosis. J Dairy Sci 62:1804, 1979
66. Frye TM: Vitamin compatibility in custom premixes. In Proceeding of the Vitamin Nutrition Update: Seminar Series 2, Nutley, 1978, p 70
67. Galio-Torres HE: Transport and metabolism. In Machlin LJ (ed): Vitamin E: A Comprehensive Treatise. New York, Marcel Dekker, 1980, p 193
68. Gallop PM, Lian JB, Hauschka PU: Carboxylated calcium-binding protein and vitamin K. N Engl J Med 302:1460, 1980
69. Garabedian M, Tanaka Y, Holick MF, et al: Response of intestinal calcium transport and bone calcium mobilization to 1,25-dihydroxyvitamin D₃ in thyroparathyroid-ectomized rats. Endocrinology 94:1022, 1974
70. Giausddin ASM, Diplock AT: The influence of vitamin E on membrane lipids of mouse fibroblasts in culture. Anal Biochem Biophys 210:348, 1981
71. Giesecke D: Nicotinic acid or nicotinamide: The biochemical significance of these vitamins and the differences in their metabolic activity. Ubers Tierernahrung 11:133, 1983
72. Gill DR, Smith RA, Hicks RB, et al: The effect of vitamin E supplementation on the health and performance of newly arrived stocker cattle. Oklahoma Agr Exp Sta Res MP 118:240, 1986
73. Goff JP, Horst RL, Littledike ET: Effect of sow vitamin D status at parturition on the vitamin D status of neonatal piglets. J Nutr 114:163, 1984
74. Golub MS, Gershwin ME: Stress-inducted immunomodulation: what is it, if it is? In Moberg GP (ed): Animal Stress, Bethesda, Am J Physiol Soc, 1985, p 177
75. Gonnerman WA, Toverud SV, Ramp WK, et al: Effects of dietary vitamin D and calcium on lysyl oxidase activity in chick bone metaphyses. Proc Soc Exp Biol Med 151:453, 1976

76. Goplen BP, Bell JM: Dicumarol studies IV: Antidotal and antagonistic properties of vitamin K_1 and K_3 in cattle. Can J Anim Sci 41:91, 1967
77. Griminger P, Donis O: Potency of Vitamin K_1 and two analogues in counteracting the effects of dicumarol and sulfaquinoxaline on the chick. J Nutr 70:361, 1960
78. Griminger P: Vitamin K in animal nutrition: Deficiency can be fatal, Part 1. Feedstuffs 56(38):25, 1984
79. Griminger P, Brubacher G: The transfer of vitamin K_1 and menadione from the hen to the egg. Poultry Sci 45:512, 1966
80. Guilbert HR, Howell CE, Hart GH: Minimum vitamin A and carotene requirements of mammalian species. J Nutr 19:91, 1940
81. Hadden JW: Neuroendocrine modulation of the thymus-dependent immune system. Ann NY Acad Sci 496:39, 1987
82. Hale WH, Hubbert F, Taylor RE, et al: The effect of feeding high levels of vitamin A to beef cattle upon performance and tissue vitamin A levels. J Anim Sci 20:668, 1961
83. Hankes LU: Nicotinic acid and nicotinamide. In Machlin LJ (ed): Handbook of Vitamins: Nutritional, Biochemical and Clinical Aspects. New York, Marcel Dekker, 1984, p 329
84. Harman D, Heidrick ML, Eddy DE: Free radical theory of aging effect of free-radical-reaction inhibitors on the immune response. J Am Geriatr Soc 25:400, 1977
85. Harrison JH, Hancock DD, Conrad HR: Vitamin E and selenium for reproduction of the dairy cow. J Dairy Sci 67:123, 1984
86. Harvey JD, Bieber-Wlaschny M: Vitamin E availability to livestock varies dramatically. Feedstuffs 60(12):15, 1988
87. Hemming BC, Gubler CJ: Separation of thiamin, thiamin antagonists and their phosphate esters by high-performance liquid chromatography. J Liq Chromatogr 3:1697, 1980
88. Henderson LM, Gross CJ: Metabolism of niacin and niacinamide in perfused rat intestine. J Nutr 109:654, 1979
89. Hidiroglou M, Hoffmann I, Jenkins KJ: Selenium distribution and radiotocopherol metabolism in the pregnant ewe and fetal lamb. Can J Physiol Parmacol 47:953, 1969
90. Hidiroglou M, Jenkins KJ, Lessard JR, et al: Metabolism of vitamin E in sheep. Br J Nutr 24:917, 1970
91. Hill GM: Vitamin E and selenium supplementation of cattle. In Proceedings 1987 Georgia Nutrition Conference For the Feed Industry, Atlanta, 1987
92. Hirsch A: Vitamin D—History, Manufacture, Analysis and Metabolism: An Overview. In Vitamins—The Life Essentials. Des Moines. National Feed Ingredients Association, 1982
93. Hoekstra WG: Biochemical function of selenium and its relation to vitamin E. Fed Proc 34:2083, 1975
94. Hoffmann-La Roche: Vitamin E/Se in ruminants. News and Reviews, 1972
95. Hoffmann-La Roche: Roche Technical Bulletin: Vitamin B_{12}. Nutley, Hoffmann-La Roche Inc, 1984
95a. Hoffmann-La Roche: Vitamin Fortification Guidelines: Update 2. Nutley, Hoffmann-La Roche Inc, 1989
96. Hoffsten PE, Hunter FE, Gebicki JM, et al: Formation of lipid peroxide under conditions which lead to swelling and lysis of rat liver mitochondria. Biochem Biophys Res Commun 7:276, 1962
97. Hollander D: Vitamin K absorption by everted intestinal sacs of the rat. Am J Physiol 225:360, 1973
98. Hutcheson DP, Cole NA: Vitamin E and selenium for yearling feedlot cattle. Fed Proc 44(3):549, 1985
99. Hutchinson LJ, Scholz RW, Drake TR: Nutritional myodegeneration in a group of Chianina heifers. J Am Vet Med Assoc 181:581, 1982
100. Imawari M, Kida K, Goodman DS: The transport of vitamin D and its 25-hydroxy metabolite in human plasma. J Clin Invest 58:514, 1976
101. International Union of Pure and Applied Chemistry—International Union of Bio-

chemistry Commission on Biochemical Nomenclature: Tocopherols and Related Compounds, Recommendations. Eur J Biochem 46:217, 1973

102. Jenkins KJ, Hidiroglou M: A review of selenium/vitamin E responsive problems in livestock: A case for selenium as a feed additive in Canada. Can J Anim Sci 52:591, 1972

103. Johnson AB, Krautmann BA: Water soluble vitamins for ruminants. *In* Proceedings of the 24th Pacific Northwest Animal Nutrition Conference, Boise, 1989, p 81

104. Johnson BC, Hamilton TS, Nevens WB, et al: Thiamine deficiency in the calf. J Nutr 35:137, 1948

105. Julien WE, Conrad HR: Selenium and vitamin E and incidence of retained placenta in parturient dairy cows. II. Prevention in commercial herds with prepartum treatment. J Dairy Science 59:1960, 1976

106. Kelley K, Easter R: Nutritional factors can influence immune response of swine. Feedstuffs 59(22):14, 1987

107. Kimura M, Fujita T, Nishida S, et al: Differential fluorometric determination of program levels of thiamine, thiamine monophosphate, diphosphate and triphosphate using high-performance liquid chromatography. J Chromatogr 188:417, 1980

108. Kimura M, Fujita T, Hokawa Y: Liquid-chromatographic determination of the total thiamin content of blood. Clin Chem 28:29, 1982

109. King MM, Lai EK, McCay PB: Singlet oxygen production associated with enzyme-catalysed lipid J Biol Chem 250:6496, 1975

110. Kodicek ED, Ashby DR, Muller M, et al: The conversion of bound nicotinic acid to free nicotinamide on roasting sweet corn. Proc Nutr Soc 33:105A, 1974

111. Kung L Jr, Gubert K, Huber JT: Supplemental niacin for lactating cows fed diets of natural protein or nonprotein nitrogen. J Dairy Sci 63:2020, 1980

112. Lake AM, Stuart MJ, Oski FA: Vitamin E deficiency and enhanced platelet function: Reversal following E supplementation. J Pediatr 90:722, 1977

113. Lauriault LM, Dougherty CT, Bradley NW, et al: Thiamin supplementation and the ingestive behavior of beef cattle grazing endophyte-infected tall fescue. J Anim Sci 68:1245, 1990

114. Lee RW, Stuart RL, Perryman KR, et al: Effect of vitamin supplementation on the performance of stressed beef calves. J Anim Sci 61 (Suppl 1):425, 1985

115. Lewis JM, Wilson LT: Vitamin A requirement in calves. J Nutr 30:467, 1945

116. Littledike ET, Horst RL: Vitamin D_3 toxicity in dairy cows. J Dairy Sci 65:749, 1982

117. Loew FM, Dunlop RH: Induction of thiamin inadequacy and polioencephalomalacia in adult sheep with amprolium. Am J Vet Res 32:2195, 1972

118. Lotthammer KH: Importance of B-carotene for the fertility of dairy cattle. Feedstuffs 51(43):16, 37, 1979

118a. Lotthammer KH, Ahlswede HL, Meyer H: Untersuchungen uber eine spezifische Vitamin-A-unabhangige wirkung des B-carotenes aus die fertilitat des Rindes z. mitt. Weitere Klinische betunde und Besamungsengebnisse. Dtsch Tieraerztl Wochenschr 83:353, 1976

119. Lusby KS: Hyperalimentation in lambs: A model for the study of polioencephalomalacia. MS Thesis, Manhattan, Kansas State University, 1971

120. Lynch GP: Changes of tocopherols in blood serum of cows fed hay or silage. J Dairy Sci 66:1461, 1983

121. Maas JP, Bulgin MS, Anderson BC, et al: Nutritional myodegeneration associated with vitamin E deficiency and normal selenium status in lambs. J Am Vet Med Assoc 184:201, 1984

121a. Machlin LJ: Vitamin E. *In* Machlin LJ (ed). Handbook of Vitamins: Nutritional, Biochemical and Clinical Aspects. New York, Marcel Dekker, 1984, p 99

122. Mann SO, Wilson AB, Barr M, et al: Thiaminase activity in the gut of cobalt-deficient sheep. Aust J Agric Res 34:211, 1983

123. Manoukas AG, Ringrose RC, Toori AE: The availability of niacin in corn, soybean meal and wheat middlings for the hen. Poultry Sci 47:1836, 1968

124. Marks J: Thiamine: *In* A Guide to the Vitamins: Their Role in Health and Disease. Lancaster, Medical and Technical Publishing Co Ltd, 1975, p 73

125. Marks J: Vitamin D — Calciferol. *In* A Guide to the Vitamins: Their Role in Health and Disease. Lancaster, Medical and Technical Publishing Co Ltd, 1979, p 52
126. Martin MM, Hurley LS: Effects of large amounts of vitamin E during pregnancy and lactation. Am J Clin Nutr 30:1629, 1977
127. Martinez FE, Goncalves AL, Jorge SM: Vitamin E in placental blood and its interrelationship to maternal and newborn levels of vitamin E. J Pediatr 99:298, 1981
128. Marusich WL: Vitamin E as an in vivo lipid stabilizer and its effect on flavor and storage properties of milk and meat. *In* Machlin LJ (ed): Vitamin E: A Comprehensive Treatis. New York, Marcel Dekker, 1980, p 445
129. Marusich WL, DeRitter E, Ogrinz EF, et al: Effect of supplemental E in control of rancidity in poultry meat. Poultry Sci 54:831, 1975
130. Massey JB, She HS, Pownall HJ: Interaction of vitamin E with saturated phospholipid bilayers. Biochem Biophys Res Commun 106:842, 1982
131. Mathison GW: B-vitamins, choline, inositol and paraminobenzoic acid for ruminants. *In* Proceedings of the 21st Northwest Animal Nutrition Conference, Vancouver, 1986, p 107
132. May T, Preston RL, Fick TP, et al: Vitamin E as a receiving treatment for feedlot cattle. Texas Tech Univ Anim Sci Rep, 1987, p 52
133. Maynard LA, Loosli JK, Hintz HF, et al: The Vitamins. *In* Animal Nutrition, ed 7. New York, McGraw-Hill Book Co, 1979, p 229
134. McCay PB, Gibson DD, Hornbrook KR: Glutathione dependent inhibition of lipid peroxidation by a soluble heat-labile factor not glutathione peroxidase. Fed Proc 40:199, 1981
135. McCay PB, King MM: Vitamin E: Its role as a biological free radical scavenger and its relationship to the microsomal mixed function oxidase system. *In* Machlin LJ (ed): Vitamin E: A Comprehensive Treatise. New York, Marcel-Dekker, 1980, p 289
136. McDonald JW: Mortality and ill-thrift associated with thiamine deficiency in lambs. Aust Vet J 58:212, 1982
137. McDowell LR: Vitamin A: *In* Vitamins in Animal Nutrition: Comparative Aspects to Human Nutrition. San Diego, Academic Press Inc, 1989, p 10
138. McDowell LR: Vitamin E. *In* Vitamins in Animal Nutrition: Comparative Aspects to Human Nutrition. San Diego, Academic Press Inc, 1989, p 93
139. McDowell LR: Thiamin. *In* Vitamins in Animal Nutrition: Comparative Aspects to Human Nutrition. San Diego, Academic Press Inc, 1989, p 155
140. McDowell LR: Niacin. *In* Vitamins in Animal Nutrition: Comparative Aspects to Human Nutrition. San Diego, Academic Press Inc, 1989, p 210
141. McGinnis CH Jr: New concepts in vitamin nutrition. *In* Proceedings 1988 Georgia Nutrition Conference, Athens, 1988, p 1
142. McMurray CH, Rice DA: Vitamin E and selenium deficiency diseases. Irish Vet J 36:57, 1982
143. Millar KR, Craig J, Dawe I: Tocopherol and selenium levels in pastuerised cow's milk from different areas in New Zealand. New Zealand J Agric Res 16:301, 1973
144. Miller BE, Norman AW: Vitamin D. *In* Machlin LJ (ed): Handbook of Vitamins: Nutritional, Biochemical, and Clinical Aspects. New York, Marcel Dekker, 1984, p 45
145. Mitchell GE: Vitamin A nutrition of ruminants. J Vet Med Assoc 151:430, 1967
146. Moore LA: Carotene intake, levels of blood plasma carotene and the development of papillary edema and nyctalopia in calves. J Dairy Sci 22:803, 1939
147. Moore LA: Some ocular changes and deficiency manifestation in mature cows fed a ration deficient in vitamin A. J Dairy Sci 24:893, 1941
148. Morrill JL, Reddy PG: Effects of vitamin E on immune responses and performance on dairy calves. *In* Proceedings Roche Technical Symposium: The Role of Vitamins on Animal Performance and Immune Response, Daytona Beach, 1987, p 34
149. Muralt A: The role of thiamin in neurophysiology. Ann NY Acad Sci 98:499, 1962
150. Muth OH: White muscle disease (myopathy) in lambs and calves. I. Occurrence

and nature of the disease under Oregon conditions. J Am Vet Med Assoc 126:355, 1955

151. Nakajama N: Studies on the metabolism of thiamine in cattle: Blood level and urinary excretion after intravenous administration of thiamine preparations. J Japan Vet Med Assn 37:99, 1984

151a. National Research Council: Atlas of Nutritional Data on U.S. and Canadian Feeds: Washington National Academy of Science, 1971

152. National Research Council: Nutrient Requirements of Dairy Cattle, ed 5. Washington, National Academy Press, 1978

153. National Research Council: Nutrient Requirements of Beef Cattle, ed 6. Washington, National Academy Press, 1984

154. National Research Council, Subcommittee on Vitamin Tolerance: Vitamin Tolerance of Animals. Washington, National Academy Press, 1987

154a. National Research Council: Nutrient Requirements of Dairy Cattle, ed 6. Washington National Academy Press, 1988

155. Newlander JA, Jones CH, Foote MW: Barn-cured and field-cured hays as sources of vitamin D and carotene (Vitamin A) for dairy cattle from birth to first freshening. Vermont Experiment Station Bulletin 561:3, 1950

156. Nockels CF: Protective effects of supplemental vitamin E against infection. Fed Proc 38:2134, 1979

157. Nockels CF: Stress, disease and vitamin E requirements. In Proceedings of the Twentieth Annual Convention of American Association of Bovine Practitioners. Kansas City, 1989, in press

158. Norman AW, DeLuca HF: The preparation of H^3-Vitamins D_2 and D_3 and their localization in the rat. Biochemistry 2:1160, 1963

159. Olson JA: Vitamin A. In Machlin LJ (ed): Handbook of Vitamins. New York, Marcel Dekker, 1984, p 1

160. Panganamata RV, Cornwell DC: The effects of vitamin E on arachidonic acid metabolism. Ann NY Acad Sci 393:376, 1982

161. Panush RS, Delafuente JC: Vitamins and immunocompetence. In Bourne GH (ed): World Nutritional Determinants. Basel, Karger, 1985, p 97

162. Parrish DB, Wise GH, Hughes JS: Properties of the colostrum of the dairy cow. J Dairy Sci 30:849, 1947

163. Parrish DB, Wise GH, Latschar CE, et al: Effect of prepartal diet of the cow on placental and mammary transfer of tocopherol to the calf. J Nutr 40:193, 1950

164. Perry TW: Vitamin requirements of beef cattle. In Animal Feeding and Nutrition. New York, Academic Press Inc, 1980, p 23

165. Pruiett SP, Morrill JL, Blecha F, et al: Effect of supplemental vitamin C and E in milk replacer on lymphocyte and neutrophil function in bull calves. J Anim Sci 67 (Supp 1):243, 1989

166. Quackenbush FW: Corn carotenoid: Effect of temperature and moisture on losses during storage. Cereal Chem 40:266, 1963

167. Rammell CG, Hill JH: A review of thiamine deficiency and its diagnosis, especially in ruminants. New Zealand Vet J 34:202, 1986

168. Rammell CG, Thompson KG, Bentley GR, et al: Selenium, vitamin E and polyunsaturated fatty acid concentrations in goat kids with and without myodegeneration. New Zealand Vet J 37:4, 1989

169. Reddy MU, Pushpamma P: Effect of storage and insect infestation on thiamin and niacin content in different varieties of rice, sorghum and legumes. Nutr Rep Int 34:393, 1986

170. Reddy PG, Morrill JL, Minocha HC, et al: Effect of supplemental vitamin E on the immune system of calves. J Dairy Sci 69:164, 1986

171. Reddy PG, Morrill JL, Minocha HC, et al: Vitamin E requirements of dairy calves. J Dairy Sci 70:123, 1987

172. Reddy PG, Morrill JL, Minocha HC, et al: Vitamin E is immunostimulatory in calves. J Dairy Sci 70:993, 1987

173. Reinhardt TA, Hustmyer FG: Role of vitamin D in the immune system. J Dairy Sci 70:952, 1987

174. Rice DA, Blanchflower WJ, McMurray CH: The effects of moisture, propionic

acid, sodium hydroxide and anaerobiasis on the stability of vitamin E in stored barley. J Agric Sci (Cambridge) 105:15, 1985

175. Riddell DO, Bartley EE, Dayton AD: Effect of nicotinic acid on rumen fermentation in vitro and in vivo. J Dairy Sci 63:1429, 1980

176. Ronning ME, Berousek R, Kuhlman AH, et al: The carotene requirements for reproduction in guernsey cattle. J Dairy Sci 36:52, 1953

177. Rousseau JE Jr, Dicks MW, Teichman R, et al: Relationships between plasma, liver and dietary tocopherol in calves, lambs and pigs. J Anim Sci 16:612, 1957

178. Roussel JD, Patrick TE, Kellgren HC, et al: Influence of high levels of vitamin A supplementation on semen characteristics and blood composition of breeding bulls. J Dairy Sci 46:583, 1963

179. Rowland R: Vitamin D function. In Vitamins—The Life Essentials. Des Moines. National Feed Ingredients Association, 1982

180. Sapienza DA: An hypothesis for the etiology of polioencephamalacia. PhD Dissertation, Manhattan, Kansas State University, 1981

181. Sauberlich HE: Biochemical alterations in thiamine deficiency—their interpretations. Am J Clin Nutr 20:528, 1967

182. Schaefer DM, Scheller KK, Arp SC, et al: Growth of Holstein steers and beef color as affected by dietary vitamin E supplementation. J Anim Sci 67 (Supp 1):501, 1989

183. Schaefer DM, Scheller KK, Arp S, et al: Slaughter weights and dietary vitamin E supplementation for enhanced viability of finished Holstein steer production systems. In Proceedings Arlington Cattle Feeders Day, Arlington, 1989, p 29

184. Schendel HE, Johnson BC: Vitamin K deficiency in the baby pig. J Nutr 76:124, 1962

185. Schingoethe DJ, Parsons JG, Ludens FC, et al: Vitamin E status of dairy cows fed stored feeds continuously on pasture during summer. J Dairy Sci 61:1582, 1978

186. Scott ML, Nesheim MC, Young RJ: The Vitamins. In Nutrition of the Chicken, ed 3. Ithaca, M. L. Scott and Associates, 1982, p 119

187. Shearer MJ, Barkhan P, Webster GR: Absorption and excretion of an oral dose of tritiated vitamin K_1 in man. Br J Hematol 18:297, 1970

188. Sheffy BE, Schultz RD: Influence of vitamin E and selenium on immune response mechanisms. Fed Proc 38:2139, 1979

189. Shields RG, Campbell DR, Hughes DM, et al: Researchers study vitamin A stability in feeds. Feedstuffs 54(7):22, 1982

190. Sipocz J, Schmidt J: Effect of niacin (nicotinic acid) addition on milk production, milk constituent and various blood plasma parameters. Kraftfutter 68:253, 1985

191. Smith KL, Conrad HR: Vitamin E and selenium supplementation for dairy cows. In Proceedings Roche Technical Symposium: The Role of Vitamins on Animal Performance and Immune Response, Daytona Beach, 1987, p 47

192. Smith KL, Harrison JH, Hancock DD, et al: Effect of vitamin E and selenium supplementation on incidence of clinical mastitis and duration of clinical symptoms. J Dairy Sci 67:1293, 1984

193. Smith MC: Polioencephalomalacia in goats. J Am Vet Med Assoc 174:1328, 1979

194. Spatling FR: Experimental hypovitaminosis A in calves. Clinical and gross postmortem findings. Vet Rec 77:1532, 1965

195. Stafford JW, Swingle KF, Marsh H: Experimental tocopherol deficiency in young calves. Am J Vet Res 15:373, 1954

196. Steele P, Peet RL, Skirrow S, et al: Low alpha-tocopherol levels in livers of wether sheep with nutritional myopathy. Aust Vet J 56:529, 1980

197. Stuart RL: Factors affecting the vitamin E status of beef cattle. In Proceedings Roche Technical Symposium: The Role of Vitamins on Animal Performance and Immune Response, Daytona Beach, 1987, p 67

198. Sturen M: Serum 25-hydroxyvitamin D concentrations in beef cattle herds in which ruptures of the achilles tendon has occurred. Acta Vet Scand 26:169, 1985

199. Suttie JW, Jackson CM: Prothrombin structure, activation and biosynthesis. Physiol Rev 57:1, 1977

200. Tanphaichair V: Thiamin. In Hegsted DM, Chichester CO, Darby WJ, McNutt

KW, Stalvey RM, Stotz EH (eds): Nutrition Reviews' Present Knowledge in Nutrition, ed 4. New York, The Nutrition Foundation Inc, 1976, p 141
201. Taylor SI, Lambden MP, Tappel AL: Sensitive fluorometric method for tissue tocopherol analysis. Lipids 11:530, 1976
202. Tengerdy RP: Disease Resistance: Immune Response. In Machlin LJ (ed): Vitamin E: A Comprehensive Treatise. New York, Marcel Dekker, 1980, p 429
203. Tengerdy RP, Mathias MM, Nockels CF: Vitamin E, immunity and disease resistance. In Phillips M, Baetz A (eds): Diet and Resistance to Disease. New York, Plenum Press, 1981, p 27
204. The United States Pharmacoepial Convention. The United States Pharmacopeia. The National Formulary. ed 20. Easton, Mack Publishing Co, 1980
205. Thomas KW: Thiaminase in sheep. Victorian Vet Proc 39:24, 1981
206. Thomas KW: Oral treatment of polioencephalomalacia and subclinical thiamine deficiency with thiamine propyl disulphide and thiamine hydrochloride. J Vet Pharmacol Therap 9:402, 1986
207. Thornber EJ, Dunlop RH, Gawthorne JM: Thiamin deficiency in the lambs: Changes in thiamin phosphate esters in the brain. J Neurochem 33:713, 1980
208. Thornber EJ, Dunlop RH, Gawthorne JM, et al: Polioencephalomalacia (cerebrocortical necrosis) induced by experimental thiamine deficiency in lambs. Res Vet Sci 26:378, 1979
209. Thornber EJ, Dunlop RH, Gawthorne JM, et al: Induced thiamin deficiency in lambs. Aust Vet J 57:21, 1981
210. Trinder N, Hall RJ, Renton CP: The relationship between the intake of selenium and vitamin E on the incidence of retained placenta in dairy cows. Vet Record 93:641, 1973
211. Ullrey DE: Biological availability of fat-soluble vitamins: Vitamin A and carotene. J Anim Sci 35:648, 1972
212. Ullrey DE: Vitamin E for swine. J Anim Sci 53:1039, 1981
213. Van Saun RJ, Herdt TH, Stowe HD: Maternal and fetal vitamin E concentration and Se-Vitamin E interrelationship in dairy cattle. J Nutr 119:1156, 1989
214. Verbeeck J: Vitamin behavior in premixes. Feedstuffs 47(36):4, 1975
215. Vermeer C: The vitamin K-dependent carboxylation reaction. Mol Cellu Biochem 61:17, 1984
216. Völker L, Steinberg R: Recent findings of vitamin E in dairy cows and sheeps. In Roche Vitamin E Workshop, Salamanca, 1985
217. Wallis GC: Vitamin D deficiency in dairy cows: symptoms, causes and treatment. South Dakota Experiment Station Bulletin 372:3, 1944
218. Weichenthal BA, Emerick RJ, Whetzal FW et al: Influence of sodium nitrate vitamin A and protein level on feedlot performance and vitamin status of fattening cattle. J Anim Sci 22:979, 1963
219. Weiss WP, Hogan JS, Smith KL: Relationship among selenium, vitamin E and mammary gland health in commercial dairy herds. J Dairy Sci 73:381, 1990
220. Whitting F, Loosli JK: The placental and mammary transfer of tocopherols (vitamin E) in sheep, goats and swine. J Nutr 36:721, 1948
221. Wielders JPM, Mink CJK: Quantitative analysis of total thiamine in human blood, milk and cerebrospinal fluid by reversed-phase ion-pair high-performance liquid chromatography. J Chromatogr 277:145, 1983
222. Yen JT, Jensen AH, Baker DH: Assessment of the availability of niacin in corn, soybean and soybean meal. J Anim Sci 45:269, 1977
223. Zintzen H: Vitamin B$_1$ (thiamin) in the nutrition of the ruminant. Basel, F. Hoffmann-La Roche Co Ltd, 1974

Address reprint requests to

Dr. Thomas W. Graham
Department of Nutrition
University of California
Davis, CA 95616

0749–0720/91 $0.00 + .20

Toxic Effects of Trace Element Excess

Larry J. Thompson, DVM,* Jeffery O. Hall, DVM,†
and Gavin L. Meerdink, DVM‡

Trace elements are those mineral elements that occur in living tissues in such minute amounts that early analytical methods could not measure them precisely. These elements, once reported only as "trace," can now be measured into the parts per million (ppm) and parts per billion (ppb) range. The term trace element remains an accepted descriptive term for those elements that are not major mineral elements in the diet, such as calcium, phosphorus, magnesium, potassium, sodium, sulfur, and chloride. The trace elements covered in this article are aluminum, arsenic, boron, chromium, copper, fluoride, iodine, iron, lead, manganese, mercury, molybdenum, selenium, vanadium, and zinc.

Many trace elements have been shown to be essential for life and health in plants, animals, and humans while other trace elements have no clear biological function.[59] An important concept is that an essential trace element can also be a toxic trace element. The toxicity is inherent in the element and is a function of the level of exposure of the animal to that element.

A deficiency of a trace element can either be primary or secondary. A primary deficiency is that caused by an inadequate intake due to a low dietary level of that element. A secondary deficiency is when an adequate level of that trace element is present in the diet but there are one or more dietary components which inhibit utilization of the first element. One example would be a secondary copper deficiency caused by the decreasing availability of copper in the diet due to increasing

---

*Diplomate, American Board of Veterinary Toxicology; Clinical Toxicologist, Diagnostic Laboratory, New York State College of Veterinary Medicine, Cornell University, Ithaca, New York

†Research Associate, Department of Veterinary Biosciences, University of Illinois at Urbana-Champaign, Urbana, Illinois

‡Diplomate, American Board of Veterinary Toxicology; Clinical Toxicologist, Laboratories of Diagnostic Veterinary Medicine, University of Illinois at Urbana-Champaign, Urbana, Illinois

amounts of molybdenum.[30] As will be discussed, the toxic effect of a trace element present in great excess can often be to cause a secondary deficiency of another trace element.

ALUMINUM

Aluminum is the third most abundant element on the earth's crust, exceeded only by oxygen and silicon.[68] Although aluminum occurs in great abundance in the environment, water sources as well as animal tissues generally have very low aluminum concentrations. The concentration of aluminum can increase in water with a pH of 5 or less, as is commonly found in industrial waste discharge, mine leachate or volcanic regions.[3] Normal grass and clover aluminum content is in the range of 10 to 50 ppm which would be considered low in light of the much greater environmental concentrations of aluminum, including soils. Plants can contain extremely high concentrations of aluminum, with as great as 8000 ppm having been reported in mixed pasture plants.[84] Aluminum in plant material may undergo a seasonal variation with peak concentrations being achieved during the winter months.[3]

Aluminum has a very low potential for direct toxic effects and very little information is available on acute lethality in the ruminant. High concentrations of aluminum may cause gastrointestinal irritation.[84] Aluminum sulfate at 1.5% of the diet resulted in decreased feed intake suggestive of a low palatability.[7] Beef steers have been supplemented with aluminum chloride at concentrations of 300, 600, and 1200 ppm with no adverse effects on feed consumption, bodyweight or feed conversion.[106] No changes were noted in the plasma concentrations of phosphorus, calcium, magnesium, or aluminum.

The primary toxic effect of aluminum seems to be its interactions with other essential nutrients rather than a direct mechanism of action, but the ruminant does not appear to be as susceptible to these interactions as monogastrics. Aluminum incorporated into the diet has been shown to decrease fluoride uptake from the digestive tract and has been reported to be beneficial in treating fluorosis.[3,68] The most significant effect of a high aluminum diet is seen in monogastrics, where hypophosphatemia develops and can result in the development of rickets.[68] High aluminum diets have been implicated as a cause of hypomagnesemic tetany, but this theory needs further investigation. The toxicity of aluminum is increased by deficiencies of copper, iron, magnesium, or zinc.[84] Increased dietary aluminum will result in increased intestinal absorption of both zinc and iron.[3,84]

Ruminants are less susceptible to the toxic effects of aluminum and in cattle aluminum appears not to play a major role as a dietary toxicant. A diagnosis of toxic aluminum interaction would be based upon feed and forage analysis for total aluminum content. Based on previously described dietary levels, the maximum tolerable dietary concentration of aluminum for cattle is suggested to be 1000 ppm.[68]

ARSENIC

With the decreased use of arsenical herbicides, arsenic poisoning in cattle has been reduced. Arsenic is, however, ubiquitous and most foods contain minute amounts (average 0.02 ppm). Beef (muscle) usually has less than 0.5 ppm. Seafood is higher and bottom-dwelling marine organisms may contain up to 50 ppm. Trivalent herbicides and fungicides (copper acetoarsenite or Paris green, arsenic trioxide, lead arsenate), defoliants (MSMA, DSMA), oil drilling materials, and ashes from arsenic-treated lumber may contain hazardous levels of arsenic. Treated lumber, per se, does not contain sufficient concentrations of arsenic to be hazardous to livestock.

Organic arsenicals (phenylarsonic compounds) are pentavalent and cause a distinctly different syndrome than do the inorganic arsenic compounds. Organic arsenicals are used as feed additives. Cattle are tolerant to pentavalent arsenicals and feed levels of 500 ppm fed for several weeks have caused no harmful effects.[39,78]

The toxicity of arsenic depends on the formulation. Either 33 to 45 mg/kg bodyweight arsenic trioxide, 7.5 mg/kg sodium arsenite, 10 mg/kg MSMA for 5 days, or 25 mg/kg DSMA for 6 days can be lethal to cattle.[78] The trivalent arsenicals produce most of their effects by reaction with sulfhydryl (-SH) groups. This results in the blockage of carbohydrate metabolism and cellular respiration. Tissues rich in oxidative systems (e.g., alimentary tract, kidney, liver, lung, and epidermis) are affected to the greatest degree. The subsequent capillary damage and dilatation results in transudation of plasma into the intestinal tract and reduced blood volume. The usual lesions in cattle range from edema and reddening of the gastrointestinal (GI) epithelium to necrosis with sloughing. The fluid GI contents are usually foul smelling and may contain blood or shreds of mucosa. A soft pale yellow liver and pulmonary congestion or generalized congestion is usually evident. In addition to the gross GI lesions, histopathologic changes may include renal tubular degeneration, hepatic fatty change and necrosis, capillary degeneration in vascular beds of GI tract, skin, and other organs.[39] Pentavalent arsenicals will affect myelin sheaths, resulting in peripheral nerve paralysis which is a syndrome reported in swine but not cattle. Arsenicals are excreted rapidly by the kidney and meat residues are unlikely in exposed cattle.[78]

Arsenic can cause sudden death but not without some clinical signs associated with severe abdominal pain and GI tract damage. Cattle will often show clinical signs of depression, anorexia, rumen atony, and dehydration due to watery or bloody diarrhea. Signs may progress to hematuria, extreme weakness, and seizures. Body temperatures may be above or below normal.

Dimercaprol (British anti-Lewiste or BAL) is considered the treatment of choice for arsenic poisoning but its use is often disappointing in cattle and other supportive therapy must be included (e.g., fluid electrolyte therapy).[19] Combinations of BAL and thioctic acid have been found to be more beneficial than BAL alone.[12] Treatment details for arsenic-poisoned cattle can be found elsewhere.[78]

Arsenic tends to concentrate in liver and kidney and analysis of these body tissues, along with other tissues and rumen contents, is required for diagnostic confirmation of arsenic poisoning. These tissues should be collected at necropsy as well as rumen contents for analysis.[84] Urine and blood can be analyzed from the antemortem patient.

BORON

Boron is a non-metallic trace element that is commonly combined in a variety of chemical formulations to provide a vast array of useful products. When added to steel in very small concentrations, boron provides an increase in hardness and heat resistance but can also be added to other metals such as titanium for the same purpose.[68] Boron is utilized in manufacturing of glass, soaps, enamels, wood preservatives, abrasives, high energy fuel, deoxidizing agents, fertilizers, and pigments. Borax, a compound containing boron, is utilized as a pH modifier in drilling muds for oil field purposes.[11]

Boron is found at varying concentrations in relatively all plant material, soils, and water sources. Localized water sources may contain greater than the 5 ppm boron suggested as an allowable maximum in water for livestock, as is seen in several water sources in Nevada.[33,68] Water concentrations of boron have been found as high as 80 ppm in the borax flats of Nevada. Boron has been shown to be an essential nutrient for proper growth of higher plants and boron deficiencies can be seen in a variety of plants when the dry matter boron concentration is less than 15 ppm.[68] However, it should be noted that monocotyledon plants generally require and contain less boron than dicotyledons.[59] Since boron can also be toxic to plants at high concentration and boron is of low toxicity to mammals, the accumulation of boron in plants would not be expected to result in naturally occurring toxicoses.

Although boron has not been proved to be an essential element in animals there are some indications that boron may play an important physiologic role in animals. It has been suggested that boron plays a role in cholecalciferol metabolism as well as the metabolism of calcium, phosphorus, and magnesium.[59] Boron is also reabsorbed by the kidneys after filtration, which is considered unusual for an ion that is not of physiologic need.[33]

Boron is of low toxicity but marginally high boron intake can cause chronic adverse effects. Cattle supplemented with 150 ppm and 300 ppm boron in the water displayed a decrease in feed consumption and weight loss.[33] These findings may be a result of a direct gastric irritation or renal damage which has been seen in laboratory animal experiments at dosages below an acute lethal dose.[59,68] A testicular degeneration with sperm agenesis has also been described from high dietary boron in both the rat and the dog.[109] Cattle ingesting water containing 150 and 300 ppm boron have developed swelling and irritation of the skin around the dewclaws and were lethargic with a mild diarrhea at the higher dose.[109]

Cattle erroneously exposed to high concentration boron materials can develop acute boron toxicosis. The two types of high concentration boron materials associated with cattle deaths have been boron fertilizers[83,94] and borax utilized as a pH modifier for oil field drilling muds.[11] Both sources of high concentration boron material have resulted in similar clinical signs associated with a gastroenteritis and neurologic problems. The GI syndrome has been described as a severe hemorrhagic gastroenteritis accompanied with a greenish diarrhea and dehydration.[83,94] Affected animals also develop weakness and incoordination that progresses to recumbency and death. In these two acute boron poisonings there were no significant gross necropsy lesions.

The diagnosis of boron toxicoses is based upon chemical analysis of tissues for boron content. It is also beneficial to have an adequate history of potential boron exposure and analysis of suspect sources. Boron ingestion can be approximated by analysis of urine.[108]

CHROMIUM

Chromium is widely distributed in both the environment and animal tissues.[59,68] Chromium is used extensively in industry for chrome plating, leather tanning, steel fabrication, production of paints and pigments, wood treatment, and as corrosive inhibitors in the oil field industry.[50,59,68,101] Trivalent chromium as chromic oxide has also been utilized as a fecal marker in digestibility and absorption studies for many species.[44]

Chromium functions in several key metabolic processes. The trivalent form of chromium is necessary for the proper metabolic functioning of glucose. Chromium has also been shown to be essential for proper lipid metabolism, amino acid metabolism, and nucleic acid metabolism.[59,68]

Chromium toxicosis in cattle is probably of minimal concern in all but the most unusual circumstance. Plant material has been shown to contain chromium at 0.1 to 5.0 ppm, but concentrations as great as 3000 ppm have been reported.[84] Hexivalent chromium is considered to be much more toxic than trivalent chromium and may be a direct result of its increased systemic absorption.[59] Both hexivalent chromium and dichromate are easily converted to trivalent chromium in mammalian systems,[68] but the burning of chromium treated wood does not produce heat of the magnitude necessary to convert dichromate to trivalent chromium.[101] Acute chromium toxicoses are associated with severe congestion and inflammation of the digestive tract, kidney damage, and liver damage. Chronic toxicosis is associated with digestive irritation, scouring, and dermatitis.[50,59,68,84] The precipitating and oxidizing properties are thought to be the basis of chromium associated tissue damage. The damage to the digestive mucosa can be severe enough to result in complete sloughing of the gastric mucosa. In severe acute toxicoses, death can be rapid without the appearance of struggle.[50]

Chromic oxide has been used as a fecal digestion marker in cattle at levels of up to 3000 ppm for extended periods of time without adverse effects and therefore 3000 ppm chromium as the oxide has been suggested to be the maximum tolerable dietary level. It has also been suggested that chromic chloride have a maximum tolerable dietary concentration of 1000 ppm.[68] Although the maximum safe dietary concentration of hexivalent chromium has not been established, it has been observed that oral administration of 50 ppm of hexivalent chromium has been associated with growth depression, liver damage, and kidney damage in experimental animals.[59] Oil field contamination with hexivalent chromium has been associated with cases of cattle death.[50] Cattle exposed to ammonium chromate, with a chromium concentration of 436,000 ppm, were found to have severe inflammation and reddening of the abomasum on gross necropsy and severe hepatic congestion on histopathologic examination. The death of two heifers having access to an oil field drilling site was attributed to the exposure to zinc chromate that contained chromium at 10,800 ppm.[50] A clinical case of arsenic toxicosis and suspected chromium toxicosis in a herd of cattle exposed to ashes of chromium and arsenic treated wood has been reported.[101] Since gross and histopathologic changes associated with chromium toxicosis and arsenic toxicosis are indistinguishable, and the ashes of the treated wood were high in concentrations of both elements, it could not be discerned which element was the primary cause of death or if the elements acted synergistically.

Chromium has interactions with other metals such as zinc, iron, and vanadium.[59,68] These interactions appear to be of a competitive nature at the sites of absorption. However, it is possible that chromium also interacts at the molecular level with proteins in enzyme systems when ingested at excessive concentrations.

COPPER

Copper has been shown to be an essential trace element for both plants and animals but can be toxic under certain conditions. A deficiency of copper has been associated with cardiac lesions and sudden death or "falling disease" in cattle,[9] achromotrichia, bone disorders, reproductive failure, and poor growth.[105] Copper has a complex relationship with molybdenum and sulfur and when high dietary concentrations of molybdenum are present relative to that of copper, a progressive copper depletion occurs. In the rumen molybdenum and sulfur combine to form thiomolybdates that can be absorbed and combine with copper to hold it in a biologically unavailable form.[46,99] The optimum dietary copper to molybdenum ratio (Cu : Mo) in cattle is between 6 : 1 and 10 : 1. A Cu : Mo ratio less than 2 : 1 could result in a copper deficiency while increasing the Cu : Mo over 10 : 1 will increase the risk of developing copper toxicosis, particularly in sheep.[78] Different species of animals show varying responses to dietary copper, with cattle being sensitive to deficiencies of copper while sheep are more sensitive to copper excesses on both an acute and chronic basis. Copper in livestock feed is generally recognized as safe by the FDA and although the NRC places the requirement at 10 ppm[70,71] cattle rations are routinely supplemented in the 30 to 40 ppm range. Specific recommendations for the treatment of animals with copper toxicosis can be found elsewhere.[78]

Inorganic sources of copper used in feed supplements include the sulfate, carbonate, and oxide forms with the sulfate in most common usage. Chelated sources of copper are also available. Although many injectable sources of copper have been tested, copper glycinate and copper EDTA are most widely accepted.[45] Copper-containing glass pellets and copper oxide needles are given orally and remain in the GI tract to slowly release copper. Copper concentrations in plants are generally in the range of 2 to 20 ppm dry matter and vary with the plant age and species, soil content, and environmental conditions.[46] Normal drinking water sources rarely contain significant amounts of copper and 0.5 ppm is the recommended safe upper limit for livestock.[78] Water can be a significant source of copper when treated with copper-based algaecides, contaminated with older pesticides such as Bordeaux mixture, or when copper sulfate is added for use as a footbath. Local contamination from mining waste or industrial activity can also occur. Other sources of excess copper may be poultry or swine waste as these two species are often supplemented with high dietary levels of copper and are relatively resistant to copper toxicosis.

Acute copper toxicosis in cattle can occur in two ways. The first is the ingestion of large amounts of copper salts over a short period of time. This is a relatively rare occurrence in cattle but can occur as the result of gross feed or mineral mix misformulation, contamination of feed with copper compounds, or when animals are forced to drink water treated with copper sulfate or other copper compounds.[56] When dissolved in water, copper sulfate is more toxic than an equal amount in the dry crystalline form.[18] The excess copper will cause a gastroenteritis and clinical signs may include abnormal pain, diarrhea, and death with post mortem findings of congestion and hemorrhages in the GI tract and a blue-green coloration of the gut contents.[45] Copper concentrations in serum and gut contents will be greatly elevated with liver and kidney concentrations varying from normal to elevated.

A second type of acute copper toxicosis has occurred following the use of injectable copper preparations. In one clinical case animals become weak and lethargic within 24 hours after injection of cupric hydroxyquinoline and many showed hemoglobinuria and icterus.[67] Severely affected animals died in 3 to 12 days following the injection. Those dying at 5 to 7 days after injection had fluid accumulation in the body cavities. In another case clinical signs of hindlimb weakness, ataxia, excess salivation, and hyperexcitability developed in 15 of 40 yearling calves dosed with 120 mg of copper disodium edetate.[15] Massive hepatic necrosis was found in animals that died. Animals from the herd were shown to be deficient in both copper and selenium and had been injected with sodium selenate at the same time. Although both copper/selenium and copper/iron interactions have been shown, their relationship in acute copper toxicosis is unknown. Clinical cases of acute copper toxicosis from injectables remain uncommon, especially in light of the great number of animals treated. One side effect of parenteral copper administration that is not uncommon is the swelling and formation of sterile abscesses at the injection site.[22,23] In this regard copper disodium EDTA generally causes less localized reaction but is potentially more toxic than copper glycinate.[10] Subcutaneous injection using aseptic technique, in the brisket, is the preferred method of administration.[1]

Chronic copper toxicosis may develop over a period of weeks to months but the onset of clinical signs is usually very rapid. With dietary excess, copper will slowly accumulate in the liver until stress and a sudden release of copper into the bloodstream occurs, causing hemolysis, methemoglobinemia, hemoglobinuria, and kidney damage.[78] Other liver insults or pre-existing liver dysfunction will cause increased sensitivity to elevated dietary copper. The preruminant calf is most sensitive to excess dietary copper and tolerance appears to increase with age.

Weight gains and feed efficiency were similar in young calves fed milk replacer containing 10 ppm or 50 ppm dietary copper but were reduced in calves fed over 200 ppm copper. Calves survived 500 ppm copper for 6 weeks but deaths occurred after 21 days of 1000 ppm copper. Clinical signs of anorexia, icterus, and hemoglobinuria were seen in affected calves. Post mortem findings included generalized icterus and darkly discolored kidneys with liver copper concentrations of 3855 ppm DM.[49] Clinical cases of chronic copper toxicosis were reported in 10 to 12 week old calves fed milk replacer containing 115 ppm copper.[91] Subsequent experiments using milk replacers containing 72 ppm or 115 ppm copper produced no health problems in the calves but after 13 weeks histologic changes in the liver and kidneys were seen in both groups along with greatly elevated copper concentrations. With elevated liver copper concentrations and liver damage evident a hemolytic crisis could have likely been triggered by a stress such as weaning.[91] Calves fed 300 ppm copper sulfate for 2 weeks developed clinical signs of excessive thirst and lethargy along with evidence of hemolysis and liver damage, including hemoglobinuria and icterus.[110]

Older cattle appear to be more resistant to excess dietary copper, although clinical cases and experimental studies both vary widely in results and are difficult to standardize into a final recommendation. Swine feed containing 200 to 250 ppm copper was reported to cause typical clinical signs of chronic copper toxicosis and death in a heifer and a Jersey cow.[102] The animals had been receiving the diets for 5 to 6 months and elevated serum and liver copper concentrations were found. Experimentally, copper sulfate was dosed at 0.5 to 8.0 g per day to 200 kg steers and no effects or differences were seen after 16 months.[18] Yearling steers dosed with 12 g per day of copper sulfate in a gelatin capsule showed elevated liver copper concentrations after 65 days but no abnormal clinical signs or performance. However, steers given 12 g per day of copper sulfate in a water drench died at 65 days after developing typical clinical signs.[18] Deaths were reported in dairy cattle after receiving either 11 or 22 g day of copper sulfate for 6 months.[98] In addition to icterus and liver damage, intestinal hemorrhage was also reported. Two of 80 dairy cattle fed a ration containing chicken litter for 10 days developed clinical signs of icterus and hemoglobinuria and died within 48 hours.[8] Both serum and liver concentrations of copper were greatly elevated. The chicken litter contained 620 ppm copper, which elevated the complete diet to 300 ppm copper. Adjusting the Cu:Mo ratio to 9:1 with sodium molybdate prevented further problems.

The current maximum tolerable level of dietary copper for cattle is 100 ppm.[68] Adult cattle appear to be able to tolerate higher levels for several weeks to months before developing clinical signs. Consideration must be given to other dietary elements, especially molybdenum and sulfur, which act to decrease copper absorption and thus protect the animal from chronic copper toxicosis. Young calves appear to be more sensitive to excess dietary copper than adult cattle and a maximum tolerable level of 50 ppm or less of dietary copper is suggested.

FLUORINE

Fluorine or its chemically bound form, fluoride (as found in nature), causes chronic toxicosis in the bovine from the gradual accumulation of the element in osseous tissues. Forage contamination has been associated with the manufacturing processes of smelter operations and rock phosphate for fertilizers. Water levels may also be increased by industrial or natural bedrock contamination. Plant uptake of the element is usually not an important source for cattle but plant uptake is greater in acid soils and can be decreased by liming.

Table 1. *Relationship Between Fluoride Content of the Diet and the Development of Various Symptoms in Cattle*[*]

	Total Fluorine in Diet (ppm)			
CLINICAL SIGNS	20–30	30–40	40–50	50
Discernible dental mottling[†]	yes	yes	yes	yes
Enamel hypoplasia score No. 4[†]	no	no	yes	yes
Slight gross periosteal hyperostosis	no	yes	yes	yes
Moderate gross periosteal hyperostosis	no	no	yes	yes
Significant incidence of lameness	no	no	no	yes
Decreased milk production	no	no	no	yes
Skeletal fluorine equal to 5000 ppm at 5 years[‡]	no	no	no	yes

*Adapted from National Research Council: Effects of Fluorides in Animals. Washingon, DC, National Academy of Science, 1974
†Only if fluoride is present during formation period of the tooth
‡Measurement of metatarsal bone, fat free basis

Acute fluoride poisoning is rare but can occur in cattle with a single dose in the range of 50 to 70 mg/kg bodyweight or 6 to 20 mg/kg for several days.[84] Table 1 lists the chronic effects associated with dietary levels.

About half of the fluorides absorbed from the intestinal tract are excreted in the urine. The remainder is taken up by bone and teeth. The release of fluoride from osseous tissues is very slow after intake is reduced. Fluoride affects osteoblastic activity and/or hydroxyapatite crystalline structure which results in sclerosis and exostosis and occasionally osteoporosis. Teeth become less resistant to wear and appear chalky, mottled, or stained because of softened enamel. Tooth changes, particularly in the enamel, occur during the time of tooth development.[78]

Acute fluorosis will cause a rapid onset of GI irritation with diarrhea, muscle weakness, dyspnea, and possible respiratory and cardiac failure. Most often fluorosis is a chronic disease which gradually develops by the slow accumulation of the element from high dietary intake. Tooth lesions will be evident and cattle may lap water because of dental pain. Lameness may be evident due to exostosis and mineralization of ligaments and muscle insertions. Fluoride does not affect articular cartilage and does not accumulate in soft tissues. Poor reproductive performance, anemia, and hypothyroidism have been associated with excess fluoride intake and many of these sequelae are likely due to impaired mobility and inanition.[93]

Dietary additions of some aluminum salts and defluorinated rick phosphate may increase the excretion of excess fluorides from tissues. Other treatment involves removal of the source of fluoride and relief of the skeletal pain. A diagnosis of fluorosis is based upon chemical analysis of urine and bone. Urine values should be adjusted to a specific gravity of 1.04 to reduce comparison error. Rib or mandible have become standards for the measurement of body burdens of fluoride. A diagnosis of fluorosis should not be based only upon tooth changes. If due to fluoride, the tooth lesions occur at the time of development and remain regardless of the body burden of the element.[78,84,93]

IODINE

Iodine is essential for normal synthesis of thyroid hormones and a deficiency of iodine can result in thyroid enlargement or goiter, stunted growth, weak calves, and reproductive problems.[13] Deficiencies may occur from eating feeds grown on iodine deficient soils, such as occurs in the northwestern United States and areas surrounding the Great Lakes, or from the presence of goitrogenic substances.[40] Iodine is widely distributed in nature but present in only small amounts in common feedstuffs. The requirement for dietary iodine is given at 0.5 ppm or approximately 1 mg/day for a 500-kg cow.[70] Toxic effects in cattle have only been reported for iodine-containing feed additives. Two common dietary sources of iodine are iodized salt and ethylenediamine dihydriodide (EDDI) but other sources can include potassium and sodium salts. Iodized salt can contain 0.01% iodine (100 ppm). Continuous feeding of EDDI at 50 mg/head/day has been recommended to prevent foot rot and lumpy jaw, with levels of 400 to 500 mg/head/day EDDI for 2 to 3 weeks recommended for treatment of foot rot or lumpy jaw.[78]

Iodine has a very wide range between the minimum daily required dose and the acute toxic dose. Younger animals seem to be more susceptible than adults to the effects of excess iodine. Calves 10 to 14 weeks of age had depressed feed intake and weight gain when dietary levels of iodine exceeded 50 ppm.[72] After 14 days at 100 or 200 ppm dietary iodine calves exhibited chronic coughing and shortly thereafter exhibited profuse nasal discharge. No deaths occurred and some calves receiving 100 ppm recovered by the end of the 144 day trial. When fed to calves weighing approximately 200 kg, EDDI at either 50 mg/head/day or 500 mg/head/day had no effect on weight gain or response to experimentally induced infectious bovine rhinotracheitis.[88] However, the calves at 500 mg/herd/day coughed more and produced more nasal discharge.

In clinical cases where dairy herds were receiving from approximately 68 up to 600 mg/head/day EDDI, clinical signs included respiratory tract disease, naso-ocular discharge, dry hair coat, increased calving interval and non-responsive hock lesions.[77] When iodine content of the diets was reduced to 12 mg/head/day, within 1 to 4 weeks respiratory and naso-ocular signs resolved and most herds experienced a milk production increase with no other changes in diet. Dairy cattle receiving a calculated 12,000 mg/head/day iodine as EDDI for 30 days showed clinical signs of decreased feed intake, nasal and lacrimal discharge, rapid breathing and decreased milk production.[65] There was also a high abortion rate occurring in cows that were in the first trimester of pregnancy when the high iodine intake began. Because of higher milk production these cows that receiving more iodine-containing concentrate than cows that were later in gestation. Iodine freely crosses the placenta and concentrates in the fetus due to lack of efficient urinary excretion by the fetus.[63] Residual effects on reproduction following iodine withdrawal from the feed could not be detected and other clinical signs resolved rapidly.[65] Another survey of herds with chronic iodine intakes in excess of 164 mg/head/day showed scaly dermatitis, coughing, nasal discharge, lacrimation, conjunctivitis, and loss of hair around the eyes to be common clinical signs.[42] Decreases in cell-mediated and humoral immune responses have also been reported.[34]

Because of its expectorant action the use of iodine as EDDI in mild respiratory infections has been suggested.[41] However, the use of EDDI can be detrimental to some cattle exposed to stress and infectious agents[58] and currently there is no clear efficacy of iodine administration in bovine respiratory disease.

A tentative diagnosis of iodine toxicosis can be made by the presence of compatible clinical signs and evidence of high levels of dietary iodine. Total serum iodine in normal cattle is usually $25-50$ $\mu g/100$ ml ($0.25-0.50$ ppm) but can range up to 300 $\mu g/100$ ml.[13,84] Serum levels of iodine over 1600 $\mu g/100$ ml have been reported in clinically affected animals.[78,78a] EDDI intake can be estimated if serum iodine concentration is known.[2] Treatment of affected animals should include removal of excess iodine from the diet and supportive care as needed.

IRON

Iron is one of the most abundant trace elements and is essential for all plants and animals. Iron is an integral part of many oxidation/reduction reactions and is required for hemoglobin, myoglobin, cytochromes, and other enzyme systems. Iron deficiency is associated with the lack of oxygen carrying capacity caused by a decrease in red blood cell production and function.[59,68] Animals deficient in iron will exhibit reduced growth rate, anorexia, and pale mucous membranes. Mild anemias occur in iron deficient neonates but cattle under natural field conditions will generally not exhibit clinical anemia from iron deprivation unless they have also experienced a loss of blood. Blood loss sufficient to produce iron deficiency can occur from direct loss as a result of lacerations or from external or internal parasites. Animals with blood loss are highly susceptible to iron deficiency because a majority of body iron is associated with the red blood cell.

Iron can be found in relatively all potential nutrient sources but can occur at very low concentrations in some materials. The iron content of plant material is dependent upon the plant, soil type, and total iron content of the soil. Plant material can contain iron in a range from 40 to 3850 ppm.[59] Cereal grains can contain 30 to 60 ppm while normal leguminous plants contain 200 to 400 ppm. Feed materials of animal origin are generally higher in iron content than those of plant origin.[68] Water can also contain significant amounts of iron, although most water supplies contain less than 1 ppm. Some water sources have been found to contain as much as 180 ppm iron.[31]

Iron is poorly eliminated from the body and the normal homeostatic regulation of iron occurs at the intestinal epithelium.[59,68] Ruminants appear to be able to increase the intestinal absorption of iron in the presence of low iron intake.[5] The chemical form of the iron will affect the systemic absorption and plays an important role in the absorption of potentially toxic amounts of iron. Ferrous compounds (water soluble iron) are generally much more bioavailable than ferric compounds. Ferrous chloride, ferrous sulfide, and ferrous carbonate were each well absorbed systemically while ferric oxide did not appear to have systemic absorption and had a much longer GI transit time.[5] Toxic effects associated with chronic high iron intake include decreased feed intake, decreased weight gain, and decreased feed efficiency. In experiments to determine minimum toxic dietary iron concentrations, calves were fed total dietary iron concentrations of 100, 500, 1000, and 2000 ppm in the form of iron citrate.[51] Although there was a trend for the iron to decrease average daily gain and decrease feed efficiency, the results were not considered statistically significant. In a second experiment, calves were fed dietary concentrations of 1000, 2500, and 4000 ppm iron as iron citrate. At the highest dietary iron level (4000 ppm) the calves developed a severe diarrhea along with decreased feed intake and were then switched to a diet containing 2000 ppm iron. As in the first experiment, there was decreased average daily gain, decreased feed intake, and decreased feed efficiency. Significant changes in average daily gain and feed efficiency were observed at the 2500 and 4000 ppm supplemental iron levels. A tendency to decrease the average daily gain and feed efficiency was observed with total dietary iron as low as 500 ppm although the decreases were of marginal significance. The highest dietary iron also caused an increase in serum iron and blood hemoglobin, while serum phosphorus was decreased.[51] Dietary iron fed to beef steers at 400, 1600, and 3200 ppm as ferrous sulfate produced severe weight loss at the 3200 ppm level.[97] This study also showed the correlation between increased supplemental iron and decreased feed intake, average daily gain, and feed efficiency. Dietary iron concentrations over 1600 ppm produced significant decreases in the above parameters but at the 400 ppm level only feed efficiency showed a significant depression. There was a significant decrease in liver concentrations of copper and zinc while liver iron concentrations increased proportionally to the dose.[97]

Cattle have the possibility of being exposed to high concentrations of soluble iron in water or in other unusual circumstances such as high iron in plants. The use of irrigation water with a high iron content (17 ppm iron) has resulted in iron concentrations as high as 9980 ppm in the forage plants exposed.[21] Dairy cattle ingesting the forage with high iron content developed a dark colored, malodorous, frothy feces and had a severe decline in milk production, bodyweight, and general condition. Subsequent dosing of ferric iron at rates of 15, 30, and 60 g per day for 10 days also produced a decrease in milk production, milk fat, and bodyweight. It should be noted that the experiment used iron in the ferric form, which is much less bioavailable than ferrous iron.[59,68] In a clinical case in the Ohio valley, water iron content of greater than 80 ppm was associated with decreased water intake, severe decrease in milk production, poor reproductive performance, weight loss, and marginal deficiency of selenium and copper (Hall, unpublished data).

Iron has interactive effects with a number of essential nutrients in cattle. A high dietary iron content decreased phosphorus absorption while an increase in dietary phosphorus decreased iron absorption.[96] Increases in iron and phosphorus resulted in decreased tissue concentrations of copper and zinc. High dietary iron also decreased kidney magnesium concentration. Ascorbic acid, certain sugars, several amino acids, and vitamin E may also enhance systemic iron absorption.[68] High dietary iron may have an impact on copper status in beef cattle, causing a severe depletion of copper stores.[16] It has also been suggested that high dietary iron will inhibit selenium absorption. Thus, high dietary iron may result in deficiencies of selenium, copper, and other essential nutrients.

A diagnosis of iron toxicosis would be uncommon and would be a detailed undertaking. Because excess iron in the diet results mainly in a decreased feed efficiency and feed intake as well as potentially causing deficiencies in other nutrients, it would be necessary to analyze all dietary components for iron content. In situations of selenium and copper deficiencies in the presence of adequate dietary intake, iron should be analyzed in the feed in order to determine whether potential interactive effects are occurring.

If high dietary iron is encountered, the main treatment would be to remove the cattle from the high dietary iron source. Treatment for systemic iron toxicity can be accomplished with treatments of desferrioxamine but would be extremely costly. Phlebotomy also results in depletion of iron, but would not be useful for therapy of acute cases. It has been suggested that increased phosphorus in the diet may be beneficial in decreasing systemic iron stores.[96]

In light of the available information, it is suggested that dietary iron in excess of 400 ppm could result in less than optimal feed utilization. However, the suggested dietary maximum iron concentration for cattle has been given as 1000 ppm.[68] Maximum water iron content for cattle should be less than 10 ppm.[103]

LEAD

Lead is one of the most common causes of poisoning in cattle and cases of lead toxicosis appear to be more common in late winter and spring. Discarded batteries, paint, pipe joint compounds, used motor oil, and grease are some common sources.[79] Lead-free paint may contain up to 1% lead.[84] Plants may contribute to lead intake by aerial fallout or other direct contamination. Translocation of lead to plants from soil does not contribute more than 15 μg lead/g dry weight of forage even when plants are grown in soil containing up to 700 to 3000 μg lead/g.[6]

Apparent toxicity of lead is increased by other dietary factors such as a deficiency of calcium, ascorbic acid, or nicotinic acid. An excess of zinc or cadmium will also increase the apparent toxicity of lead.[79] Lethal single doses of lead in cattle have been reported at 200 to 800 mg/kg body weight.[78,84] A daily intake of approximately 6 mg lead/kg bodyweight has been estimated to be the minimum dose that will eventually poison cattle.[6,78] A toxic cumulative dose for calves on milk is approximately 2.5 mg/kg/day for 1 to 8 weeks and a milk diet will enhance lead absorption.[84] Lead is poorly absorbed from the intestinal tract, however, solubilized forms are apparently more available and may result in more rapid onset of poisoning. Upon absorption the element combines with erythrocytes and eventually has detrimental effects in multiple body sites. A number of enzyme systems are affected, particularly those of hematopoiesis. Aminolevulinic acid (ALA) metabolism is inhibited, causing increased delta-ALA levels in urine and plasma. Lead readily crosses the placenta and has produced embryopathic effects and infertility. Abortions have been documented; however, permanent reproductive effects or teratogenic or mutagenic effects have not been described.[79] Gross lesions are usually not observed in lead toxicosis and have only been associated with ancillary effects such as anorexia or recumbency. A post mortem examination should include a thorough examination of the ingesta for evidence of source material such as oil or grease, lead plates from batteries, or paint.

Clinical signs of lead poisoning in cattle consistently involve the nervous and digestive systems. Signs may vary from blindness and depression to hyperexcitability, bellowing, and convulsive seizures. Muscle twitching (especially face and ears), grinding of teeth, excessive salivation, anorexia, and constipation or diarrhea may be observed.[79] Clinical pathologic changes are of little help early in the syndrome. A normocytic normochromic anemia develops with increased blood lead levels.

Treatment of lead toxicosis involves chelation by CaEDTA (calcium disodium edetate) at 70 to 110 mg/kg per day in divided doses for 5 days. This may be repeated after 2 days' rest.[78,79] Thiamine hydrochloride has been suggested as additional treatment at doses of 250 to 1000 mg per day. Oral magnesium sulfate might assist in hastening removal from the intestinal tract as well as limiting further absorption of the element.

Whole blood (not serum or plasma) lead levels generally provide reliable evidence of lead exposure in the antemortem animal. Cattle whole blood lead background concentrations are usually less than 0.1 ppm. Greater than 0.3 ppm suggests excessive exposure and greater than 1 ppm indicates severe exposure and a guarded prognosis.[78] Post mortem tissue analysis for lead should include liver and kidney and perhaps ingesta. When blood lead levels are questionable, erythrocyte ALA dehydrase may be useful. Calf erythrocyte ALA dehydrase increases two to threefold from 1 week to 9 weeks of age then drops to adult levels by 9 months. ALA dehydrase levels will not return to normal until the lead excretion is nearly complete.[84]

Violative lead residues in muscle are not likely from a healthy beef animal. However, milk levels could be a concern in some situations and analyses might be advisable. In one study cows with blood lead levels of 0.28 to 0.58 ppm excreted levels of 0.034 to 0.25 ppm in milk as opposed to a background of 0.06 to 0.13 ppm in milk and 0.06 to 0.18 ppm in blood.[26]

MANGANESE

Manganese is a gray/silver metal utilized in history in the production of steel to increase its strength as well as to remove the impurities of oxygen and sulphur from the iron. Manganese is also utilized in the production of cast iron, alloys of copper and aluminum, color pigments, dry cell batteries, feed supplements, and fertilizer.[68]

Both plants and animals require manganese for proper growth and function, however many plants and most animals retain minimal concentrations of manganese.[59] The concentration of manganese in plant material varies with the type of plant as well as the manganese concentration in the soil and type of soil. Most forage plants will contain from 60 ppm to greater than 800 ppm. Protein supplements of animal origin are generally low in manganese, with concentrations of 5 to 15 ppm being common. Cereal grains contain marginal to adequate manganese concentrations.[59,68]

Manganese is an essential nutrient, a constituent of several metalloenzymes, and is necessary for proper bone growth, reproductive function, lipid metabolism, carbohydrate metabolism, pancreatic function, and possibly immune function.[59] Deficiencies of manganese in cattle can result in calves born with weak or deformed legs as well as delayed estrus and poor conception rates.[86]

Manganese has a low potential for toxicity due to its poor intestinal absorption[59,112] and its efficient biliary elimination.[35,100] Feedlot calves supplemented with 0, 250, 500, and 1000 ppm manganese as manganese sulfate did not show a decrease in weight gain or feed efficiency. Blood analysis showed no effect on hematocrit, hemoglobin, plasma iron, calcium, or phosphorus content.[85] There was an increase in manganese storage in the liver and depletion of iron. The excess manganese also decreased the ability of the rumen microorganisms to digest cellulose in vitro. Young male calves were given a basal diet containing 12 ppm manganese or were supplemented with 820, 2460, or 4920 ppm added manganese.[24] At the two highest dosages the calves had decreased feed intake, feed efficiency, and weight gain. In a subsequent trial, calves were pair fed to eliminate the effects of decreased feed intake. Mild decreases in weight gain and feed efficiency still occurred which were greater at the higher manganese levels.[24] The high dietary manganese also caused an alteration in rumen bacteria, resulting in a change in volatile fatty acid production.

Manganese interacts with several other dietary nutrients. Manganese and iron appear to share a similar uptake mechanism from the digestive tract and tend to compete for intestinal absorption sites.[43,85] Manganese also exacerbates iron deficiencies which can be corrected by increasing the iron supplementation. Manganese absorption is inhibited by excess dietary calcium, cobalt, and protein.[59] The reverse is also true, where low dietary levels of these competing nutrients can enhance the toxic effects of a manganese excess.

Manganese toxicosis is not thought to occur naturally but does have the potential to be caused by feed mixing error. Minimum dietary recommendations for manganese range from 10 ppm for growing and finishing cattle to 40 ppm for dairy cattle.[59] Due to the low order of toxicity, 1000 ppm dietary manganese is the recommended maximum tolerable level.[68] Maximum water content of manganese has not been set for livestock. However, it has been recommended at less than 0.05 ppm for humans to avoid palatability problems.[31] Since manganese can adversely affect the taste of water it is suggested that excess concentrations of manganese may also decrease voluntary water consumption in livestock. Because manganese is not retained in the body to any appreciable degree, there is little concern for potential transfer into the human food chain.

MERCURY

Few sites exist in the earth's crust where mercury is found in amounts exceeding 30 ppb. mercury poisoning in cattle has become less common mainly because mercurial fungicides (e.g., Ceresan) are no longer used as seed treatment. Sources of environmental pollution, such as sewage sludge and industries using mercury, can provide opportunity for poisoning. Microorganisms are capable of converting inorganic forms of mercury to the more dangerous organic compound, methyl mercury.[17,114]

Organic mercury compounds are more readily absorbed than inorganic forms and will accumulate in tissues rapidly but inconsistently.[114] Toxic doses range from several grams of mercury salts to fractions of milligrams of organic forms if ingestion occurs continuously over several weeks. Large amounts of the inorganic mercurials can cause arsenic-like lesions of coagulative necrosis of the alimentary mucosa and blood vascular system. In cattle the more soluble forms of mercury will primarily affect vascular walls and eventually nervous tissue. Lesions can appear as interstitial nephritis, lymphadenopathy, focal hepatic necrosis, and multiple hemorrhages in serosal linings.[78]

Clinical signs can vary with and depend on the amount and type of mercury as well as the duration of exposure. Acute clinical signs from high exposures to mercury may resemble inorganic arsenic poisoning, with violent abdominal pain, epistaxis, hematuria, and bloody diarrhea.[17] Anorexia, fever, lymph node swelling, depilation (especially tailhead), salivation and lacrimation, dyspnea, eczema, skin pustules and ulcers, muscular incoordination, and lameness have been observed.[78,114]

Treatment for mercury poisoning is not specific and often unrewarding, especially in protracted cases with permanent damage to nervous and other tissues. The use of BAL (dimercaprol) has been suggested in mercury as well as arsenic poisoning. In addition, sodium thiosulfate in an aqueous solution at up to 30 g given intravenously followed by up to 60 g given orally to an adult cow at 6 hour intervals for 2 to 3 days has shown beneficial results in the early stages of poisoning.[17]

Blood, urine, feces, and milk mercury levels may not reveal elevations of the element, particularly if poisoning is recent.[84] Mercury concentrations above 100 mg/L in the urine are indicative of an excessive exposure.[17] The highest tissue levels of mercury from inorganic compounds are usually found in the kidney cortex. Kidney mercury concentrations above 3 ppm are suspicious if clinical signs and lesions are compatible.[17] Cattle poisoned with mercury likely contain significant tissue residues and would not be acceptable for human consumption.

MOLYBDENUM

Although molybdenum is known to be an essential trace element, as a constituent of xanthine oxidase and other enzymes, a deficiency of molybdenum under natural conditions has not been reported.[105] Molybdenum has a complex relationship with copper and sulfur. When high dietary concentrations of molybdenum are present relative to that of copper a progressive copper depletion occurs. In the rumen molybdenum and sulfur combine to form thiomolybdates which can be absorbed and combine with copper to hold it in a biologically unavailable form.[46,99] The optimum dietary copper to molybdenum ratio (Cu:Mo) is between 6:1 and 10:1. A Cu:Mo ratio less than 2:1 will result in a copper deficiency while increasing the Cu:Mo over 10:1 will increase the risk of developing copper toxicosis, particularly in sheep.[78] This relationship between molybdenum and copper was first reported when "Teart scours" in England was shown to be caused by excess molybdenum in pasture herbage. The severe diarrhea was controlled when the cattle were supplemented with copper.[28] At about the same time it was also discovered that the chronic copper toxicosis of sheep could be alleviated by the addition of molybdenum to the diet.[25]

Potential sources for molybdenum include air, water, soil, plant material, and feed supplements. Emissions and airborne dust in the vicinity of industrial complexes can contribute excess molybdenum to soil and herbage.[107] Although water can contribute to molybdenum intake, no confirmed cases of molybdenum toxicosis were related to contaminated drinking water[107] and currently there is no suggested maximum limit of concentration.[78]

Acute molybdenum toxicosis can occur when the diet contains 20 ppm or greater of molybdenum. Young animals and lactating cows appear more susceptible. Clinical signs include a severe diarrhea containing gas, bubbles, anorexia, emaciation, and the development of a dry haircoat with achromotrichia.[59,78] More common is the occurrence of chronic molybdenum toxicosis involving a relative deficiency of copper. Molybdenum concentrations above 5 to 6 ppm can cause a toxicosis in cattle if the Cu:Mo ratio is below 2:1 and adequate or high sulfur/sulfate is present in the diet.[113] This chronic situation involves a relative excess of molybdenum and deficiency of copper that can result in depressed growth, anemia, bone disorders, and achromotrichia. Additional problems that have been reported include impaired reproduction performance, cardiovascular defects, and GI disorders.[59,78]

A diagnosis of molybdenum toxicosis is based upon the presence of compatible clinical signs and analysis of the diet for molybdenum and copper. In certain instances the levels of sulfur or sulfate in the diet and water should be evaluated also.[53] Tissue levels of molybdenum will be increased and copper levels will be decreased. In the live animal, urine and milk concentrations will increase with increasing molybdenum in the diet.[84] Treatment of molybdenum toxicosis involves removing the source of excess molybdenum (if possible) and supplying additional copper to the animal, either in the diet or parenterally. Dietary additions of copper should be directed at obtaining adequate copper supplementation, including an optimum Cu:Mo ratio.[78]

NICKEL

Nickel is an essential element with a low potential for deficiency under natural conditions. Dietary absorption is less than 10% and urinary elimination appears to be equal to absorption.[75] The dietary nickel requirements for cattle have been estimated to be 0.3 to 0.35 ppm since rumen bacteria may require nickel as an enzyme co-factor.[59] Nickel occurs very commonly in pasture plant material at concentrations of 0.5 to 3.5 ppm on a dry matter basis[59] and is probably related to soil content.[74] Other common components of cattle diets that have been tested include corn, 0.4 ppm; oats, 1 ppm; soybean meal, 3.6 ppm; alfalfa meal, 1.4 ppm; cottonseed hulls, 0.6 ppm;[75] wheat, 0.08 to 0.3 ppm; sunflower cake, 7.78 ppm.[59] Since most of the potential dietary sources of nickel have concentrations greater than the proposed minimum dietary requirement, it seems unlikely that a naturally occurring nickel deficiency would be encountered.

The interaction of nickel with other dietary materials has been shown to occur, including the antagonism of iron, zinc, and copper.[59] Deficiencies in iron, zinc, or copper can increase the potential toxic effects of high dietary nickel, while high dietary nickel enhances the deficiencies of these nutrients. As with other metal interactions, nickel probably interacts with iron, zinc, and copper by competing for binding sites on enzymes and for sites of absorption.

Natural dietary nickel intake has a low potential for causing overt toxicosis. Experimentally, very high dietary nickel content primarily causes a decrease in feed palatability[74] and a direct GI irritation.[59] Elemental nickel as nickel carbonate supplemented at 62.5 or 250 ppm in the diet of calves did not produce adverse health effects but at 1000 ppm there was a significant decrease in daily rate of gain and total daily feed consumption.[75] At the 1000 ppm dietary concentration there was an increase in percent nickel absorbed, suggesting that an inherent absorption control mechanism had been overcome. Elemental nickel, as nickel carbonate, at 50 or 250 ppm in adult lactating dairy cow rations had no adverse health effects.[73] Nickel chloride was shown to be more toxic than nickel carbonate in palatability studies of dairy heifers.[74] Both nickel chloride and nickel carbonate had a linear depression of palatability as concentrations increased, with nickel chloride being approximately five times greater in preventing voluntary feed intake.

The nonspecific clinical signs of feed refusal and decreased weight gain that have been associated with excessive nickel in the diet make it difficult to diagnose nickel toxicosis. However, as with most feed refusal cases, of primary importance is removal of the feed source. Calves experiencing severe weight gain and feed intake depression caused by elevated dietary nickel responded by simply placing these animals on rations without elevated nickel.[75] The only way to diagnose a nickel toxicosis associated with feed is to analyze the feed for total nickel content; however, it must be stressed that the chemical nature of the nickel also plays a key role. Nickel chloride at concentrations greater than 50 ppm and nickel carbonate at concentrations greater than 250 ppm could result in a nickel toxicosis.

SELENIUM

The trace element selenium has gained widespread attention as an essential micronutrient that has complex interactions with vitamin E and other dietary components. A deficiency of selenium has been shown to cause specific disorders in cattle such as muscular dystrophy as well as general problems such as poor production and increased susceptibility to disease.[54] In 1973, a biological role for selenium was established when it was found to be an essential component of the enzyme glutathione peroxidase which functions to protect the cell from oxidative damage.[89] Selenium has a fairly narrow safety range with toxic levels only 10 to 50 times greater than the dietary requirements.[68] Selenium toxicosis (selenosis) is a world wide problem and both the acute and chronic poisoning of cattle have been reported.

Selenium can be present in soils at levels that may allow plants to accumulate selenium in quantities that can be toxic to animals. Certain selenium accumulator plants (indicator plants) may contain greater than 1000 ppm selenium.[87] These plants include some species of Astragalus, Stanleya, Haplopappus, and Machaeranthera. Other plants may accumulate selenium to a lesser degree. Those that contain 25 to 100 ppm selenium are often called secondary accumulators or facultative indicator plants and include certain species of Aster, Atriplex, Castelleja, and Gutierrezia.[48] Nonaccumulator plants growing on seleniferous soils may contain 1 to 25 ppm selenium.[37]

Inorganic forms of selenium that are used as feed sources include sodium selenite and sodium selenate. Although the selenite form appears most available to the animal, it may be more readily reduced to the poorly available elemental form of selenium. Organic forms of selenium are generally more bioavailable than inorganic forms. Injectable forms of selenium are also available, as well as slow-release bolus forms.[69]

Cattle can be acutely poisoned by ingestion of selenium accumulator plants, the ingestion of large amounts of selenium compounds, or the misuse of injectable selenium preparations. The ingestion of selenium accumulator plants is rare under field conditions because the plants are not considered palatable and many have an offensive odor. Toxicoses can occur under conditions such as limited pasture.[76] Clinical signs include abnormal posture, ataxia, dyspnea, diarrhea, prostration, and death. Abdominal pain is often apparent and bloating may occur. The clinical time course may range from several hours to several days. Treatment is supportive in nature and usually unrewarding.[68,78] A post mortem examination may show enteritis and petechial hemorrhages in the intestine and endocardium as well as congestion in the lungs and liver. A diagnosis is based upon evidence of ingestion of accumulator plants and the presence of compatible clinical signs. Analysis of the rumen contents or suspect plants for selenium content may be helpful.

Selenium supplements added in excess to complete feeds or mineral supplements can also result in acute selenosis. The single acute oral minimum lethal dose in cattle is reported at between 5 mg/kg[78] and 11 mg/kg.[66] Selenium concentrations in the diet above 25 ppm may be sufficient to produce acute poisoning in most animals.[14] Clinical signs are similar to the acute toxicosis situation caused by accumulator plants. High concentrations of selenium salts will have a direct irritant effect on mucous membranes and the GI tract similar to several other trace elements discussed in this article.

The misuse of injectable selenium preparations can also cause acute problems. In one report, 557 6-month-old calves were administered sodium selenite IM or SQ. An error in preparation resulted in the calves receiving 100 mg selenium, or approximately 0.5 mg/kg, which was over eight times the intended dose. Within 2 hours many calves showed clinical signs of severe depression, dyspnea, and excess salivation. Several calves died within 2 hours. A total of 75 calves died within 72 hours and over a period of 5 weeks a total of 376 calves died. Dyspnea was the most obvious clinical sign in calves that died later over the course of the episode.[92] A post mortem examination showed the lungs to be dark red, firm, and edematous with the interlobular septa distended by serous fluid. The heart was pale with ecchymotic hemorrhages on the epicardial surface and red streaking to the myocardium. In another report, neonatal calves tolerated 1 mg/kg IM selenium as sodium selenite.[55] However, at 2 mg/kg the calves showed clinical signs of depression, anorexia, and weakness 3 to 6 hours post injection. The calves subsequently developed dyspnea and death occurred in less than 12 hours following injection. Post mortem examination showed only mild pulmonary edema and congestion.

Chronic selenium poisoning, also known as alkali disease, was first described by Marco Polo as a necrotic disease of horses that occurred in thirteenth century China.[20] The recognition of selenium compounds as the toxic principles occurred in the early 1930s at the South Dakota State Experiment Station[29] after it was recognized that the distribution of this disease was associated with particular soil types now known to be seleniferous.[47] In cattle, chronic selenosis results from ingesting forage containing 4 to 40 ppm selenium for prolonged periods of time. The amount of selenium and the time period needed for toxic effects to be exhibited vary with individual animals. Young animals are more susceptible to selenium poisoning than older animals. Clinical signs associated with chronic selenium poisoning include loss of hair, deformities of the hoof beginning at the coronary band which can lead to sloughing of the entire hoof, decreased appetite, emaciation, and death.[48,76,78] Gross post mortem changes may include cirrhosis and atrophy of the liver and atrophy of the heart, often described as a "dishrag heart."[27,54] Signs of chronic selenosis may be expected in cattle with whole blood selenium concentrations greater than 2 ppm.[48] Treatment of chronically poisoned animals involves removal of selenium source and supportive care. Control measures should be initiated to regulate and limit selenium intake.

A paralytic syndrome in swine after chronic exposures to 19 to 24 ppm sodium selenite in the feed has been reported.[38] Similar problems in cattle have not been observed.

VANADIUM

Vanadium is a bright white metal in the pure state and occurs in a large number of naturally occurring mineral compositions. Often referred to as being rare, vanadium is actually one of the more prevalent trace elements.[68] Vanadium is utilized in the manufacture of many tools, cutting and die steels, high strength structural steels, and wear resistant cast metals.

Vanadium may be an essential element that is required at very low concentrations but the essential nature of vanadium is questioned due to an inability in many instances to reproduce findings showing a deficiency.[59] It has been suggested that vanadium is required for adequate growth and reproductive performance and may also play a role in lipid metabolism, bone development, and hematopoiesis.[4,59,68] Although vanadium is more toxic to growing animals than many other trace elements, the potential of exposure is considered minimal. It is possible, however, for animals to be exposed to high concentrations of vanadium. Dietary phosphorus supplements may contain as high as 1400 ppm vanadium.[4,59] Vanadium has also been detected in relatively high concentrations in coal, petroleum, and asphalt ash, with concentrations as great as 12% vanadium reported.[4] Plant and animal tissue generally contain very low concentrations of vanadium.

Little information is available on the potential toxicity of vanadium to cattle. No adverse effects were seen in calves given vanadium at 1, 3, 5, and 7.5 mg/kg of body weight.[82] However, vanadium at 10, 15, and 20 mg/kg bodyweight resulted in the calves exhibiting clinical signs, with a more rapid onset at the higher dosage levels. The initial clinical signs included diarrhea, anorexia, dehydration, and depression. The affected calves became emaciated, very weak, and recumbent prior to their death. Gross necropsy findings included congestion of the liver and lung, petechiation of the heart and kidney, rumenal ulcers, and hemorrhagic gastroenteritis. Cows exposed to vanadium from fuel oil ash deposited on grazing areas displayed weakness and incoordination.[68] Even though vanadium is relatively toxic, most animals appear to absorb very minimal amounts of vanadium from the digestive tract and thus have minimal systemic exposure.[4,68] In studies utilizing laboratory animals, vanadium absorption was greater than in ruminants and the variation in absorption may be due in part to the chemical nature of the vanadium used in dosing.[59] In calves dosed with vanadium as ammonium metavanadate, the highest no-effect level of 7.5 mg/kg body-weight would equal approximately 250 ppm in the diet while the lowest dosage resulting in adverse clinical effects (10 mg/kg body-weight) would equal 333 ppm, assuming a 3% bodyweight dry matter intake per day. In sheep, feed refusal and diarrhea were seen at 400 and 800 ppm dietary vanadium as ammonium metavanadate.[36] The sheep eventually refused to consume the experimental diet and were switched back to a normal diet with feed consumption returning to normal within 5 to 6 days. Both laboratory animals and poultry have demonstrated the ability to acclimate to high dietary vanadium if increased slowly over time.[59] It has also been suggested that young animals are more susceptible to vanadium toxicity than adult animals.

Vanadium has antagonistic interactions with chromium, iron, copper, chloride, and mercury.[4,68] Thus, elevated dietary levels of these minerals would decrease the toxic potential of vanadium. However, deficiencies in the essential metals would result in an increased susceptibility to vanadium toxicosis. There is evidence that the protein content of the diet and ascorbic acid may also have antagonistic relationships to vanadium.

Because vanadium is poorly absorbed and fairly rapidly excreted in the urine, the potential for bioaccumulation or a residue problem is minimal.[95] Increased dietary levels of vanadium will result in increased tissue concentrations in ruminants but the minimal elevation of vanadium in these tissues would not be of human health concern.[36,82] The potential exposure of humans from tissue residues has been thoroughly evaluated but is thought to be of minimal concern.[95]

A diagnosis of vanadium toxicosis is based upon chemical evaluation of tissues along with feed and other source material. In cases of acute exposure to vanadium the tissue of choice for analysis is kidney.[82] After an exposure to vanadium, the kidney vanadium content will decrease over time with subsequent increases in liver and bone vanadium, content.[59] To provide a margin of safety, the recommended dietary maximum of vanadium has been placed at 50 ppm.[68]

ZINC

Zinc is a bluish white metallic element which is utilized for many commercial uses including metal alloys, dry cell batteries, printing plates, and galvanized iron. Compounds of zinc are used in the manufacture of products such as cosmetics, rubber goods, wood preservatives, antibacterials, fungicides, and medicinal agents.[68]

Zinc is an essential element and is necessary for a wide variety of physiologic functions. Primary clinical manifestations of zinc deficiencies are seen as decreased weight gain, decreased feed efficiency, and parakeratosis.[57,60,90] However, it has been noted that zinc deficiencies can cause poor testicular development in growing bulls as well as the cessation of spermatogenesis.[103] Other clinical signs that have been described in zinc deficiencies include stiffness and swelling of joints, cracking and poor healing of the skin, thickening of the skin, excessive salivation, unthrifty appearance, and inflammation of the nose and mouth.[60] Zinc plays an active role in a large number of metalloenzymes, as well as a number of other zinc associated enzymes.[60,68] Many of these enzymes play important functions in carbohydrate, DNA, RNA, and amino acid metabolism. Zinc requirements for domestic animals range from 40 to 100 ppm in the diet.[68]

Zinc is common in most dietary components. Dietary components of animal origin may contain 90 to 100 ppm zinc. Normal pasture herbage ranges between 17 and 60 ppm zinc on a dry weight basis.[68] However, grass material grown on industrially contaminated soil has been found to contain as great as 7300 ppm zinc.[111]

Zinc homeostasis appears to be regulated primarily at the site of absorption in the duodenum and small intestine.[60,68] Regulation in the absorbence of zinc occurs such that deficient animals will preferentially absorb more dietary zinc while in animals with adequate zinc intake the absorption rate will be lower. Zinc excretion from the body is minimal, with small amounts being lost in the urine, bile and pancreatic secretions. There is also zinc lost from the digestive tract by sloughing of mucosal epithelium cells. Ruminants do not appear to have appreciable body stores of zinc necessary to meet their requirements in times of deficiency. Cattle experiencing deficiency for even such short periods as 2 to 3 weeks develop clinical manifestation of zinc deficiencies.[90]

Chronic zinc excess appears to primarily affect the digestive tract. Marginally high elevations in zinc have caused decreased feed consumption, decreased feed efficiency, and decreased weight gain.[68] Beef calves fed zinc in the diet at 0, 1000, 2000, and 3000 ppm showed no clinical signs of toxicosis but did have decreased feed consumption and average daily gain.[80] The average daily gain, average daily feed intake, and feed-to-gain ratio showed significant depressions at the two higher concentrations while the average daily gain and feed-to-gain ratio were only marginally affected at the 1000 ppm zinc concentration. It was also determined that concentrations of 100 or 500 ppm zinc as zinc oxide produced no adverse effects on feed intake, weight gain, or feed efficiency.[80] Zinc oxide fed to lactating dairy cows at concentrations of 0, 500, 1000, and 2000 ppm had no adverse effects on milk production or blood chemistries.[62] There was an increase in milk zinc that was not proportional to the elevations in plasma zinc. Lactating dairy cattle fed supplemental zinc at 0, 1000, and 2000 ppm in the form of zinc sulfate monohydrate had decreased milk yield and feed intake after several weeks.[52] It was also observed that removal of the high supplemental zinc allowed the animals to return to normal feed intake and milk yield, with the exception of having lower calf weights at their next parturition.

A severe acute toxicosis can occur in cattle exposed to high dietary zinc. Feed mixing errors and herbage contamination from zinc metal processing facilities have resulted in clinical signs of severe diarrhea, anorexia, weight loss, and decreased milk production.[2,111] A case of zinc toxicosis associated with industrial contamination of forage reported submandibular edema, ulcerations of the esophagus, and chronic gastritis.[111] Elevations in tissue zinc were found as well as increases in lead and decreases in copper. Herbage from the contaminated farm was found to contain 3000 to 7300 ppm zinc. There was also excess lead in the herbage, which is not unexpected, as lead is found with zinc in several ores and is a common contaminant of zinc materials. Another case of zinc toxicosis was associated with zinc oxide added to a feed, in place of magnesium oxide, at a final concentration of 20,000 ppm.[2] Post mortem findings revealed a pulmonary emphysema, pale myocardium, hemorrhaging in the cortex and medulla of both kidneys, and degenerative changes in the liver. The cattle showed a dramatic decrease in milk production, severe diarrhea, and icterus. The animals had a 10-fold increase in liver and kidney zinc concentrations as well as decreased copper concentrations. Some cattle had pale mucous membranes due to anemia as has been reported in other animals exposed to very high dietary zinc.[68] A case of zinc toxicosis due to excess zinc sulfate in milk replacer reported a concentration of 706 ppm, which is below the concentration in a number of studies that resulted in no adverse effects.[32] Young calves in a veal operation where dietary iron is usually restricted may be more sensitive to the toxic effects of excess zinc.

Zinc has a profound interactive effect with a number of essential nutrients. Zinc has been shown to decrease the absorption of copper and thus over time the excess zinc can cause a gradual depletion of the body reserve of copper.[61,81,104] A number of studies have shown that excess zinc can decrease hepatic concentrations of iron and copper[68] but others have shown an actual increase in liver iron.[81] Calcium and phosphorus have been shown not to play a dramatic role in the metabolism of zinc but increased dietary phosphorus did improve both feed intake and feed efficiency in zinc dosed calves.[52] Excess dietary cadmium can decrease zinc absorption in calves[60] and deficiencies in selenium may increase the potential toxicity of excess zinc in the diet.[68]

A diagnosis of zinc toxicosis is based upon compatible clinical signs and the finding of high concentrations of zinc in the tissues and diet of affected animals. A problem associated with the analysis of serum or plasma is contamination with zinc stearate from the rubber parts of most disposable syringes and blood collection tubes.[64] The use of all-plastic disposable syringes and special trace element blood collection tubes or plastic screw-top tubes will avoid this rubber-associated zinc contamination. Zinc concentrations in serum samples can also be elevated due to hemolysis.

Based on the available information, it would be unusual to experience a severe zinc toxicosis in adult cattle. A toxicosis would be anticipated with diets that contain greater than 2000 ppm zinc while marginal problems may be caused by as low as 1000 ppm zinc. It has been suggested that the maximum tolerable dietary level of zinc for cattle is 500 ppm.[68] It has also been suggested that water zinc content should be limited to 25 ppm.

REFERENCES

1. Allcroft R, Uvarov O: Parenteral administration of copper compounds to cattle with special reference to copper glycine (copper amino-acetate). Vet Rec 71:797–810, 1959
2. Allen GS: An outbreak of zinc poisoning in cattle. Vet Rec 83:8–9, 1968
3. Allen VG: Influence of dietary aluminum on nutrient utilization in ruminants. J Anim Sci 59:836–844, 1984
4. Ammerman CB, Fick KR, Hansard SL, et al: Toxicity of certain minerals to domestic animals: A review. Fla Agric Exp Stn Res Bull AL73-6:1-36-6:1–36, 1973
5. Ammerman CB, Wing JM, Dunavant BG, et al: Utilization of inorganic iron by ruminants as influenced by form of iron and iron status of the animal. J Anim Sci 26:404–410, 1967
6. Aronson AL: Outbreaks of plumbism in animals associated with industrial lead operations. In Oehme FW (ed): Toxicity of Heavy Metals in the Environment. New York, Marcel Dekker, 1978, pp 173–177
7. Bailey CV: Influence of aluminum hydroxide on the solubility of silicic acid in rumen fluid and the absorption of silicic acid from the digestive tract of ruminants. Can J Anim Sci 57:239–244, 1977
8. Banton MI, Nicholson SS, Jowett PLH, et al: Copper toxicosis in cattle fed chicken litter. J Am Vet Med Assoc 191:827–828, 1987
9. Bennetts HW, Beck AB, Harley R: The pathogenesis of falling disease. Studies on copper deficiency in cattle. Aust Vet J 24:237–244, 1948
10. Bohman VR, Poole SC, Kvasnicka WG, et al: The toxicology and composition of bovine tissues after parenteral administration of high levels of copper salts. Vet Hum Toxicol 29:307–312, 1987
11. Brockman RP, Audette RJ, Gray M: Borax toxicity. Can Vet J 26:147–148, 1985
12. Buck WB: Toxicity of inorganic and aliphatic organic arsenicals. In Oehme FW (ed): Toxicity of Heavy Metals in the Environment. New York, Marcel Dekker, 1978, pp 357–374
13. Buck WB: Iodine. In Howard JL (ed): Current Veterinary Therapy: Food Animal Practice 2. Philadelphia, WB Saunders Co, 1986, pp 357–359.
14. Buck WB, Ewan RC: Toxicology and adverse effects of mineral imbalance. Clin Toxicol 6:459–485, 1973
15. Bulgin MS, Maas J, Anderson BC, et al: Death associated with parenteral administration of copper disodium edetate in calves. J Am Vet Med Assoc 188:406–409, 1986
16. Campbell AG, Coup MR, Bishop WH, Wright DE: Effect of elevated iron intake on the copper status of grazing cattle. NZ Agric Res 17:393–399, 1974
17. Cassidy DR, Furr AA: Toxicity of inorganic and organic mercury compounds in animals. In Oehme FW (ed): Toxicity of Heavy Metals in the Environment. New York, Marcel Dekker, 1978, pp 303–330
18. Chapman HL Jr, Nelson SL, Kidder RW, et al: Toxicity of cupric sulfate for beef cattle. J Anim Sci 21:960–962, 1962
19. Clarke ML, Harvey DG, Humphreys DJ (eds): Veterinary Toxicology, ed 2. Baltimore, MD, Williams & Wilkins, 1981
20. Combs GF Jr, Combs SB: Effects of selenium excesses. In Combs GF Jr, Combs SB (eds): The Role of Selenium in Nutrition. New York, Academic Press, 1986, pp 463–525
21. Coup MR, Campbell AG: The effects of excessive iron intake upon health and production of dairy cows. NZ J Agric Res 7:624–638, 1964
22. Cummins LJ, Harris DJ: Temporary infertility possibly associated with parenteral copper therapy in cattle. Aust Vet J 61:164–165, 1984
23. Cunningham IJ: Parenteral administration of copper as cerate to cattle and sheep. NZ Vet J 5:9–16, 1957
24. Cunningham GN, Wise MB, Barrick ER: Effect of dietary levels of manganese on the performance and blood constituents of calves. J Anim Sci 25.532–538, 1966
25. Dick AT, Bull LB: Some preliminary observations on the effect of molybdenum on copper metabolism in herbivorous animals. Aust Vet J 21:70–71, 1945

26. Dorn RC, Pierce JO, Chase GR, et al: Report for Environmental Protection Agency, Univ Missouri, Contract 68-02-2292, 1972
27. Ewan RC: Toxicology and adverse effects of mineral imbalance with emphasis on selenium and other minerals. In Oehme FW (ed): Toxicity of Heavy Metals in the Environment. New York, Marcel Dekker, 1978, pp 445–489
28. Ferguson WS, Lewis AH, Watson SJ: The teart pastures of Somerset. 1. The cause and cure of teartness. J Agri Sci 33:44–51, 1943
29. Franke KW: A new toxicant occurring naturally in certain samples of plant foodstuffs. I. Results obtained in preliminary feeding trials. J Nutr 8:597–608, 1934
30. Gawthorne JM: Copper interactions. In Howell J McC, Gawthorne JM (eds): Copper in Animals and Man, Volume 1. Boca Raton, FL, CRC Press, 1987, pp 79–99
31. Grace ND (ed): The Mineral Requirements of Grazing Ruminants. New Zealand, NZ Society of Animal Production, 1987
32. Graham TW, Thurmond MC, Clegg NS, et al: Epidemic study of mortality in veal calves subsequent to an episode of zinc toxicosis in a California veal calf operation using zinc sulphate supplemented milk replacer. J Am Vet Med Assoc 190:1296–1301, 1987
33. Green GH, Weeth HJ: Responses of heifers ingesting boron in water. J Anim Sci 46:812–817, 1977
34. Haggard DL, Stowe HD, Conner GH, et al: Immunologic effects of experimental iodine toxicosis in young cattle. Am J Vet Res 41:539–543, 1980
35. Hall ED, Symond HW, Mallinson CB: Maximum capacity of bovine liver to remove manganese from portal plasma and the effect of the route of entry of manganese on its rate of removal. Res Vet Sci 33:89–943, 1982
36. Hansard SL, Ammerman CB, Fick KR, et al: Performance and vanadium contents of tissues in sheep as influenced by dietary vanadium. J Anim Sci 46:1091–1095, 1978
37. Harr JR, Muth OH: Selenium poisoning in domestic animals and its relationship to man. Clin Toxicol 5:175–186, 1972
38. Harrison LH, Colvin BM, Stuart BP, et al: Paralysis in swine due to focal symmetrical poliomalacia: Possible selenium toxicosis. Vet Pathol 20:265–273, 1983
39. Hatch RC, Clark JD, Jain AV: Use of thiols and thiosulfate for treatment of experimentally induced acute arsenic toxicosis in cattle. Am J Vet Res 39:1411–1414, 1978
40. Hemken RW: Iodine. J Dairy Sci 53:1138–1143, 1970
41. Herrick JB: What role for EDDI (ethylene diamine dihydriodide) in bovine respiratory disease complex. Vet Med Small Anim Clin 67:480–482, 1972
42. Hillman D, Curtis AR: Chronic iodine toxicity in dairy cattle: Blood chemistry, leukocytes, and milk iodide. J Dairy Sci 63:55–63, 1980
43. Ho SY, Miller WJ, Gentry RP, et al: Effects of high but non-toxic dietary manganese and iron on their metabolism by calves. J Dairy Sci 67:1489–1495, 1984
44. Hopper JT, Holloway JW, Butts WT J.: Animal variation in chromium sesquioxide excretion patterns of grazing cows. J Anim Sci 46:1096–1102, 1978
45. Howell J McC, Gawthorne JM (eds): Copper in Animals and Man, Volume 2. Boca Raton, FL, CRC Press, 1987
46. Howell J McC, Gawthorne JM (eds): Copper in Animals and Man, Volume I. Boca Raton, FL, CRC Press, 1987
47. Hutton JG: The correlation of certain lesions in animals with certain soil types. J Am Soc Agron 23:1076–1082, 1931
48. James LF, Shupe JL: Selenium accumulators. In Howard JL (ed): Current Veterinary Therapy, Food Animal Practice 2. Philadelphia, WB Saunders Co, 1986, pp 394–396
49. Jenkins KJ, Hidiroglou M: Tolerance of the calf for excess copper in milk replacer. J Dairy Sci 72:150–156, 1989
50. Kerr LA, Edwards WC: Chromate poisoning in livestock from oil field waste. Vet Hum Toxicol 23:401–402, 1981
51. Koong LJ, Wise MB, Barrick ER: Effect of elevated dietary levels of iron on the performance and blood constituents of calves. J Anim Sci 31:422–427, 1970
52. Laflamme DP, Miller WJ, Neathery NW, et al: The effects of low to normal dietary

phosphorus levels on zinc metabolism and zinc tissue distribution in calves. J Anim Sci 61:525–531, 1985

53. Lamand M: Influence of molybdenum and sulfur on copper metabolism in sheep: Comparison of elemental sulfur and sulfate. Ann Rech Vet 20:103–106, 1989

54. Levander OA: Selenium. In Mertz, W, (ed): Trace Elements in Human and Animal Nutrition, ed 5, Vol 2. Orlando, FL, Academic Press, 1986, pp 209–279

55. MacDonald CW, Christian RG, Strausz KI, et al: Acute selenium toxicity in neonatal calves. Can Vet J 22:279–281, 1981

56. Marshall DR, Todd JR: A case of acute copper oxychloride poisoning in cattle. Vet Rec 69:77–78, 1957

57. Mayland HF, Rosenau RC, Florence AR: Grazing cow and calf responses to zinc supplementation. J Anim Sci 51:966–974, 1980

58. McCauley EH, Johnson DW: The role of EDDI (ethylene diamine dihydriodide) in bovine respiratory disease complex: Another point of view. Vet Med Small Anim Clin 67:836–838, 1972

59. Mertz W (ed): Trace Elements in Human and Animal Nutrition, ed 5. Orlando, FL, Academic Press, 1986

60. Miller WJ: Zinc nutrition of cattle: A review. J Dairy Sci 53:1123–1135, 1970

61. Miller WJ, Amos HW, Gentry RP, et al: Long term feeding of high zinc sulphate diets to lactating and gestating dairy cows. J Dairy Sci 72:1499–1508, 1989

62. Miller WJ, Clifton CM, Fowler PR, et al: Influence of high levels of dietary zinc on zinc in milk, performance, and biochemistry of lactating cows. J Dairy Sci 48:450–453, 1965

63. Miller JK, Swanson EW, Aschbacher PW, et al: Iodine transfer and concentration in the prepartum cow, fetus, and neonatal calf. J Dairy Sci 50:1301–1305, 1967

64. Minnick PD, Braselton WE, Meerdink GL, et al: Altered serum element concentrations due to laboratory usage of Vacutainer tubes. Vet Hum Toxicol 24:41–42, 1982

65. Morrow DA, Edwards L: Effects of acute iodine toxicity on reproduction in a dairy herd. Bovine Practice 16:114–118, 1981

66. Moxon AL, Rhian M: Selenium poisoning. Physiol Rev 23:305–337, 1943

67. Mylrea PJ, Byrne DT: An outbreak of acute copper poisoning in calves. Aust Vet J 50:169–172, 1974

68. National Research Council: Mineral Tolerance of Domestic Animals. Washington, DC, National Academy of Sciences, 1980

69. National Research Council: Selenium in Nutrition. Washington, DC, National Academy Press, 1983

70. National Research Council: Nutrient Requirements of Beef Cattle, ed 6. Washington, DC, National Academy Press, 1984

71. National Research Council: Nutrient Requirements of Dairy Cattle, ed 6. Washington, DC, National Academy Press, 1988

72. Newton GL, Barrick ER, Harvey RW, et al: Iodine toxicity. Physiological effects of elevated dietary iodine on calves. J Anim Sci 38:449–455, 1974

73. O'Dell GD, Miller WJ, King WA, et al: Effects of nickel supplementation on production and composition of milk. J Dairy Sci 53:1545–1547, 1970a

74. O'Dell GD, Miller WJ, Moore SL, et al: Effects of nickel as chloride or the carbonate on palatability of cattle feed. J Dairy Sci 53:1266–1269, 1970b

75. O'Dell GD, Miller WJ, Moore SL, et al: Effects of dietary nickel level on excretion and nickel content of tissues in male calves. J Anim Sci 32:769–773, 1971

76. Olson OE: Selenium in plants as a cause of livestock poisoning. In Keeler RF, VanKampen KR, James LF, (eds): Effects of Poisonous Plants on Livestock. New York, Academic Press, 1978, pp 121–133.

77. Olson WG, Stevens JB, Anderson J, et al: Iodine toxicosis in six herds of dairy cattle. J Am Vet Med Assoc 184:179–181, 1984

78. Osweiler GD, Carson TL, Buck WB, (eds): Clinical and Diagnostic Veterinary Toxicology, ed 3. Dubuque, IA, Kendall/Hunt Publishing Co, 1985

a. Maas J, Berg JN, Petersen RG: Serum distribution of iodine after oral administration of ethylnediamine dihydriodide in cattle. Am J Vet Res 50:1758–1759, 1989

79. Osweiler GD, VanGelder GA, Buck WB: Epidemiology of lead poisoning in ani-

mals. *In* Oehme FW (ed): Toxicity of Heavy Metals in the Environment. New York, Marcel Dekker, 1978, pp 143–171.

80. Ott EA, Smith WH, Harrington RB, et al: Zinc toxicity in ruminants. 2. Effect of high levels of dietary zinc on gains, feed consumption, and feed efficiency of beef cattle. J Anim Sci 25:419–423, 1966a

81. Ott EA, Smith WH, Harrington RB, et al: Zinc toxicity in ruminants. 4. Physiological changes in tissues of beef cattle. J Anim Sci 25:432–438, 1966b

82. Platonow N, Abbey HK: Toxicity of vanadium in calves. Vet Rec 82:292–293, 1968

83. Pottenger RC: Boron toxicity in cattle. Diag Forum Purdue Univ; April 1990

84. Puls R (ed): Mineral Levels in Animal Health. Clearbrook, BC, Canada, Sherpa International, 1988

85. Robinson NW, Harsard SL, Johns DM, et al: Excess dietary manganese and feedlot performance of beef cattle. J Anim Sci 19:290, 1960

86. Rojas MA, Dyer IA, Cassatt WA: Manganese deficiency in the bovine. J Anim Sci 24:664–667, 1965

87. Rosenfeld I, Beath OA, (eds): Selenium: Geobotany, Biochemistry, Toxicity and Nutrition. New York, Academic Press, 1964

88. Rosiles R, Buck WB, Brown LN: Clinical infectious bovine rhinotracheitis in cattle fed organic iodine and urea. Am J Vet Res 36:1447–1453, 1975

89. Rotruck JT, Pope AL, Ganther HE, et al: Selenium: Biochemical role as a component of glutathione peroxidase. Science 179:588–590, 1973

90. Schwarz WA, Kirchgessner M: Experimental zinc deficiency in lactating dairy cows. Vet Med Rev 1:19–41, 1975

91. Shand A, Lewis G: Chronic copper poisoning in young calves. Vet Rec 69:618–621, 1957

92. Shortridge EH, O'Hara PJ, Marshall PM: Acute selenium poisoning in cattle. NZ Vet J 19:47–50, 1971

93. Shupe JL, Peterson HB, Leone NC (eds): Fluorides. Effects of Vegetation, Animals and Humans. Salt Lake City, Utah, Paragon Press, 1983

94. Sisk DB, Colvin BM, Bridges CR: Acute, fatal illness in cattle exposed to boron fertilizer. J Am Vet Med Assoc 193:943–945, 1988

95. Spivey-Fox MR: Assessment of cadmium, lead, and vanadium status of large animals as related to the human food chain. J Anim Sci 65:1744–1752, 1987

96. Standish JF, Ammerman CB, Palmer AZ, et al: Influence of dietary iron and phosphorus on performance, tissue mineral composition, and mineral absorption in steers. J Anim Sci 33:171–178, 1971

97. Standish JF, Ammerman CB, Simpson CF, et al: Influence of graded levels of dietary iron, as ferrous sulphate, on performance and tissue mineral composition of steers. J Anim Sci 29:496–503, 1969

98. Stogdale L: Chronic copper poisoning in dairy cows. Aust Vet J 54:139–141, 1978

99. Suttle NF: Recent studies of the copper-molybdenum antagonism. Proc Nutr Soc 33:299–303, 1974

100. Symond HW, Hall ED: Acute manganese toxicity and the absorption and biliary excretion of manganese in cattle. Res Vet Sci 35:5–13, 1983

101. Thatcher CD, Meldrum JB, Wikse SE, et al: Arsenic toxicosis and suspected chromium toxicosis in a herd of cattle. J Am Vet Med Assoc 187:179–182, 1985

102. Todd JR, Gribben HJ: Suspected chronic copper poisoning in a cow. Vet Rec 77:498–499, 1965

103. Towers NR, Grace ND: Minimum requirements of grazing livestock. *In* Grace ND (ed): The Mineral Requirements of Grazing Ruminants. New Zealand Society of Animal Production, 1987, pp 76–79.

104. Towers NR, Young PW, Wright DE: Effects of zinc supplementation on bovine plasma copper. NZ Vet J 29:113–114, 1981

105. Underwood EJ: *In* Underwood EJ (ed): Trace Elements in Human and Animal Nutrition, ed 4. New York, Academic Press, 1977

106. Valdivia R, Ammerman CB, Wilcox CJ, et al: Effect of dietary aluminum on animal performance and animal tissue mineral levels in growing steers. J Anim Sci 47:1352–1356, 1978

107. Ward GM: Molybdenum toxicity and hypocuprosis in ruminants: A review. J Anim
     Sci 46:1078–1085, 1978
108. Weeth HJ, Speth CF, Hanks DR: Boron content of plasma and urine as indicators of
     boron intake of cattle. Am J Vet Res 42:474–477, 1981
109. Weir RJ Jr, Fisher RS: Toxicologic studies on borax and boric acid. Toxicol Appl
     Pharmacol 23:253–264, 1972
110. Weiss E, Baur P: Experimentelle untersuchungen zur chronischen kupfervergif-
     tung des kalbes. Zentralblatt Vet 15:156–184, 1968
111. Wentink GH, Spierenburg TJ, de Graff GJ, et al: A case of chronic zinc poisoning in
     calves fed with zinc-contaminated roughage. Vet Q 7:153–157, 1985
112. Wilson WD, Ward GM: Transfer of fallout manganese-54 from feed to milk. J Dairy
     Sci 50:592–593, 1967
113. Wittenberg KM, Boila RJ: Supplementary copper for growing cattle consuming
     diets high in molybdenum or molybdenum plus sulfur. Can J Anim Sci 68:1143–
     1154, 1988
114. Wright FC, Riner JC, Hufler M, et al: Toxicity and residual aspects of alkylmercury
     fungicides in livestock. In Oehme FW (ed): Toxicity of Heavy Metals in the
     Environment. New York, Marcel Dekker, 1978, pp 331–355

Address reprint requests to

Larry J. Thompson, DVM
Diagnostic Laboratory
New York State College of Veterinary Medicine
Cornell University
Ithaca, NY 14853

Index

Note: Page numbers of article titles are in **boldface** type.

Changing Your Address?

Make sure your subscription changes too! When you notify us of your new address, you can help make our job easier by including an exact copy of your Clinics label number with your old address (see illustration below.) This number identifies you to our computer system and will speed the processing of your address change. Please be sure this label number accompanies your old address and your corrected address—you can send an old Clinics label with your number on it or just copy it exactly and send it to the address listed below.

We appreciate your help in our attempt to give you continuous coverage. Thank you.

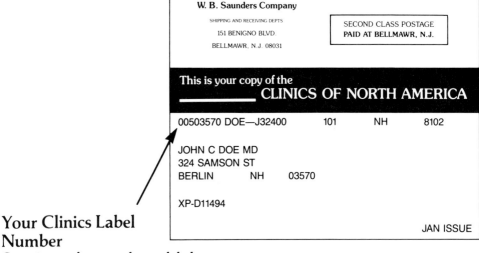

Your Clinics Label Number
Copy it exactly or send your label along with your address to:
W. B. Saunders Company, Customer Service
Post Office Box 6467
Duluth, MN 55806-9854
Call Toll Free 1-800-654-2452

Please allow four to six weeks for delivery of new subscriptions and for processing address changes.